TEACHERS COLLEGE
LIBRARY
ADELAIDE NUTTING
HISTORICAL NURSING COLLECTION
COLUMBIA UNIVERSITY

This book belongs to:

Joan Snyder

Nursing
THE FINEST ART · SECOND EDITION

An Illustrated History

Thomas Webster, *Sickness and Health*, 1843. *(Copyright The Board of Trustees of the Victoria & Albert Museum, London, England.)*

Nursing
THE FINEST ART SECOND EDITION

An Illustrated History

M. Patricia Donahue, PhD, RN, FAAN
Professor
College of Nursing
The University of Iowa
Iowa City, Iowa

with *441* illustrations, including *229* in full color

 Mosby

St. Louis Baltimore Boston Carlsbad Chicago Naples New York Philadelphia Portland
London Madrid Mexico City Singapore Sydney Tokyo Toronto Wiesbaden

Mosby
Dedicated to Publishing Excellence

A Times Mirror
Company

Publisher: *Nancy L. Coon*
Editor: *N. Darlene Como*
Developmental Editor: *Dana L. Knighten*
Project Manager: *Patricia Tannian*
Senior Production Editor: *Ann E. Rogers*
Manuscript Editor: *Mary McAuley*
Book Design Manager: *Gail Morey Hudson*
Book Design and Layout: *Jeanne Wolfgeher Design*
Manufacturing Manager: *Theresa Fuchs*

Cover Image: Edvard Munch, The Sick Child, 1907. *(Copyright 1995 Munch Museum/Munch-Ellingsen Group/Artists Rights Society [ARS], New York, New York.)*
Marble Paper: *Susan Pogany, Lawrence, Kansas*

SECOND EDITION
Copyright © 1996 by Mosby–Year Book, Inc.

Previous edition copyrighted 1985

Printed in the United States of America.
Composition by Black Dot Graphics.
Printing/binding by RR Donnelley & Sons, Inc.

Mosby–Year Book, Inc.
11830 Westline Industrial Drive
St. Louis, MO   63146

Library of Congress Cataloging in Publication Data
Donahue, M. Patricia.
     Nursing, the finest art: an illustrated history / M. Patricia
Donahue.—2nd ed.
        p.   cm.
     Includes bibliographical references and index.
     ISBN 0-8151-2727-8
     1. Nursing—History.   2. Nursing—United States—History.
3. Nursing in art.   I. Title.
RT31.D66   1996
610.73'09—dc20   96-26093
                                                             CIP

95 96 97 98 99 / 9 8 7 6 5 4 3 2 1

── *The Shell* ──

Sometimes I feel like a shell
Cast out by the sea,

An empty vessel without a purpose,
Awash in the surf is Me

Yet, I know if you lift the shell that is Me
and hold it close to your ear

You will hear my song
One of Joy, Love, and Life.

My shell will sing
And you will know
I was here.

— PETER TYREE

For My Daughter and Son,
Erin Marie and Mark Joseph

For My Parents,
Joseph Edward and Mary Theresa Rohovsky

Foreword

s the profession of nursing moves into the rapidly changing health care arena of the twenty-first century, it is imperative that we have a firm sense of the art and science of our history.

This magnificent volume presents an exhilarating visual and literary perspective on the evolution of nursing. Through more than four hundred illustrations presented in a wide variety of artistic media, it provides a dramatic interpretation of the joy and pain inherent in nursing's work.

While it is nearly impossible for any one publication to capture all the emotion of a profession as varied and rich as nursing, Dr. Donahue has provided us with a passionate testament to the value and rich heritage of the oldest and finest healing art. Not by coincidence, she also has presented us with a magnificent vision for our future.

Represented here are materials that portray the lives of contemporary practicing nurses and nursing pioneers, as well as the monumental social movements that have affected the multitude of ways nursing has contributed to the well-being of humanity.

Not only does this collection provide a stunning visual portrayal of the history of nursing, but it also serves as a precious scholarly chronicle of our past. Dr. Donahue's work is a gift to all of us—nurses, historians, artists, professional colleagues, and laypersons—and will be cherished by all who have been touched by the expert care, kind words, and warm hands of a nurse.

Norma M. Lang, PhD, RN, FAAN, FRCN
Margaret Bond Simon Dean
Professor of Nursing
University of Pennsylvania
Philadelphia, Pennsylvania

Preface to the First Edition

It is something to be able to paint a picture, or to carve a statue, and to make a few objects beautiful. But it is far more glorious to carve and paint the atmosphere in which we work, to effect the quality of the day—This is the highest of the arts.

— HENRY DAVID THOREAU

Nursing has long been defined as both an art and a science. The primary emphasis, however, has been on the scientific aspects of nursing with little consideration given to its state as an art. Nursing is a fine art. According to Florence Nightingale, it is "the finest of the fine arts." Nursing is not merely a technique but a process that incorporates the elements of soul, mind, and imagination. Its very essence lies in the creative imagination, the sensitive spirit, and the intelligent understanding that provide the very foundation for effective nursing care. These have been captured consistently in a wide range of illustrative material that can greatly enhance the study of nursing history through visual representation. Every art gallery has its nursing saints, nurturing mothers, healing miracles, sick beds, and lying-in chambers. Many of the finest paintings and sculptures dealing with nursing subjects have been done by the "great masters" and contemporary artists. All of these serve to capture the art of nursing.

Nursing: The Finest Art: An Illustrated History has been a labor of love and a realization of a dream. It has been a labor because I have struggled to portray effectively the eloquent beauty of nursing and nursing care so that all who read the words and see the illustrations will appreciate its vitality. My love of both history and nursing provided the motivation to demonstrate the historical development of nursing through an integration of a variety of selected illustrations and written text. The dream that this book would be written and published initially belonged to Dr. Teresa E. Christy, who died "too young and too soon" but not before she had nurtured my interest in nursing history and had become my mentor as I began my journey into historical research. The words of this history are mine, but the spirit is Terry's.

This book is intended to provide an illustrated history of nursing from primitive times to the present. It is written for nurses, other interested professionals, and the layman. Various forms of art are used to depict the particular shifts and changes in the roles and functions of the nurse as they have been created and influenced by major social, political, and historical forces in society. Alterations in the image of nursing are also portrayed, since nursing has progressed through an evolutionary process. Although this book is referenced, it is *not* a comprehensive text of nursing history. It can, however, be used to augment both nursing courses and art courses. Most important is its aesthetic value not only for nurses but for all lovers of art.

It can be argued that some significant events, persons and places were omitted from the text. Indeed, I have chosen specific occurrences in an attempt to balance the artwork with the text and yet render a fair appraisal of nursing's journey through time. Selected events, topics, and individuals important to the development of nursing have been highlighted. These represent a larger body of information that could be used to demonstrate nursing's struggles, growth, challenges, dilemmas, humanitarianism, and beauty. All would reinforce the recurring themes evident in the text and reaffirm the need to effectively communicate the essence of nursing.

> We need to realize and to affirm anew that nursing is one of the most difficult of arts. Compassion may provide the motive, but knowledge is our only working power. Perhaps, too, we need to remember that growth in our work must be preceded by ideas, and that any conditions which suppress thought, must retard growth. Surely we will not be satisfied in perpetuating methods and traditions. Surely we shall wish to be more and more occupied with creating them.
>
> — *M. Adelaide Nutting, 1925*

Many individuals have been involved with this project in different ways. To all of them I extend my sincere appreciation. Those persons who are not identified know of their invaluable assistance and unique contributions.

It is impossible to give adequate thanks to my daughter and my son, Erin and Mark, who freely and unselfishly gave of themselves during this period of writing, when I frequently did not have time to be their mother. Once again they have respected and accepted my need to do what I think I must. To my son Johnny, who throughout his short life provided a living example of unselfishness, patience, love, and a courage to attempt the "impossible," I give thanks. Finally, I acknowledge the interest of my parents, who often did not always understand my excitement about this book or my drive to accomplish but who patiently endured.

My deepest gratitude is extended to my research assistant, Patricia A. Russac, who taught me about the subtleties of art. Her expertise, determination, and precision were a primary factor in the completion of this work. To the many individuals at The C.V. Mosby Company who assisted with this project I extend grateful appreciation, particularly Julie Cardamon, my first Editor, who initiated my contract; Nancy L. Mullins, Editor, Nursing Division, who inherited the project and assisted with the steady progression necessary for completion; and Bess Arends, Developmental Editor, who provided sustained support, encouragement, interest, and understanding throughout all of the difficult phases.

I am deeply indebted to my support network whose members probably do not even recognize their significant contributions in the development of this manuscript. Particular thanks are due to LTC Sarah A. Balkema, U.S. Army (ret.); LTC Joan K. Cotter, U.S. Army (ret.); Karen A. O'Heath; Sandra R. Powell; Dr. Imogene M. King; and Steven Warner. Finally, the support of Dean Geraldene Felton, The University of Iowa College of Nursing, facilitated the progress of the project.

M. Patricia Donahue

Preface to the Second Edition

Ten years have passed since the publication of the first edition of *Nursing: The Finest Art: An Illustrated History*. During that time society has witnessed a number of conflicts and crises, as well as the information revolution. Health care delivery systems worldwide have been caught in a web of social problems, financial crises, and scarce resources that is forcing a major transformation in the rendering of care. Nursing practice must adapt to these shifting realities as it has in the past while taking into account the need for internal change to meet new opportunities created by such upheaval. Challenges and visions once again have become important components in the fostering of nursing's future evolution.

Several years ago an interesting article appeared in the local newspaper, "Refuge Named for Eagle-Watcher." It was the story of Elton Fawks from East Moline, Illinois, who waged a one-man campaign environmentalists say helped to save the bald eagle from extinction. He took up birdwatching after childhood polio kept him from more active pursuits, and bald eagles became his passion. With a pair of binoculars and a keen curiosity about nature, he noticed in the 1950s a marked decrease in the number of immature bald eagles that nested around the river's locks and dams. He took it upon himself to confer with Charles Broley, an ornithologist who was among the first to determine that DDT damages the eagle's egg shells. Fawks then began a lobbying campaign for tough state laws to control pesticides. In the 1960s the Illinois general assembly adopted measures based on his proposals, and DDT was banned nationwide in the 1970s. What started as the effort of one human being escalated into nationwide involvement, the result being the removal of the bald eagle from the endangered species list. Challenges and visions are a part of Fawks' story just as they are a part of nursing's heritage. Elton Fawks had challenges and a vision; early nurses and nursing leaders also had challenges and visions. I hope that they have been adequately represented in this work. Now it is up to each of us—to all nurses—not only to meet challenges but also to create visions.

It is difficult to capture the totality of nursing in a book of this type, which attempts to portray not only nursing's history but also its eloquent beauty and vitality as represented by the written word and a variety of art forms. As in the first edition, art has been used to depict the particular shifts and changes in the roles and functions of the nurse and the effects of major social, political, and historical forces in society. Some artwork that appeared in the first edition has been eliminated; some that was black and white is now reproduced in color. A variety of new artwork is integrated throughout. The historical content in Units 1 through 9 remains essentially the same, with some editing and some additional content added.

Units 10 and 11 are new and explicate the current status of the nursing profession with particular emphasis on the global scene. Each of the units taken alone is a compelling story, while all units taken together create an epic tale of nursing's struggles and successes in the quest for quality patient care. Because any history book must be selective, the printed text represents a much larger body of information relative to nursing's history. Some later sections of the book concentrate more heavily on western civilization. This in no way is meant to diminish the importance of nursing history in other countries but instead reflects my thought that American nursing frequently mirrors the evolution of that in other countries. The ideal situation would be to give a brief and concise account of nursing's history in all countries, but that is not feasible in a book of this type.

Although much about nursing will have changed by the beginning of the twenty-first century, much will also remain constant. Still, as these words and works of art tell us, there was a great deal of dignity in nursing's past. These pages inform us not only about what nursing was, but what it still is, and will always be. They provide a moving and informative view of people and events that made nursing unique in "the care of strangers." Through visual images and the written word, those traditional attributes of compassion, humanity, advocacy, commitment, and caring that are so important to nursing and its structure are revealed. Numerous resources were used to provide information for the timelines, including Ira Rutkow's *Surgery: An Illustrated History*; *Smithsonian Timelines of the Ancient World*; *A Visual Chronology From the Origins of Life to AD 1500*; Bernard Grun's *The Timetables of History*, new third revised edition; and a variety of historical works. The intent of these timelines is to provide the reader with an overview of significant global and nursing events that have occurred; they represent only a fraction of the material that could have been included.

I am indebted to many individuals who have assisted with this project in different ways, particularly to family and friends. To all of them I extend my sincere appreciation. My deepest gratitude is extended to my research assistant, Erin M. Donahue, who taught me about the subtleties of the computer. Her particular expertise with information systems and data bases was a primary factor in the completion of this work at a much earlier date than anticipated. Nell Andrew gave many hours to the project before leaving to pursue her own career development. Fortunately, Evea Wenger stepped in to replace her. Evea has performed innumerable tasks with persistent enthusiasm for the project. Her influence in the development of the timelines has been immeasurable. Many individuals at Mosby were instrumental in pushing this project forward. However, my editor, N. Darlene Como, and developmental editor, Dana Knighten, provided the sustained support, encouragement, understanding, and caring necessary to carry us through the particularly difficult aspects of the project. I would be remiss if I did not mention Ann Rogers, senior production editor at Mosby, and Jeanne Wolfgeher of Jeanne Wolfgeher Design, who together had the most difficult task of unifying all the materials to enhance the book's character and appearance.

I also wish to acknowledge the support services provided by the Obermann Center for Advanced Studies at The University of Iowa. This Center actually became the hub of the wheel that moved production along its journey toward completion of the book.

M. Patricia Donahue
Coralville, Iowa
August, 1995

Contents

4 *Nursing in a Changing World*
Aristocratic and Military Influences, 111

5 *Nursing in Transition*
The Dark Period and the Dawn of Modern Times, 151

6   *The Development of Nursing in America,* 213

7   *Advancing Toward New Frontiers,* 293

8 *Nurses in Action*
Wars of the Twentieth Century, 349

9 *The Age of Expansion, 405*

Nursing

THE FINEST ART SECOND EDITION

An Illustrated History

U N I T   1

The Origin of Nursing

Woman is an instinctive nurse, taught by Mother Nature. The nurse has always been a necessity, thus lacked social status. In primitive times she was a slave, and in the civilized era a domestic. Overlooked in the plans of legislators, and forgotten in the curricula of pedagogues, she was left without protection and remained without education. She was not an artisan who could obtain the help of an hereditary guild; there was no Hanseatic League for nurses. Drawn from the nameless and numberless army of poverty, the nurse worked as a menial and obeyed as a servant. Denied the dignity of a trade, and devoid of professional ethics, she could not rise above the degradation of her environment. It never occurred to the Aristotles of the past that it would be safer for the public welfare if nurses were educated instead of lawyers. The untrained nurse is as old as the human race; the trained nurse is a recent discovery. The distinction between the two is a sharp commentary on the follies and prejudices of mankind.

– VICTOR ROBINSON

Margo Mandette, *Desert Mother and Child,* 1994. Oil on canvas, approx. 76.2 × 101.6 cm. *(By permission of Margo Mandette, Jerome, Arizona.)*

*A*n adequate identification and description of the exact origin of nursing is difficult because nothing is known about the actual work of the nurse in prehistory. Everything that has been written about nursing during this period is merely inference based on the discoveries of prehistorians, archaeologists, and anthropologists. Yet early records do provide information about the legacy left to civilized humans from primitive societies. From the dawn of civilization, evidence prevails to support the premise that *nurturing* has been essential to the preservation of life. Survival of the human race, therefore, is inextricably intertwined with the development of nursing.

THE NURSING IMPULSE

It is difficult at times to distinguish nursing from medicine in this evolutionary process, since the early stages of each are so closely interwoven. Although some individuals believe that nursing began with Florence Nightingale, nursing is as old as and actually predates medicine. An interdependence of the two is evident throughout history and has produced a unique and curious relationship. At some periods, such as the Hippocratic era, rational medicine functioned without nursing, whereas at other times, for example, the Middle Ages, nursing was practiced without rational medicine. According to Davison (1943), who identified four main cycles of medicine (primitive, Renaissance, pharmacy, and modern), nursing approached adequacy in three (not pharmacy), and only in these did medicine progress. Davison believes that nursing merits recognition as the "cornerstone of its [medicine's] foundation." Certainly the mother-nurse must have preceded the magician-priest or the medicine man. It is even possible that these two types of service were at first united but eventually divided to produce two practitioners of the healing art—the medicine giver and the caretaker (Stewart and Austin, 1962). Indeed, the modern doctor has the aura of the medicine man, but the seeds of medical knowledge were sown by the natural remedies of the mother.

Nursing has been called the oldest of the arts and the youngest of the professions. As such, it has gone through many stages and has been an integral part of societal movements. Nursing has been involved in the existing culture—shaped by it and yet helping to develop it. The history of nursing has been one of frustration, ignorance, and misunderstanding. It is a great epic involving trials and triumph, romance and adventure. Most important, it is the story of an occupational group whose status has always been affected by the prevalent standards of humanity. The great turning points in world progress have also been important turning points in nursing. Events that give rise to "higher degrees of consideration for those who are helpless or oppressed, kindliness and sympathy for the unfortunate and for those who suffer, tolerance for those of differing religion, race, color, etc.—all tend to promote activities like nursing which are primarily humanitarian" (Dock and Stewart, 1925, p. 3).

In any text concerning the genesis of nursing, there is considerable content that refers to the history of nursing as an episode in the history of woman. In fact, one historian described this phenomenon with a clear and emphatic statement: "The nurse is the mirror in which is reflected the position of woman through the ages" (Robinson, 1946, p. vii). During those periods when women were closely restricted to the home by social convention and their energies were limited to family life, nursing must have had the character of a household art. The duties of women, their degree of economic independence, the freedom of women outside the family, and other factors have seriously influenced the progress of nursing. The fullest development of nursing was not possible without emancipation from the conditions of subjection endured by women. Ultimately, the full demands of nursing could not be

John Henry Twachtman, *On the Terrace*, c. 1890-1900. Canvas, approx. 64.8 × 76.2 cm. *(Gift of John Gellatly, National Museum of American Art, Washington, D.C./Art Resource, New York.)*

realized without education and knowledge of the social conditions and needs of the day.

Confusion exists regarding the proper role or function of the nurse, since the connotations of the word *nurse* have changed over the course of human history. *Nurse* and *nursing* currently have many meanings, a condition that causes varying interpretations of the appropriate work and function of the nurse. Throughout history the development of nursing has been closely related to the evolution of the word *nurse*, specific definitions of which are dependent upon the major social forces of the day. It is apparent that the meaning of the word has progressed from a term indicating a woman who performed the basic unlearned human activity of suckling an infant to one describing a person who is part of a highly learned, sophisticated profession. These shifts in meaning are clearly reflected in changes in the nursing role.

Nursing has its origin in the mother-care of helpless infants and must have coexisted with this type of care from earliest times. The word *nursing* is derived from the Latin *nutrire*, "to nourish." The word *nurse* also has its roots in Latin in the noun *nutrix*, which means "nursing mother." Frequently this referred to a woman who suckled a child who was not her own, that is, a wet nurse. Eventually the term *nutrix* was used to identify a female who nourished, which provided a broader yet still gender-related definition. The Latin words were the basis for the French *nourrice*, which also referred to a woman who suckled a child, particularly the child of another. The original meaning of the English word was the same, a wet nurse. The term was first used in

Norman Rockwell, *The Nanny,* October 24, 1936, cover of the *Saturday Evening Post. (Copyright 1936, The Norman Rockwell Family Trust. Printed by permission of the Norman Rockwell Family Trust, Poughkeepsie, New York.)*

The nurse was portrayed in a variety of ways while functioning in different roles. The "child nurse," "nursemaid," or "nanny" fulfilled an important role throughout history. A girl or woman was regularly employed to look after children through sickness and health. Rockwell capitalized on this practice.

English in the thirteenth century, and its spelling underwent many forms, from *norrice, nurice,* or *nourice* to the present *nurse.* Through this evolution of the word, another dimension was added to its meaning: a woman who cares for and tends young children.

Nurse has also been used as a verb, still having its original roots in the Latin *nutrire,* which meant to suckle and to nourish. Again the Latin word transferred into French as *nourir* ("to nourish") and into English as *nurshen, nourishen,* and *norissen.* Abbreviated it became *nursh* and finally led to the present-day usage, *nurse.* The meaning of both the noun and the verb continued to broaden to encompass more and more functions related to the care of all humanity. By the sixteenth century, meanings of the noun included "a person, but usually a woman, who waits upon or tends the sick." It was not until the eighteenth century that the meanings of the verb included "to wait upon or tend a person who is sick." During the nineteenth century two more components were added: the training of those who tend the sick and the carrying out of such duties under the supervision of a physician.

Although the aspect of nurturing has long been identified with nursing, it has been even more closely associated with education, particularly with respect to the rearing, training, and general upbringing of the young.

> This accounts for the two kinds of helpers who appeared quite early in some households—child-nurses and sick-nurses. Sick-nurses became more closely associated with the healing arts and child-nurses with the teaching and training of children. Often, the two functions were combined.
>
> — *Stewart and Austin, 1962, p. 4*

The words *nursemaid* and *governess* thus emerged and became titles for the young girl or woman who functioned in the role of the child-nurse.

The origin of the nurse as mother perpetuated the idea that nursing could be done only by women. The maternal instinct provided that strong impulse or motive necessary to care for those who were suffering or helpless. Women, because of their maternal instinct, were considered "born nurses." Consequently, the nurse as a loving mother who intuitively comforts and renders care continues to be a popular image. The parental instinct more accurately describes this strong motive and is present in both sexes of all races and within different age-groups. It is, however, generally thought that women possess a greater degree of this instinct because of their traditional role in the family, a position that has provided greater experiences in parental activities. Yet the timeless spirit of nursing contains no sexual boundaries. Human beings of both sexes have a natural tendency to respond to helplessness or to a threat to life from disease or injury. Men and women have functioned as nurses throughout various periods in history.

The role of the nurse gradually expanded from that of a mother whose biological function included the nourishing of infants and the nurturing of young children to one with a much broader scope. Care of the sick, the aged, the helpless, the infirm, and the handicapped and promotion of health became vital components of the whole of nursing. In addition, "care" eventually encompassed affection, concern, and solitude, as well as responsibility for individuals in need. In the ancient periods the woman cared for her own kin. As the nursing concept broadened, she also took care of the members of her own tribe. With the development of early civilizations, slaves and servants of households and estates also received care and nursing began to be performed outside the home. As nursing care became more complex, it became apparent that factors other than a strong motive were necessary to do the work of a nurse. Yet this motivation continued to be a vital component of

I Did Not Marry to Become a Wet Nurse, c. 1830-1840. *(From the book* Grandville's Animals, *published by Thames and Hudson.)*

Jean-Baptiste Greuze, *The Nursemaids,* late eighteenth century. Oil on canvas, approx. 31.8 × 39.37 cm. *(Copyright 1990 Nelson-Atkins Museum of Art, Kansas City, Missouri [Nelson Fund].)*

John Rogers, *Weighing the Baby*, 1876. Plaster, approx. 50.8 cm high. *(Collection of the New York Historical Society.)*

Below, Abraham Bosse (French, 1602–1676), *Childbirth,* 1633. (Previously titled *L'Accouchement.*) Etching, 26 × 33.7 cm. *(Philadelphia Museum of Art: Purchased: Smith Kline Beecham Corporation Fund.)*

6

nursing's development and prompted one to care for the suffering or the help-less. In its fullest development it produced altruism or humanitarianism, the noblest forms of love and kindness. Compelling societal forces such as reli-gious fervor reinforced this motive at different historical eras and paved the way for people to lead lives of service and self-sacrifice for the sake of others.

As time progressed, it became apparent that love and caring alone were not sufficient to nurture health or overcome disease. The development of nursing depended on two additional essential ingredients—skill and expert-ness, and knowledge. Great manual dexterity in the carrying out of specific procedures was evident even among primitive tribes and continued to be per-fected through experience. As more and more information about illness and disease became available, emphasis on the necessity of knowledge began to emerge. Knowledge of facts and principles would provide the initiating force for nursing to become both an art and a science (Dock and Stewart, 1925). The head, the heart, and the hands became truly united to provide the strong foundation for modern-day nursing. These three essentials were also referred to as the science, spirit, and skill of nursing and, at still another point, became synonymous with the theoretical, practical, and moral and ethical aspects of nursing (Stewart, 1918, 1921). The neglect or overemphasis of any one of these would cause for an imbalance in care.

The concept of nursing that has been evolving throughout the ages has not yet reached its fullest maturity. It continues to grow and develop to include widening spheres of nursing service and practice and expanding func-tions. It can never, however, "rise higher than the human instruments by which it is administered and the resources they are able to draw upon in the culture of their age and their group" (Stewart and Austin, 1962, p. 10).

Edgar Degas, *Nursemaid in the Luxembourg Gardens,* c. 1871-1872. Canvas. *(Photo Claude O'Sughrue, Musée Fabre, Montpellier, France.)*

Mary Cassatt, *Maternal Kiss,* 1897. Pastel on paper, approx. 56.8 × 46.3 cm. *(Philadelphia Museum of Art: Bequest of Anne Hinchman.)*

Everyday moments between mothers and children were eloquently portrayed by Mary Cassatt. The intimacy depicted in this pastel can almost be felt. The little girl's distress is alleviated by the mother's comforting embrace. Cassatt captures the child's brimming eyes and downturned mouth as well as her trust in her mother's unconditional love.

Limited Edition collector's plate entitled "Office Hours" in the *Friends I Remember* series by Jeanne Down. *(The Edwin M. Knowles China Company, Niles, Illinois.)*

The quote on the reverse side of the plate reads: "Playing nurse was one of my favorite games when I was growing up. . . We must have been pretty good at thinking up cures—we never lost a patient!"

NURSING: THE SEED OF EARLY COMMUNITY SERVICE

Early in its history, nursing can be distinguished as a form of early community service. This service was originally related to a strong instinct for preservation and protection of the tribe and its members. Love and concern for family and tribe extended to neighbors and strangers. One rudimentary way to assist with this effort was through the nursing of individuals who became ill. As more sophisticated civilizations developed, the care of the sick expanded to include concern for other human conditions. Methods for dealing with problems such as poverty, prevention of disease, and any type of helplessness added a social dimension to the nursing work. Those functions commonly associated with present-day social workers were incorporated into the role of the nurse. Historically, the nurse and social worker were one. This phenomenon continued until another group of workers was trained to handle the problems associated with the social ills of society. Even then, as now, nurses were still in a sense true social workers, constantly battling adverse social conditions directly affecting the health and welfare of society.

> When we consider the whole movement of social progress—the breaking down of the spirit of hatred and prejudice, the promotion of kindlier and more humane relations between human beings, the organization of practical and effective measures for reducing human suffering and distress—it would be hard to find any group of workers, who have contributed more to the sum total of social effort.
>
> — *Dock and Stewart, 1925, pp. 374–375*

During specific periods this sense of community was influenced by waves of religious awakening, ideas of chivalry, patriotism and democracy, and social and humanitarian efforts. In these instances nursing combined with other available branches of charitable aid and kindness. The religious influence, however, was probably the strongest. For long periods nursing was regarded as a calling that could be done only by those who renounced the world. This intensely religious motive, combined with the element of self-sacrifice, provided an excellent qualification for assuming the nursing role.

Jean-Honoré Fragonard, *The Happy Family*, after 1769. Oval, 53.9 × 65.1 cm. *(Timken Collection, copyright 1995 Board of Trustees, National Gallery of Art, Washington, D.C.)*

The family constellation has always been regarded by nurses as vitally important to the health and well-being of each of its members. Thus the sick individual is not the only one being cared for by the nurse. Nursing care, health education, and health screening, as well as the welfare of the total family, including their environment, received attention.

Concern for the health of the public or the community was evident in antiquity and continued as civilizations developed. Nearly all primitive tribes fostered some type of sanitary practices in order that the environment would not be tainted. These elementary practices became more sophisticated as technological advances occurred and provided for improvements such as water drainage systems. Eventually, concern broadened to include disease and its communicability and an overall emphasis on health.

From its inception, nursing was involved in this social movement, even in that period when nursing care was integrated as part of the practice of medicine men, priests, wise women, and midwives. Service to the community as well as to the individuals within it was readily incorporated into a basic conception of nursing that included both health and illness. These early roots of public health became a prominent aspect of the nursing role and ultimately provided a variety of community services to achieve this goal. Branches of public service evolved as extensions of nursing and extended into the innermost structures of society. Visiting nurses, school nurses, public health nurses (an older term for community health nurses), nursing settlements, and other facets of community service emerged to become forever a vital and necessary component of nursing.

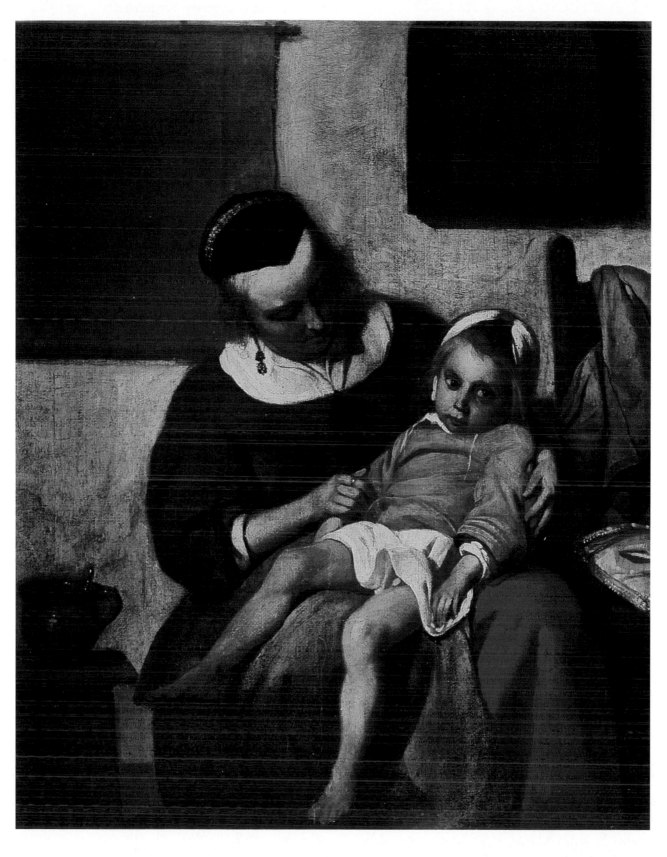

Gabriel Metsu, *The Sick Child*, c. 1660.
Canvas. *(Rijksmuseum, Amsterdam, Netherlands.)*

Nursing is a development of the mother-
care of the young, which has existed from
the earliest of times. Metsu depicts an
event that mothers know only too well—
the onset of a child's illness. The mother
gently cradles her listless child as she
closely watches for symptoms. Her love
and watchful caring are demonstrated by
her concerned expression.

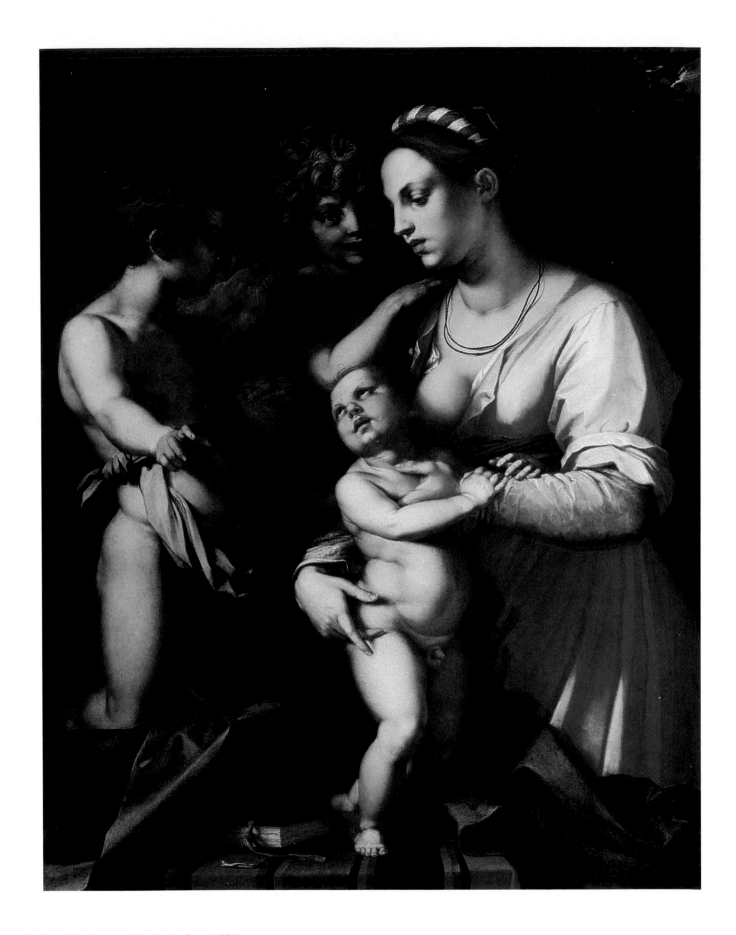

Andrea del Sarto, *Charity*, before 1530.
Oil on panel, 119.5 × 9.25 cm. *(Samuel H.
Kress Collection, 1957, National Gallery of
Art, Washington, D.C.)*

CARE OF THE SICK AMONG PRIMITIVE PEOPLE

It is possible that some of the first ideas related to medical treatment and nursing care were acquired through the observation of animals. Although it may be difficult for some to consider that simple medical and nursing procedures were prehuman in origin, support for this premise exists in natural history. The first traces of parental love, kindness, and mutual aid were exhibited by birds and other animals. The lower animals in particular subjected themselves to appropriate medical and surgical treatment when necessary, treated themselves when injured or ill, and assisted one another (Berdoe, 1893).

Primitive people, in order to escape the ravages of illness and disease, needed to learn to protect themselves and find means of treatment and cure. During this period of history people were much closer to nature and moved throughout the animal kingdom with minimal fear. They were able to readily observe and learn the animal practices associated with ailments. Even animals attempted to relieve pain and to remove the causes of infection. Animals cleansed their wounds by licking, ate grasses, leaves, and other plant life, which acted as emetics and purgatives, submerged inflamed wounds in water, and engaged in other practices that had significant effects on their well-being.

It was not possible for primitive people to find a treatment for every illness through this observational process. Nor were they able to detect more than the most obvious natural circumstances leading to illness by using such a system. Yet, instinctively aware that other causal factors of diseases existed, people turned to searching for these additional explanations. Close intimacy with nature, however, colored their ideas about myriad forms of life, of which they had no scientific knowledge. People ascribed to all such forms those qualities they identified within themselves. All natural objects—rocks, rivers, trees, mountains, the wind—were alive, or animate, and possessed a spirit or soul (psyche, anima). Natural phenomena, including those causing disaster or disease, could thus be explained. This basic belief in *animism* unlocked the door to a still greater world in the minds of humans, that of imagination.

The introduction of a belief in spirits, good and evil, profoundly affected the development of those practices related to treatments and remedies. Ideals of an occult nature, superstitions, became tightly linked to the etiology of diseases because supernatural origins for most happenings, including illness, were accepted by primitive people. Since humans lived in two worlds—the visible and the invisible—a combination of occult practices and empirical ones occurred and provided the necessary climate for the use of magic. The supernatural world could and did affect primitive humans.

Since the cause of illness and disease was attributed to evil spirits, cures were attempted through intervention with these spirits. Consequently, a great body of tribal lore arose, which included incantations, rites, rituals, and spells. In time, certain types of symptoms were ascribed to the work of particular spirits and means of driving them away were devised. The primary goal was to make the patient's body an unpleasant dwelling place for the spirit. Repeated pummeling and pounding of the inhabited area of the body were meant to dislodge the evil spirit. (It is possible that the practice of massage originated from these techniques.) Plants that had unpleasant effects were used to make concoctions that would be disagreeable to the spirits. Expulsion could occur in two ways, through the intestinal tract or through the mouth, and so appropriate herbs, which acted as either purgatives or emetics, were chosen and administered. Evil spirits lodged in the head were to be released through holes in the skull. Trephined skulls of primitive peoples give evidence of this extreme measure. Fire, hot instruments, and blistering appliances were used as counterirritants to burn out the spirits. Cold baths, sweating, starvation, bad smells, and hideous noises were all used in the attempt to expel demons from the suffering body.

The federal Republique de Cameroun, on the west coast of Africa, honored its *Croix Rouge* (Red Cross) with a set of two stamps in 1965. One shows a Red Cross station and ambulance. The companion stamp, illustrated here, honors Red Cross nurses. *(Courtesy of Howard B. Hurley.)*

This 1964 stamp issued by Papua and New Guinea pictures nurse and child. Entitled *Infant, Child and Maternal Health,* the stamp publicizes the territorial health services. *(Courtesy of Howard B. Hurley.)*

13

Paul Gauguin, *Te Pape Nave Nave (Delectable Waters)*, c. 1898. Oil on canvas, 74 × 95.25 cm. *(Collection of Mr. and Mrs. Paul Mellon, copyright 1995, Board of Trustees, National Gallery of Art, Washington, D.C.)*

A variety of techniques were used by primitive tribes to cure individuals whose bodies were believed to be inhabited by evil spirits. These techniques, in many instances, were the basis for numerous practices currently in use such as massage, ingestion of herbs for cathartics or emetics, and heat and cold applications.

The magical lore that accumulated became too complex to be understood by the ordinary tribal people. Chosen individuals who supposedly had special insight or intimate contact with the spirits devoted their time to mastering and interpreting this lore for the benefit of the tribe. These men, and sometimes women, usually went through a long and arduous training period. In addition, they might have lived through some mystical experience, spent weeks alone in fellowship with the spirits, or recovered from a critical illness or injury. In time, these "medicine men," "witch doctors," or "shamans" became the guardians and disseminators of this esoteric knowledge and skill. More important, their possession of life-giving powers granted them a place of prestige, and they were set apart from and above the rest of the tribe. "Here was the beginning of specialization in the art of healing" (Shryock, 1959).

Healers were primarily concerned with occult lore and procedures, although they undoubtedly became authorities on tribal folk medicine. In most instances the problem was not to give the illness a name but to find a cure. Consequently, this required that a magical cause be identified in order to overcome the malady. Healers were also faced with another aspect of the occult related to the cure of disease or dispelling of misfortune. They had to develop the ability to use their magic in an evil or a good way. The use of these two separate functions gave rise to a system of black magic and white magic. White magic invoked the help of good spirits to drive off evil ones and was practiced for benevolent purposes. Black magic, hostile and destructive in its aims, was used to bring disaster or disease upon enemies. This was accomplished with the aid of evil spirits, poisons, and malice.

These practices were organized into ritualistic ceremonies that eventually assumed a religious tone. The result of this union was the labeling of the medicine man as a "holy person." Primitive medicine became a mixture of magic, religion, and naturalistic remedies. According to some sources, the medicine man became the priest-physician (Dolan, Fitzpatrick, and Hermann, 1983; Jamieson and Sewall, 1950). Other authors subscribe to a belief in the development of higher and lower ranks among healers, with the priest-physician being the highest (Dock and Stewart, 1925; Stewart and Austin, 1962), or to the idea that it is unclear whether primitives made distinctions between priests and medicine men (Shryock, 1959). What is clear, however, is that both types of healers dealt with problems of life and death and were authorities on traditional lore.

The omnipotence of these early healers was supported by the use of strange disguises, elaborate ceremonies, mystical signs, charms (amulets and talismans), and fetishes. Skins, hoofs and horns of animals, feathers, grasses, and other objects adorned the ceremonial garb. Extreme drama and mystery kept the observers in awe of the medicine man. The ceremonies might last for hours or days and often included dancing, singing, and playing of instruments. The medicine man's ability to frighten off evil spirits was demonstrated by

African, Guinea Coast, Yoruba, *Divination Board.* Opo Ifa, wood, 54.6 × 3.8 cm. *(The University of Iowa Museum of Art, Iowa City, The Stanley Collection.)*

Wooden trays called *awua ifa* are used in traditional Yoruba divination ceremonies. The tray, in conjunction with the divination tapper, is used to summon the god Ifa.

these props. As late as the 1830s, an account of a medicine man's actual procedures was rendered:

> his body and head were entirely covered with the skin of a yellow bear, the head of which (his own head being inside of it) served as a mask; the huge claws of which also, were dangling on his wrists and ankles; in one hand he shook a frightful rattle, and in the other brandished his medicine spear or magic wand; to the rattling din and discord of all of which, he added the wild and startling jumps and yelps of the Indian; and the horrid and appalling grunts, and snarls, and growls of the grizzly bear, in ejaculatory and guttural incantations to the Good and Bad Spirits, in behalf of his patient; who was rolling and groaning in the agonies of death, whilst he was dancing around him, jumping over him, and pawing him about, and rolling him in every direction.

— *Catlin, 1926, p. 46*

Elon Webster, *False Face Mask,* 1957. Wood. *(Cranbrook Institute of Science, Bloomfield Hills, Michigan.)*

Iroquois peoples carved expressionistic masks for use by the False Face Society, whose ceremonies healed physical and psychological sickness and cleansed whole communities of destructive impurities.

African, Guinea Coast, Yoruba, *Divination Tapper.* Ivory, approx. 25.4 cm high. *(The University of Iowa Museum of Art, Iowa City, the Stanley Collection.)*

The divination tappers are used by the diviner priest to attract the attention of the god Ifa. The fecundity symbols of kneeling women holding their breasts are the most common ornamentations of the tappers. The Yoruba have no fertility god, and many of the clients of the diviner priest are women seeking to bear children.

José Dolores Lopez, Cordova, New Mexico, *Death Cart (Carreta de la Muerte),* c. 1930. Carved cottonwood. *(St. Louis Art Museum, St. Louis, Gift of the May Department Stores Company.)*

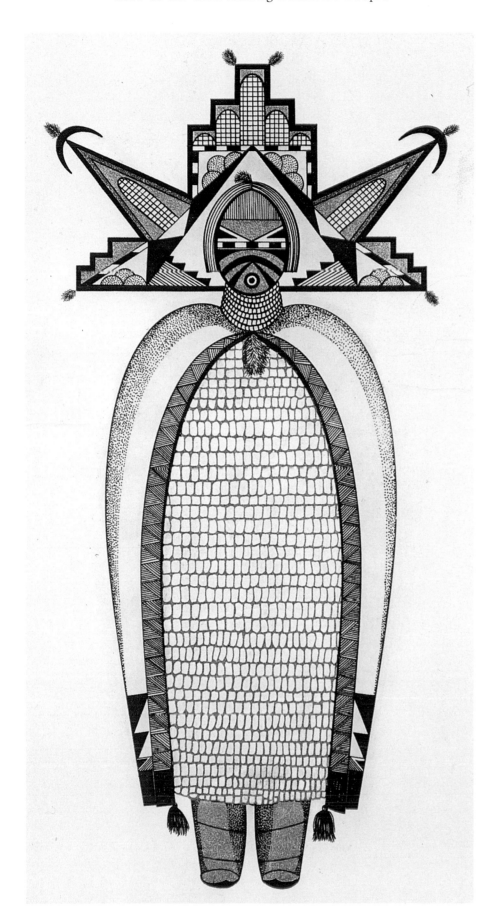

Helen Hardin, *Bountiful Mother*, 1980. Etching and intaglio printed in three colors, 45.7 × 40.64 cm. *(Copyright Helen Hardin, 1980. Photo copyright Cradoc Bagshaw, 1995. All rights reserved. Helen Hardin Estate.)*

Helen Hardin painted under her Pueblo Indian name, Tsa-Sah-Wee-Eh but she is known as "Helen Hardin." She was the daughter of Pablita Velarde, a famous Southwest painter. Corn is the foundation of Hopi and Pueblo agriculture and life. It receives a certain degree of veneration and for the Pueblo Indian was ". . . a living entity with a body similar to man's in many respects . . .the people built its flesh into their own. Hence corn was also their mother. Thus they knew their mother in two aspects which were often synonymous—as Mother Earth and the Corn Mother" (Frank Waters, *Book of the Hopi*). Hardin's *Bountiful Mother* is as convincing as the 15,000-year-old *Venus of Willendorf*. She is dressed in a snowy feminine robe; pale blue corn kernels make up the body ripe with fertility.

Venus of Willendorf, c. 30,000–20,000 BC. Limestone, 10.8 cm high. *(Naturhistorisches Museum Wien, Vienna, Austria.)*

This type of small sculpture in the full round representing the female figure is thought to have served as a fertility fetish. Her figure fits perfectly in the clasped hand. She appears to be in the late stages of pregnancy.

Indonesia, Sumatra, Batak People, *Medicine Horn,* late nineteenth century. Wood, water, buffalo horn, hair, and fiber, approx. 48.3 cm long. *(St. Louis Art Museum, St. Louis, Gift of Morton D. May.)*

Paul Gauguin, *The Invocation*, 1903. Canvas, approx. 65.5 × 75.6 cm. *(Copyright Board of Trustees National Gallery of Art, Washington, D.C. Gift from the collection of John and Louise Booth in memory of their daughter, Winkie, 1976.)*

Pieter Bruegel the Elder, *Witches of Malleghem*, 1559. Engraving. *(From H.A. Klein:* The Graphic World of Peter Bruegel the Elder, *New York, 1963, Dover Publications.)*

Dr. Syntax Turned Nurse, c. 1820. Aquatint after a drawing by Thomas Rowlandson. *(From* The Third Tour of Dr. Syntax: In Search of a Wife. *By permission of the British Library, London, England.)*

Scene when Dr. Syntax, sheltered from a coming storm,

> *"within the comfortable farm,*
> *Himself and the good dame to please,*
> *He took the children on his knees;*
> *Then danc'd the urchins to and fro, And*
> *sung as nurses often do."*

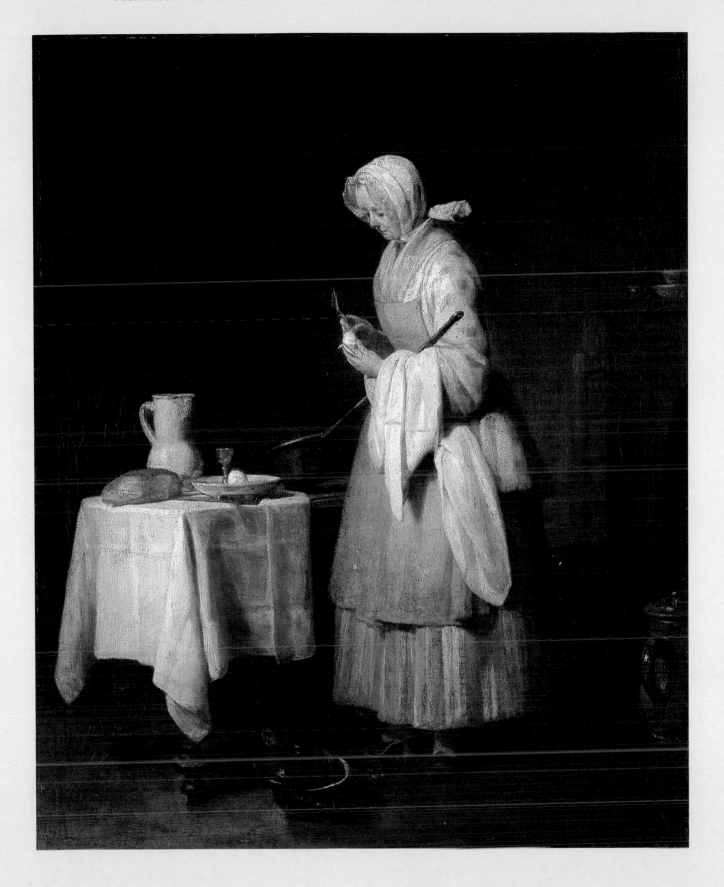

Jean–Baptiste–Siméon Chardin, *The Attentive Nurse*, c. 1738. Oil on canvas, approx. 46.2 × 37 cm. *(Samuel H. Kress Collection, copyright 1995, Board of Trustees, National Gallery of Art, Washington, D.C.)*

The attentive nurse gives special consideration to the needs, desires, and comfort of the patients. The nurse is mindful, observant, and receptive in the process of caring.

Cecilia Beaux, *Ernesta (Child With Nurse),* 1894. Canvas, approx. 128.3 × 96.5 cm. *(The Metropolitan Museum of Art, New York, Maria DeWitt Jesup Fund, 1965. All rights reserved.)*

Ernesta Drinker, the artist's niece, looks out as she grasps the hand of her nurse, Mattie. The painter cropped the nurse at the waist, giving the observer the child's view of a starched apron. The child holds hands with her nurse, symbolizing trust, protection, caring, and touch. The element of touch has proved to be extremely significant in nursing care. When no other method or technique is available, when "nothing more can be done," human touch is always available to soothe, to comfort, and to convey caring, compassion, and love.

West Mexico, Jalisco, *Pregnant Woman and Midwife Group,* Terminal Preclassic, 200 BC-AD 300. Polished gray earthenware, 21.6 cm high, 20.3 cm long. *(St. Louis Art Museum, St. Louis, Gift of Morton D. May.)*

As the caste of medicine men developed, a class of practitioners became associated with them. These individuals, most often the women of the tribe, applied the treatments, ascertained the qualities of drugs, became skillful in dressing wounds, and learned to reduce fevers. Theirs was a practical knowledge of appliances and drugs. These tribal women were the discoverers of medical herbs; they were the first empirical physicians who learned to prepare different potions to be used as remedies (Mason, 1894). Some of these women, particularly the elderly, must have been the earliest prototypes of the so-called witch. These "wise women," who were extremely knowledgeable about medicinal secrets, and who went out early and late to gather herbs, became prominent as caretakers for the sick through prehistoric ages (Alexander, 1782). In time, as a result of superstitious feelings, wise women, or witches, were credited with uncanny powers that were both good and evil, particularly the ability to cause illness and wasting diseases. Eventually, this belief led to the persecution of perhaps the first rivals of the medicine men (Dock and Stewart, 1925). Many similar superstitions still exist today in isolated communities.

The exact relationship between the practical attendants (nurses) and the medicine men or priest-physicians is not clearly understood. If the attendant received orders for the treatment of the patient from the medicine man, the relationship was probably that of physician and nurse. If the attendant prescribed the simple treatments and herbs and the medicine man limited his work to incantations, the relationship could have been the symbolic representation of the combination of the theory and practice of medicine. The latter would be indicative of the yet unspecialized department of nursing (Nutting and Dock, 1937). It is also possible that some rivalry began to occur as the struggle for a monopoly of power began to emerge.

The individuals who provided rudimentary nursing probably varied with the customs of each group or tribe. These practical tasks were first, however, the work of mothers and wives. This naturally occurred as a result of the division of labor: men hunted for the food and provided the defense for the tribe; women cared for the children and eventually for those individuals afflicted by disease, age, injury, or other incapacitating conditions. As knowledge increased, others became specialized in particular areas of medical work.

Primitive societies sowed the seeds of hygiene, sanitation, and public health as well as medicine, surgery, psychiatry, midwifery, nursing, and other branches of the healing arts. Within this structure, nursing's heritage was derived. The role of the nurse as mother, the concept of nursing as a feminine occupation, and the expansion of nursing to include people who were not related emerged and became a vital part of society. The interrelationship, yet separation, of the medical practitioner and the nursing practitioner was established.

23

UNIT 2

Ancient Civilizations

uman history has moved in a series of stages as we have tried
to understand the world around us. The first views we know
about attributed to invisible spirits all the inexplicable things
that happened. The spirits could not be dominated; they had
to be placated. Later, the idea of a multitude of animated spirits
was transformed into a vision of gods and godesses with more-
or-less human forms and superhuman attributes. They were not
indifferent to people. They could reward and punish. Then
came the idea of a single godhead, a unity of man and nature.

— FLORA LEWIS

Helen Hardin, *Medicine Woman,* 1981. Four-color copper plate etching, approx. 61 × 45.7
cm. *(Copyright Helen Hardin, 1981. Photo copyright Cradoc Bagshaw, 1995. All rights reserved.
Helen Hardin Estate.)*

This painting is a part of the "Women Series" done by Helen Hardin. The artist wanted
the series to portray women as intellectual, emotional, and sensitive. Three paintings were
included: *Changing Woman, Medicine Woman,* and *Listening Woman.* A fourth painting and
the last in the series, *Creative Woman,* died with the artist in June 1984. No sketches exist.

Medicine Woman wears feathers because she is a healer but not necessarily a nurse or a
doctor. She could be a mother nursing a child from a cold, since all women possess a healing spirit. The face is literally split in two, indicating a unique and unsettling combination
of active anguish and covert ecstasy.

According to the artist, *Medicine Woman* was derived from a 1980 kachina painting,
Arrival of Winter Messengers. "I finished *Medicine Woman* just before he [the doctor] told me
[that the biopsy results showed malignancy and that mastectomy had to be scheduled]. It
was almost as if I needed that person, that healing spirit. After I found out I had cancer,
and we were doing the print at El Cerro, I felt I had her spirit with me." The surgery
occurred in October 1981.

25

	45000 BC	30000 BC	20000 BC	10000 BC	5000 BC
DAILY LIFE				**17,000 BC** Wild grain harvesting in Middle East **13,000 BC** Earliest evidence of colonization in North America	**4000–3500 BC** First year of Jewish Calendar **6500 BC** Human populations raise sheep, goats, and cattle **5000 BC** Rice cultivation established in China **4000 BC** Babylonian civilization flourishes
SCIENCE AND TECHNOLOGY		**37,000 BC** Rudimentary counting devices used in Africa	**18,550 BC** Bone needles from wallaby shin bone used in Australia		**4241 BC** Egyptians produce 12-month calendar **4000 BC** Writing developed in Mesopotamia
THE VISUAL ARTS	**45,000 BC** Rock engravings in South Australia		**24,000 BC** First rock paintings in Africa		
MEDICINE AND HEALTH CARE					

NURSING

Nursing as a separate occupation is not well documented during this time period. The following is generally known:

- Midwives accepted as specialists to women in childbirth
- Children's nurses given some distinction in some cultures
- Priestesses believed to have performed functions that are now recognized as nursing functions

2500 BC	2000 BC	1500 BC	500 BC	80 BC

3500–3001 BC Linen produced in Middle East

2500–2000 BC Earliest Egyptian mummies

2800–2400 BC Flint widely traded

1500 BC Vedas, historical documents of India, written

1280 BC Hypostyle hall at Karnak uses 134 columns for supports

776 BC First recorded Olympic game held in Greece

550–331 BC System of roads established in Persia

469–399 BC Socrates pioneers the philosophy of Classical Greece

450–400 BC Plague in Athens

400–300 BC Open-air theaters such as Epidauros built

400–300 BC Use of chopsticks becomes common in China

250–200 BC Oil lamps introduced in Greece

200 BC Woven sandals worn by Anasazi people

3300 BC Syrian clay tablets part of earliest phase of writing

2500–2001 BC Egyptians discover use of papyrus

2000 BC Bronze used in tools in China and Europe

2000 BC Iron tools and weapons developed

1876 BC First eclipse recorded in China

1800 BC Bronze weapons used in Europe

1600 BC Glass molded to form objects and vessels

1400 BC Phonetic alphabet widely used in the Levant

800 BC Use of alphabet adopted in Greece

600 BC Earliest coins issued by kings of Lydia (modern Turkey)

80 BC Greek astronomical calculator computes changing positions of heavenly bodies

---

3000 BC First known pottery in the Americas

2650 BC Stepped pyramid of King Zoser, Egypt built

2650–2150 BC Most famous Egyptian pyramids built at Giza, Saqqara, and Dahshur

2500 BC Burial urns painted in western China

2100 BC Stonehenge reaches final form in Great Britain

2000 BC Temples and ritual centers flourish in the Huanaco Valley of Central Peru

1000–900 BC Brush-and-ink painting in China

800 BC Egyptian coffin lids decorated with painted scenes

500 BC Terra-cotta sculptures made in Northern Nigeria

500–200 BC Celtic art style becomes prominent

2900–2800 BC Imhotep identified as greatest priest physician of Egypt

2500–2001 BC Sumerian medicine discovers healing qualities of mineral springs

2000–1500 BC Contraceptives used in Egypt

1900 BC Code of Hammurabi inscribed on shaft of black stone

1800 BC Mosaic health code developed

1134 BC Asklepios is worshipped in temples in Greece

500 BC Acupuncture and moxibustion performed in China; halls of healing

460–370 BC Hippocrates credited with establishment of scientific medicine

400 BC Trephination performed to treat head injuries, migraine headaches, and seizures

300 BC Medical schools connected with temples of Asklepios in Greece

200 BC Greek physicians are made slaves and forced to practice throughout Rome

90 BC Asclepiades, Greek physician, practices nature healing in Rome

---

- ❧ Men, as well as women, function as caregivers

- ❧ Details of nursing principles and practices given in ancient writings

- ❧ Nurse, pharmacist, and physician recorded in ancient Greek mythology

Judy Chicago, "Fertile Goddess," plate from *The Dinner Party,* 1979. China-painted porcelain, 35.6 cm diameter. *(Copyright Judy Chicago, 1979. Photo copyright Donald Woodman. Through the Flower, Albuquerque, New Mexico.)*

Female goddesses are still worshipped all over the world. Their images are regarded as earth mothers, symbols of ethnic unity, creator goddesses, and objects of fertility cults. Frequently they have been referred to as fertility fetishes or symbols, and contemporary usage often stresses female sexuality. Their sole purpose, however, was not to promote fertility of the land, animals, or human beings. Rather they portrayed the fruitfulness of the earth itself. "In our own time, in our own culture, the Goddess once again is becoming a symbol of empowerment for women; a catalyst for an emerging spirituality that is earth-centered; a metaphor for the earth as a living organism; an archetype for feminine consciousness; a mentor for healers; the emblem of a new political movement; an inspiration for artists; and a model for re-sacralizing woman's body and the mystery of human sexuality." (Gadon, 1989, p. xv).

*T*he earliest thoughts of primitive humans were simple yet complex. Primitive people personified all that they saw in nature, believed that the phenomena of nature were their greatest mysteries, and developed mystical rites around the treatment and cure of illnesses and the perservation of health. These historical facts and the intimate and universal connection between religion and medicine led to a logical belief that was to permeate the majority of the ancient civilizations.

Nature worship became the basic principle upon which the mythologies and religions of the ancient civilizations were founded. The belief in evil spirits as causes of disease progressed to a belief that disease was caused by a failure to do things that the gods wished or by some moral transgression (Goodnow, 1942). Thus illness was a curse, a punishment set forth by the gods and directed at individuals, families, and their descendants, and at sinners. The many gods of ancient times "were all originally nature gods, or simply external forces of nature or attributes of the physical and intellectual man symbolised and personified" (Nutting and Dock, 1937, p. 26). Legends and myths of deities who watched over health and had powers over life and death were composed and cultivated by nations. This served to bring some order out of the old confusion about innumerable demons associated with the earlier magical medicine. Fewer beings now needed to be appeased. Furthermore, traditions of worship and methods for requesting divine aid for the sick were established. Frequently temples were built to these gods, and they became temples for healing and, ultimately, sanctuaries for the sick.

The manner of life followed by primitive tribes led to constant changes in their location. These nomadic people naturally followed the presence of food, tending to migrate toward the south, where warmth, rich soil, and vegetative growth made it possible to live with less effort and a greater degree of comfort. Evolutionary improvements such as the development of tools (Stone Age) followed by the incorporation of the use of several metals (Iron Age) occurred along with the domestication of plant and animals. These advances paved the way for tribal people to settle down as herders and farmers and to supplant the roving life with village life. Slowly, in certain fertile areas, civilization began to develop.

It is generally believed that the movement of these tribes radiated from the interior of Europe and Asia toward the warm shores of the Mediterranean Sea, India, and China. Migration of a much lesser degree evolved in the direction of western Europe and the British Isles. In most instances movement followed the shores of great rivers.

> The early civilizations on which that of the modern western world is based, were those of the eastern Mediterranean area. In Egypt, Syria, Mesopotamia, and even further east in India, oriental peoples developed cultures of a high order long before anything similar appeared in most parts of the world.
>
> — *Shryock, 1959, p. 19*

Although early civilizations also appeared in China and Japan, these exerted little influence on the Western world as a result of limited contact.

Regions bordering on the Mediterranean Sea came to form the greater part of the known world. This body of water was believed to occupy the center of the earth, as its name implies. Consequently, all areas to the east of the Mediterranean Sea became known as "eastern"; those to the west became known as "western" (Jamieson and Sewall, 1950).

The cultural patterns in these early centers of civilization exhibited an interdependence of religion, government, social welfare, and health. As in primitive tribal societies, magic, superstition, and early forms of religion were used to control the forces of nature when other measures were ineffectual. Through the use of magic and superstition government authority was enforced, property disputes were settled, woman's place was determined, social welfare was secured, and disease and injury were cured. Justice and charity toward the poor, the weak, and the sick were taught in some cultures. Human sacrifices might be demanded, and mutilation of the body was not encouraged.

> By 3000 BC or soon thereafter an advanced civilization had developed in the Near East. Buildings were constructed in brick and stone; the arch, wheel, and plow were in use; a calendar had been invented; and writing made possible the preservation of records. From this time until the fall of Rome, conventionally dated as AD 476, great kingdoms and vast empires were established, extended, and overthrown in constant shifts of power from one people to another. At different periods and in different areas many forms of government appeared. In some, the ruler's control was absolute; in others, it was restricted by custom or by the religion of the people.
>
> — *Sellew and Nuesse, 1946, p. 32*

Religious beliefs and myths were the foundations for medical practice in early civilizations. Thus religious leaders were originally given the responsibility for curing and treating the sick and the injured. As time progressed, two ideas regarding the cause of illness became accepted: illness was caused by the displeasure of the gods and all illnesses were the result of natural causes.

Judy Chicago, "Snake Goddess," plate from *The Dinner Party*, 1979. China-painted porcelain, 35.6 cm diameter. *(Copyright Judy Chicago, 1979. Photo copyright Donald Woodman. Through the Flower, Albuquerque, New Mexico.)*

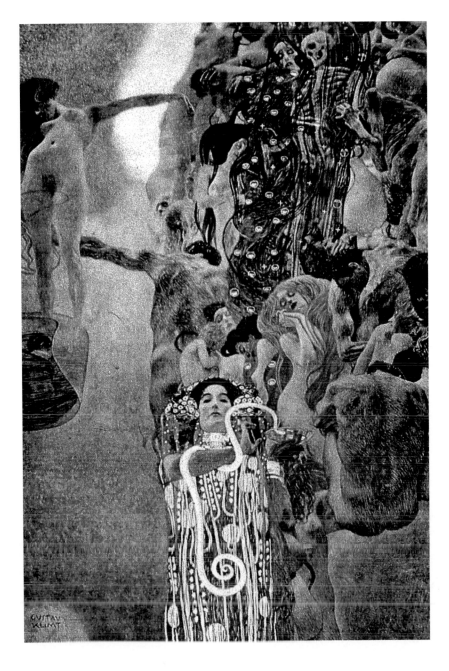

Gustav Klimt, *Medicine,* c. 1907.

Gustav Klimt, "Hygeia," detail from *Medicine*, 1900-1907. *(Schloss Immendorf, Austria/Bridgeman Art Library, London.)*

A dualism, the first step in the transition that medicine needed to make from the magical to the rational, was thus exhibited. Rational observations and treatments were preceded and followed by religious chants and rites to ensure a cure. With the development of empirical knowledge, health care was delegated to priest-physicians and eventually to secular physicians. The latter development occurred primarily in Greek and Roman civilizations. This evolution resulted in the development of significant medical contributions (special procedures, biological sciences, diagnostic measures, classification of diseases, and observation recording) that began to transform medicine from magic into a science.

A search throughout ancient history reveals little, however, about attendants to the sick—nurses. This may be so because unusual or striking events rather than ordinary ones are generally recorded in history. People have always nursed their sick as a matter of course. It was not until cities became large and problems became acute that the matter of care in illness warranted specific mention. Yet one can be reasonably sure that nurses, male or female, functioned in early civilization. From earliest times the midwife has been accepted in her role during childbirth, as has the child's nurse. Slaves, attendants, and women of good character probably cared for those with curable conditions.

> Priestesses are believed to have performed many functions now recognized as those of the nurse, for, in the temple, man's first center of community thought and activity, is disclosed the nucleus of his religious education, medicine, and nursing.
>
> — *Jamieson and Sewall, 1950, p. 52*

Indeed, the beliefs, mores, and culture of each civilization directly influenced the way in which nursing care was given. In addition, who rendered nursing care and what constituted nursing care were reflections of the prevailing society.

THE NEAR EAST

 ❧⚬❧

Egypt

One of the first civilizations to emerge clearly from barbarism was that of Egypt. The very long, narrow valley on either side of the Nile River comprised its boundaries. The people who settled on this fertile strip built a civilization that far exceeded that of other groups who settled elsewhere. Signs of prosperity became increasingly evident in Egypt: systems of irrigation were devised, roads and ships were built, trade was established, practical arts were developed, architecture became dignified, family and other social relationships were maintained through the use of accepted moral codes, and the entire society was held together by an absolute monarchy headed by the pharaoh or king. Egypt is well remembered; impressive and enduring monuments still exist to herald its glory. Pyramids, tombs, temples, and other edifices are among the wonders of the contemporary world.

More is known about Egypt than about any other ancient culture. Surviving Egyptian records are related to periods as distant as 3000 BC. A system of writing was introduced, at first in the form of pictures and later as signs or *hieroglyphics*. Formal records were carved in stone or written in inks on paper scrolls called *papyri* (writing materials made from the pith of the tall sedge plant). The papyri and the stone carvings have yielded the greatest information on certain Egyptian periods. In the dry sands of Egypt these papyri, which contained the most complete examples of ancient medical literature, were preserved. They were named after their discoverers or owners, for example, the Brugsch, Ebers, Smith, Hearst, Berlin, and London scrolls (Frank, 1953). The Ebers papyrus is known as the oldest complete medical book in the world.

> No less than five medical papyri have come down to our time, the finest being the celebrated Ebers papyrus, bought at Thebes by Dr. Ebers in 1874. The papyrus contains one hundred and ten pages, each page consisting of about twenty-two lines of bold hieratic writing. It may be described as an Encyclopedia of Medicine as known and practised by the Egyptians of the eighteenth dynasty, and it contains prescriptions for all kinds of diseases—some borrowed from Syrian medical lore, and some of such great antiquity that they are ascribed to the mythological ages, when the gods yet reigned personally upon earth.
>
> — *Edwards, 1892, p. 219*

The Smith papyrus revealed a high level of Egyptian surgical practice arranged according to the general parts of the body (only the section relating to the upper parts survives). The Hearst, London, and Berlin papyri, which focus almost entirely on the treatment of the diseases of the anus, may have been practical handbooks. The Ebers papyrus outlined many of the diseases known to modern science and minutely described their symptoms. In addition, more than seven hundred substances from the vegetable, mineral, and animal kingdom were given as drugs along with descriptions for their preparation. The complexity of these prescriptions suggests the need for specialists to compound them. The Ebers papyrus also, however, contained incantations and verbal charms.

Three elements are present in these manuscripts: religion, magic, and accounts of illness and treatments (Shryock, 1959). This is consistent with Berdoe's description:

> The art of medicine in ancient Egypt consisted of two branches, the higher, which was the theurgic part, and the lower, which was the art of the physician proper. The theurgic class devoted themselves to magic, counteracting charms by prayers, and to the interpretation of the dreams of the sick who had sought aid in the temples. The inferior class were practitioners who simply used natural means in their profession.
>
> — *Berdoe, 1893, p. 61*

Seated figure of Imhotep, Sixth Dynasty. *(Museum of Egyptian Antiquities, Staatliche Museen Preussischer Kulturbesitz, Berlin; Foto Marburg/Art Resource, New York.)*

It is possible, however, that the word *magic* did not convey the true medical state, since the Egyptians practiced hypnotism and were aware of how to control the mind and imagination. It is not clear who gave the orders for the practical treatment of the patient, the priest-magician (priests) or the priest-physician (doctors). What is clear is that two professions dealt with the sick at the same time but in different ways. In some instances the two combined to become one, commonly known as the priest-physician.

Out of this structure emerged the first physician known to history. Sometime in the Third Dynasty (c. 2900–2800 BC) Imhotep is identified as the greatest priest-physician of Egypt. His stature as a historical personage grew according to his deeds. He was recognized as a surgeon and an architect to one of the pharaohs and as a temple priest, a learned scribe, and a successful magician (priest-physician). Imhotep was noted for his great wisdom and learning in the field of health, magic, and religion. He was so successful in healing the sick that statues and temples were erected in his honor. After Imhotep's death the Egyptian people elevated him to the rank of Egyptian God of Medicine, the god of healing.

The philosophy of the Egyptians was a form of nature worship that included some aspects of animism. Diseases were believed to have partly natural, partly supernatural causes. The development of astrology also led to the belief that disease, as well as destiny, was influenced by changes in celestial phenomena, such as the movement of sun and stars and the passage of seasons. Astrological medicine arose and functioned harmoniously with mythical premises.

A spirit world inhabited by many gods developed in the Nile valley. Ultimately a trinity assumed control of bodily and spiritual welfare: Isis, Osiris, and Horus, their son. Isis (Mother Earth) and Osiris (Day or Light or Sun God) were regarded as the creators of agriculture and the medical arts. Isis gave her help to the sick most often through the medium of dreams. From his mother, Horus learned medicine as well as the gift of prophecy. Osiris sat in judgment of the souls of those who died, and immortality became an established belief. Magnificent temples emerged and became significant as molding influences in the civilization. Originally built as meager shelters to protect the gods, the temples became centers of community and national life. Priest-physicians functioned in those temples, which were frequented by individuals in search of health.

Concern for the question of life after death was especially prevalent in Egyptian society. The people hoped for personal survival beyond the grave.

Stepped Pyramid of King Zoser, c. 2610 BC, Saqqara, Egypt. *(Hirmer Verlag, Munich).*

This structure, with its temples, complex of chambered terraces, and great courtyard, is now thought to be a medical shrine built under the direction of Imhotep.

Therefore symbols of immortality, the pyramids, were erected. Bodies were skillfully embalmed so that souls could remain within or return when the afterlife began. Aromatics, resins, and other preservatives were employed in this process. The custom of embalming enabled the Egyptians to become familiar with the organs of the human body. More than two hundred fifty different diseases were identified from clinical observations. Treatments were developed that incorporated the use of drugs and procedures, including surgery. Specialization became a reality, perhaps because of the large quantity of writings that may have necessitated concentration on a limited area of knowledge. Herodotus, the Greek historian, explained:

> Medicine is practiced among them on a plan of separation; each physician treats a single disorder and no more: thus the country swarms with medical practitioners, some undertaking to cure diseases of the eye, others of the teeth, others of the head, others of the intestines, and some of those which are invisible.
>
> — *Herodotus*

Splendid examples of the art of bandaging emerged as thousands of yards of linen in various widths and patterns were used on one mummy. These bandages were hardened with a gluey substance to form an impenetrable case for an aseptically cleansed body. Safe repositories in the form of elaborate tombs were constructed to ensure the preservation of body and soul for all time.

The ancient Egyptians also established public hygiene and sanitation at a relatively high level. They appear to have had a corps of sanitary inspectors or health officers (Nutting and Dock, 1937). The Egyptians recognized the importance of an adequate drainage system, a good water supply, and the inspection of slaughter houses. They were very particular about the cleanliness of their bodies and their dress, which was always of linen. They practiced circumcision from earliest times. Strict rules were developed to regulate such matters as cleanliness, food, drink, exercise, and sexual relations. Some sources indicate that the rigid hygienic regulation of the Jews originated from these Egyptian practices (Seymer, 1932).

Modern researchers have yet to disclose evidence regarding the existence of any building identifiable as a hospital. However, according to Caton, "There is reason to believe that institutions closely related to infirmaries or

Model of Hypostyle Hall, Temple of Amen-Re, Karnak, Egyptian, Nineteenth Dynasty, c. 1350–1205 BC. *(The Metropolitan Museum of Art, New York, Purchase 1890, bequest of Levi Hale Willard.* *The Metropolitan Museum of Art.)*

hospitals existed in Egypt many centuries earlier than the Hieron of Epidauros, but no structural trace of such building has been discovered" (Nutting and Dock, 1937, p. 54). Whether there were or were not hospitals, the temples had some type of housing for the sick. In those temples frequented by individuals in search of health, priest-physicians engaged in medical practice. The existence of priestesses or "temple women" is also certain; what their duties were is not clear, although it is assumed that they performed some type of nursing functions.

The position of women in ancient Egypt was higher than in other Eastern countries. In general, women enjoyed considerable freedom and dignity. Within their own households they held a position of authority and importance. It is probable that nursing care was the chief responsibility of the mother or daughters in the home. In addition, physicians in ancient Egypt did not practice obstetrics; this field was left entirely to midwives. Wet nurses were engaged on contract to breast-feed infants for approximately six months.

In a nation as sophisticated in medicine, pharmacy, and sanitation as ancient Egypt, it is almost impossible to believe that there were no persons, male or female, who engaged in the work of nurses and nursing. History, however, fails to make this point clear.

Persia (Iran)

Persia is presently called Iran, a form of the word *Aryan*. This name indicates that the Persians spoke an Aryan or so-called Indo-European language; the Persians were related to European peoples (Shryock, 1959). The Plateau of Iran was positioned to the east of the Fertile Crescent and between the Persian Gulf and the Caspian Sea. In ancient times the land was occupied by the Medes and the Persians. However, by 500 BC the Persians had conquered the Medes, moved their borders eastward to the Indus River in India, and conquered all of the Fertile Crescent and Egypt. The energies of Persia were directed toward war, tyranny, and the acquisition of wealth and power. The result of these efforts was the founding of the most extensive empire that appeared in the Near East. Fortunately, this empire, which exerted an almost totally destructive influence, existed for only about two hundred years.

The religion of the Persians, Zoroastrianism, revolved around Zoroaster, who lived about 600 BC. This prophet wrote the sacred books of Persia, the Zendavesta, which introduced a world ruled by two creators, one producing light and good, the other darkness and evil. Although good and evil were constantly at war, good always triumphed. In addition, sacred elements were identified: fire, earth, and water, with fire described as the purest. According to the sacred books, immortality was a mental rather than a physical state. The principal virtues of veracity, virility, and hard work would enable people to achieve happiness. Thus happiness or unhappiness depended on the righteousness or evil of people on Earth with the promise of rewards after death (Jamieson and Sewall, 1950).

The Persians absorbed much of the culture of their conquered land, including the medicine and surgery of Egypt. They had great confidence in Egyptian medicine, demonstrated by the emperor Darius, who renovated an old school to be used for the training of priest-physicians. This is thought to be the first case of a medical center established as a royal or government foundation.

Three types of physicians evolved from the medical center: those who healed by the knife, those who used plants, and those who healed by exorcism and incantations (Nutting and Dock, 1937). No mention is made of nurses, although descriptions of various surgical and medical procedures are given, some of which could well have belonged to the province of nursing. In retrospect, little attention has been given to the medical history of the Persian Empire. It may be that Persia contributed little to medicine in comparison with other countries.

Facing page, Shah Nameh, The Book of Kings, *Birth of Roustem by Caesarian.* Moghul Art, sixteenth century. *(Musée Condé, Chantilly, France. Giraudon/Art Resource, New York.)*

Caesarian section became an important addition to obstetrical care during the time of the Renaissance. The surgical operation had been performed for at least two thousand years but was not acknowledged by the medical community until the latter part of the sixteenth century.

Map of the Fertile Crescent of the Pre-Christian Era.

The Fertile Crescent

A series of civilizations developed in the Fertile Crescent, an area that stretched from the Isthmus of Suez, up through Palestine and Syria, east through the region of Damascus, and down the Euphrates River valley. This land has also been called the Cradle of Civilization. In this region, thousands of years ago, the first cities in the world were built and the first attempt at developing a system of writing occurred. Three great rivers—the Tigris, the Euphrates, and the Jordan—were situated in the area. The combination of well-watered soil and a warm climate encouraged habitation. Successive peoples came and conquered their predecessors in the fertile valleys. Most of them spoke the Semitic languages.

> Sumerians, Assyrians, Babylonians, and Persians followed one another as the dominant people, in that chronological order. Conquerors took over the earlier civilizations, however, so that there was an accumulation of culture from the ancient Sumerian period about 3000 BC down to the flowering of Persian life more than two thousand years later.
>
> — *Shryock, 1959, p. 26*

Agriculture flourished in this area, and wealth and economic changes led to the building of memorable cities. Progress was similar to that of Egypt, with one significant difference: structures were built with clay or bricks instead of stone. Therefore natural phenomena and time crumbled these ancient cities into dust. Fortunately, records were kept on hardened clay tablets, and from these tablets information about religion, business, and medical practice has been deciphered. These cuneiform (wedge-shaped) writings frequently referred to practices performed by royal physicians that today would be carried out by nurses.

Babylonia.   As Egyptian civilization was developing in the Nile valley, a comparable advance was occurring in the region between the Tigris and Euphrates valleys, now known as Iraq. This area was originally known as Mesopotamia, a Greek word meaning "between the rivers." City-states that developed in southern Mesopotamia were dominated by temples where priests represented the patron deities of the city. Each ancient city was a community center with schools, libraries, granaries, and workshops. Each was governed by a divine ruler and a priest-king who was the actual ruler. The most prominent of these city states was Sumer, regarded as the finest and earliest civilization of humankind. The Sumerians made significant contributions to human civilization in the development of morals, learning, and the arts. They were eventually conquered by the Babylonians, a Semitic people. The conquered lands ultimately became known as the Babylonian Empire, which was established by about 2100 BC.

The religion of the Babylonians comprised magical and superstitious principles and a strong astral influence. These people believed in polytheism, a plurality of gods, the majority of whom were nature gods.

> The three greatest were the gods of the sky, the earth, and the sea. Next in rank were the moon god, the sun god, the god of thunder, lightning, wind, rain, and storm: of the planet Venus; Marduk or Merodak (light), (who is also called Bel), the quickener of the dead, who fought and vanquished the dragon or "Chaos" (darkness); Nebo, the god of arts, science, and letters, and others.
>
> — *Nutting and Dock, 1937, p. 57*

Local deities were also numerous. Disease was believed to be evoked by the wrath of the gods and by evil spirits; this resulted in the creation of hierarchies of good and evil spirits. Survival was dependent on securing aid from the good spirits. Ceremonies incorporating the use of fire, water, and incantations became important in this process, and various occult practices were cultivated.

The Babylonians were learned mathematicians and astronomers. They originated the division of time into months, days, and minutes, used a system of weight and measures, and followed the signs of the zodiac. Their study of sun, moon, and planets became the basis for scientific astronomy. Astrological interpretation became closely connected with physiological phenomena; the position of the stars and the motions of the planets and the moon were believed to directly affect humans. "As their lore accumulated, they began to 'cast horoscopes' in terms of an individual's birth, for the position of the planets at this time was supposed to cast a spell over a man thereafter" (Shryock, 1959, p. 28). Eventually medicine became interwoven with astrology, and the result was the practice of a magic medicine carried out by astrologer-priests. These individuals practiced medicine by using a combination of magic, religion, and science. Sources of epidemics were ascribed to inauspicious astral influences. Human ailments were diagnosed through examination of the livers of dead animals. The art of *divination* (foretelling events or discovering hidden knowledge by the interpretation of omens or by the aid of supernatural powers) was practiced through a variety of methods, including palmistry, crystal gazing, and communication with the dead.

A very primitive stage in Babylonian medicine was recorded in which the sick were brought out into the marketplace. Passers-by were required to stop and render advice based on their own personal experiences. It is difficult to determine how long this empirical stage lasted and whether it occurred before or after there were physicians. What becomes clear, however, is that lay physicians were also prominent in Babylonia. The practice of medicine by these physicians was divided into two basic areas, surgery and internal medicine. Surgery was considered to be the more advanced field. "Their surgeons understood nasal tamponing for bleeding, cataract couching, the use of facial

The Seal of Male Midwife Urlugaledinna, Sumerian, 2200 BC. *(Musée Nationale du Louvre, Paris.)*

African, Guinea Coast, Yoruba, *Divination Tray.* Wood. *(The University of Iowa Museum of Art, Iowa City, The Stanley Collection.)*

The art of divination (foretelling events or discovering hidden knowledge by the interpretation of omens or by the aid of supernatural powers) was practiced through a variety of methods. Palmistry, crystal gazing, and communication with the dead were frequently used.

applications in cases of erysipelas, and blood-letting. Bodies of sacrificed animals supplied the only opportunity for anatomical research" (Jamieson and Sewall, 1950, p. 26). Circumcision is known to have been performed by Abraham, a native of Babylonia.

Internal medicine remained primarily in the magical realm and was concerned with magical formulas to banish demons, the gods of evil spirits. Since illness was thought to be caused by sin and displeasure of the gods, methods of treatment consisted of ridding the human body of these demons through incantations and other remedies. Vile-tasting plant and mineral concoctions, powders, enemas, and human and animal excreta were used. Yet the clinical observations of the physicians were fairly accurate portrayals of symptoms, as reported in vivid descriptions such as the following:

> The sick one coughs frequently, his sputum is thick and sometimes contains blood, his respirations give a sound like a flute, his skin is cold but his feet are hot, he sweats greatly and his heart muscle is disturbed. When his disease is extremely grave his intestines are frequently opened.
>
> — *Castiglioni, 1947, p. 39*

Numerous diseases were described, including fevers, plague, abscesses, heart and skin diseases, tuberculosis, tumors, jaundice, and venereal disease.

The lay physicians and surgeons of Babylonia needed to be careful about their practice. The legal codes of this country were more advanced than those of any other ancient culture and held individuals and groups responsible for their actions. Particularly significant was the Code of Hammurabi, inscribed about 1900 BC on a single great shaft of black stone and placed in one of the temples of Babylon. This code was developed by Hammurabi, sixth king of Babylonia, who was considered the greatest king and statesman during his reign of approximately sixty years. Hammurabi collected older laws and customs and systematically arranged these into a comprehensive code of law. Justice and consideration for the poor and defenseless classes were evident in this document, which was intended to be humanitarian. The code dealt with both civil and criminal law and contained regulations for various circumstances; for

The Code of Hammurabi. (Parke-Davis Division of Warner-Lambert Co., Morris Plains, New Jersey.)

example, business contracts, thefts, rents, loans, property rights, doweries, adoption of children, employment policies, sanitation, and public health. In addition, the Code of Hammurabi contained provisions for the veterinarian, a clear indication that the two specialists (physician and veterinarian) were distinct. More important, it addressed medical and surgical practice, with control of the surgeon the most severe aspect. Fees due practitioners, severe penalties for failures in treatments, and compensations to patients injured during treatment were outlined. In essence the physician's conduct was regulated by the government, and penalties could result in cruel physical punishment:

> If a physician has treated a free-born man for a severe wound with a lancet of bronze and has caused the man to die, or has opened a tumour of the man with a lancet of bronze and has destroyed his eyes, his hands one shall cut off.
>
> — *Code of Hammurabi*

This "eye for an eye and tooth for a tooth" philosophy presumably deterred unnecessary surgeries and fostered precautionary measures among the practitioners.

A table of fees for operations was also set and varied from two shekels for surgery on a slave to ten shekels for operating on a freeman:

> If a doctor has treated a freeman with a metal knife for a severe wound, and has cured the freeman or has opened a freeman's tumour with a metal knife, and cured a freeman's eye, then he shall receive ten shekels of silver.
>
> If the son of a plebeian, he shall receive five shekels of silver.
>
> If a man's slave, the owner of the slave shall give two shekels of silver to the doctor.
>
> [For the veterinarian] If a doctor of oxen or asses has treated either ox or ass for a severe wound, and cured it, the owner of the ox or ass shall give to the doctor one sixth of a shekel of silver as his fee.
>
> — *Code of Hammurabi*

The Code of Hammurabi was the greatest legal masterpiece of ancient civilization. It advanced the common good of Babylonia, and for nearly three centuries this country experienced increasing prosperity.

The history of Babylonia gives little mention of nursing as a separate occupation. The writings, however, frequently refer to practices that are currently performed by nurses. The Babylonian nurse was probably a domestic servant or a slave, either male or female. Accounts of wet nurses, midwives, and children's nurses, who often had great affection for their charges, have been rendered. In addition, in some pictorial scenes the role of the nurse in assisting the patient has been portrayed.

Assyria. The Assyrians, who succeeded the Babylonians, were a hardened, warlike Semitic race who held the balance of power in the Near East from approximately 745 to 635 BC. Their little kingdom of Assur arose in the middle of the Fertile Crescent. Its location afforded protection of its boundaries, with mountain ranges on three sides and a river on the fourth. Nineveh, the capital city, eventually became the center of art and commerce in the Near East. Its walls, which stretched about two and one-half miles along the Tigris River, provided the setting for the ruling king.

The Assyrian laws were severe. Mutilation was inflicted as a punishment for many offenses, and the death penalty was frequently used. Absorbed in war, the Assyrians made the "god of the battlefield" their supreme god. Their intensity in military tactics resulted in the production of stronger weapons (the Assyrians were the first to use weapons made of bronze) and new techniques of warfare. However, Assyrian power was shortlived; it suddenly lost vitality, and Nineveh fell to a coalition of powers about 612 BC. "Denounced by the prophets, its name [Nineveh] has survived as a symbol of luxury for the rich and destitution for the poor, a symbol of vice and of sin" (Sellew and Nuesse, 1946, p. 34).

Stele of Hammurabi, Susa, c. 1760 BC. Basalt, approx. 220 cm high. (*Musée Nationale du Louvre, Paris.*)

At the top of the stele, which is made of black diorite and stands nearly two and a half meters tall, King Hammurabi is shown receiving the laws from the sun god, Shamash. Around the stele, in Assyrian cuneiform symbols, are engraved his 282 laws, the first to govern the practice of medicine and surgery. The Code of Hammurabi, which dealt with both civil and criminal law, was the greatest legal masterpiece of ancient civilization.

Assyria preserved the theory of demonology, which held that the sick person's body was possessed by evil spirits. Even further, the Assyrians fostered the belief that illness was a punishment for sin and could be cured only by repentance, magic, or a combination of magic and religion. The aspects of sin and repentance, however, may have been another way of stating that those who broke physiological laws would become ill and could be cured only by resuming the practice of hygienic rules (Nutting and Dock, 1937). The entire theory thus would have been predicated on the natural laws of health. Whatever is accepted as the basis for their belief, the fact remains that the Assyrians practiced only magic and empirical medicine, which was consistent with their superstitious nature. They believed in the influence of lunar changes, and charms and amulets were used extensively. Numbers were regarded as lucky and unlucky; for example, the number seven was so sacred that the seventh day was reserved for rest. Many regulations existed about the gathering of medicinal herbs: some should be gathered by night, some at dawn, and others at a certain time of the moon. Ceremonies were adopted whereby one could be purified by fire and water. Sacrifices involving the offering of human life were sometimes also required.

Medical texts were handed down by the Assyrians on clay tablets with cuneiform script. The greatest number came from Nineveh and were supposedly from the library of King Asurbanipal (668–628 BC). These texts exhibit a mixture of rational therapeutic remedies with purely magical devices:

> If a man's head is full of scabies and itch thou shalt bray sulphur, mix it in cedar oil, anoint him.
>
> . . . a thread thou shalt spin, double it twice, tie 7 knots. As thou tiest (them) thou shalt recite the charm, bind on his temples and he shall recover.
>
> If a man has a burning headache affecting his eyes, which are bloodshot, take one third of a measure of *sikhli* crushed and powdered, and knead with cassia juice; wrap it around his head, attach it (with a bandage) and do not remove it for 3 days.
>
> — *Seymer, 1932, p. 6*

Nothing about nursing is revealed in the history of Assyria, nor is there any evidence that buildings were used as hospitals. In regard to women in Assyria, it can be assumed that they did not achieve a very high status.

Palestine. As tribes of the Semitic race were moving into Babylonia and Assyria, other tribes were moving into the region of Palestine at the western side of the Fertile Crescent. The geographical position of the latter tribes, between Egypt on one side and Assyria and Mesopotamia on the other, significantly affected the development of their own culture. These people were given the name *Hebrews* by the natives whom they eventually dominated. The literal translation of the word *Hebrews* is "the people from beyond" (Reinach, 1930). The Hebrews were well established in their towns by the time Hammurabi was king of Babylonia (c. 1955 BC). Agriculture became their chief endeavor, although the mountainous character of this portion of the Fertile Crescent provided less than desirable conditions. The terrain comprised narrow, gorgelike valleys; the soil was lacking in minerals; and rainfall was inadequate, causing an insufficient water supply. The industrious Hebrew people, however, overcame these obstacles. They built towns, raised sheep, collected water in cisterns, and patiently cultivated olives and grapes. The country flourished, and the city of Jerusalem became the center of religious and political activities.

The Jews (Hebrews, or Israelites) were the first to develop the art of writing historical narratives, and their early histories are preserved in the Old Testament.

In Genesis, Exodus and other books, we are told how Abraham (Israel) first came into Palestine, how his descendants (the "Children of Israel") were made captives in Egypt, how they escaped therefrom into Palestine, how they were then conquered and taken into exile "by the waters of Babylon," and how the Persians finally restored them to Jerusalem. In the course of these adventures they absorbed much of the culture of both Egypt and Babylon, and the Bible is full of accounts of those two civilizations.

— *Shryock, 1959, p. 30*

Thus the Jews traced their descent from Abraham, who was born in Ur, Chaldea, and migrated to Palestine with his family. Abraham was the first of the patriarchs, his son Isaac was the second, and his grandson Jacob was the third. In the eighteenth century BC famine drove the Jews into Egypt, where they lived for a time in prosperity. Ultimately, they were taken into captivity, where they remained as slaves for more than four hundred years. It was not until the fifteenth century BC that the Jews left Egypt under the leadership of Moses. Their reentry into Palestine took place after forty years of wandering. At that time the people were divided into twelve tribes (from the patriarchs to the twelve tribes). Jacob had twelve sons and a daughter. However, his favorite son, Joseph, had no tribe; instead, Joseph's two sons Manasseh and Ephraim received his birthright. Because the tribe of Levi had a priestly role and did not bear arms, it was neither counted in the general census of the Israelites in the wilderness nor allotted tribal territory in the land of Canaan. State and church were under the same head, a theocratic government. The chiefs of the tribes and the elders possessed the power of civil authority. A tribal assembly approved or rejected decisions.

From approximately 1095 BC, Palestine was ruled by kings. Saul was its first king, followed by David, under whom the country flourished. David's successor was Solomon, who financed his love for luxury by burdening the people with taxes. Yet Solomon earned respect for wisdom and justice in administration. After his death the kingdom was split into two, and each of these new kingdoms fell to invading powers. Israel was conquered by Assyria in 722 BC; Jerusalem fell to Babylonia in 587 BC. From this time forward the Jews became a people without a country, since rising empires constantly seized Palestine. By AD 1, Palestine was under the rule of Rome.

The Hebrews embraced a theocentric philosophy, a belief in a personal God. This philosophy held that humans have free will and an immortal soul created by God, and that a human being is a body-mind-spirit unity. Hebrew religious belief was theocratic and monotheistic. The Hebrew people abhorred the innumerable deities of other nations. They denounced superstitious and magical practices to the extent that death was the penalty for performing them. Yet they held the extreme view that disease is a punishment for one's own sins. Their strength was derived from belief in the one true God. According to Shryock (1959), this monotheistic conception had been formed in Egypt earlier but had exerted only temporary influence there. All power over life and death was in the hands of Jehovah. God became the source of health, and its preservation was to be found in "keeping pure before the Lord." A way of living emerged that did not necessitate specific medical practices.

Religion and medicine were combined, and responsibility for the public health centered on the priest-physicians drawn from the priestly tribe of Levites. These men were held in high esteem:

Honor the physician for the need thou hast of him: for the most
    High created him.
For all healing is from God: and he shall receive gifts of the king.
The skill of the physician shall lift up his head: and in the sight of men he shall
    be praised.

— *Ecclesiastes 38:1–4*

Michelangelo Buonarroti, *Moses,* c. 1500. Marble. *(San Pietro in Vincoli, Rome, Italy. Photo copyright by Leonard von Matt-Photo Researchers, Inc., New York.)*

It is possible that much of the knowledge of the Hebrew people was borrowed from the Egyptians. Moses, the adopted son of the pharaoh's daughter, had led the enslaved people out of Egypt. Undoubtedly, he was well acquainted with Egyptian wisdom and received a sophisticated education, most likely at the University of Heliopolis (now Cairo). Although Moses' learning took place in a pagan atmosphere, he was taught the religious beliefs and traditions of his Hebrew heritage by his mother, who had been selected as his nursemaid. Mosaic Law was given to the Hebrew nation by Moses upon God's command. It contained civil specifications similar to those of the Code of Hammurabi. Yet the Mosaic Law exhibited consideration for the poor and the weak. As a result, justice became one of the most important characteristics of Hebrew social thought.

The laws ascribed to Moses, although expressed in religious terms, had definite hygienic significance. Regulations were provided for the general public health. Every detail of personal, family, and national hygiene were specified and directed toward the maintenance of health and the prolongation of life. A method for prevention of disease included personal hygiene, cleanliness, rest, sleep, and hours for work. Definite provisions were ascribed for women during menstruation, pregnancy, and childbirth. Other provisions dealt with inspection and selection of food, disposal of excreta, notification of authorities in cases of communicable disease, quarantine, and disinfection. It is interesting to note that the health regulations were planned to improve the endurance of the race, which was in keeping with the thought that the Israelites were the chosen people (Deuteronomy 14:2).

Master Hugo, *Moses Expounding the Law,*
frontispiece of the Book of Deuteronomy
of the *Bury Bible,* the abbey of Bury St.
Edmunds, early twelfth century. Illuminat-
ed manuscript, approx. 50.8 × 35.6 cm.
*(Reproduced by permission of the Master and
Fellows of Corpus Christi College, Cambridge,
England.)*

43

The priest-physicians also functioned as health inspectors. Contagious diseases had to be reported and isolation was compulsory. The orders for treatment and isolation came from the priest, who also initiated the disinfection of the body, clothing, and environment. Permission had to be secured from the priest to reenter the camp after being quarantined. The acceptance of these practices demonstrates the ancient Jewish belief in infection by contact (contagion), the idea that epidemic diseases were spread from one individual to the next:

> Thus the Jews not only pioneered in establishing the concept of contagion but also in those measures of notification and isolation which were based upon it. This approach to public health control, however, made little impression on other ancient races, and it remained for European Christians to revive it during the Middle Ages.
>
> — *Shryock, 1959, p. 32*

Dietary laws were a significant part of the Mosaic Law. Four cardinal points were to be observed about animal food. First, blood was forbidden as food. Meats were to be drained of their blood before cooking (animals were scientifically bled). Second, animals torn by wild beasts or accidentally killed were not to be used as food. Third, animals that died naturally were not to be used as food. Fourth, the pig was forbidden as unclean. Cloven-hoofed animals that chew their cud and are not scavengers, birds that are not birds of prey, and fish that have fins and scales were permitted in the diet. According to Lyons, there may have been explanations for food prohibitions other than those with a medical basis. He renders this account:

> One recent suggestion is that the taboo against pigs was originally related to their competition with humans for water and grain (scarce commodities in a barren land), in contrast to cattle and sheep which consume relatively little water and graze on forage inedible to man. Since transmissible parasitic diseases and infestations such as tapeworm are also found in sheep and cows, singling out trichinosis in pigs would not be wholly logical. However, to discourage the raising of swine so as to conserve water and grain resources for human consumption, a strict religious taboo may have been necessary—considering man's nearly universal agreement on the delectableness of pork. Medical observations may indeed have been at the core of hygienic codes, but the Biblical listing of seemingly unrelated creatures prohibited as food is difficult to associate with purposes entirely hygienic.
>
> — *Lyons, 1978, p. 71.*

Knowledge of ancient Jewish medicine is derived almost entirely from the Old Testament of the Bible and the later Talmud, the authoritative compilation of Jewish tradition. The two Talmuds, the Jerusalem and the Babylonian, were written, approximately, from the second to the sixth century AD. In addition to exhibiting remarkable medical observations, they incorporate the attitudes, influences, and methods of the various peoples with whom the Jews lived. References to nurses in the Talmud and the Old Testament suggest wet nurses or children's nurses rather than nurses who were caretakers of the sick. The Jewish midwife was important, but more attention was given to the hygiene of pregnancy than to the actual assistance of the mother at the time of delivery. A woman was usually delivered while sitting on a stool designed in a circular fashion; the midwife sat on a lower stool before her. If complications arose and all known methods failed to improve the situation, religion dictated that she be cared for and comforted until she died (Sellew and Nuesse, 1946). Deborah was the first nurse to be recorded in history, as shown in the twenty-fourth chapter of Genesis. She is included in the story of Rebekah, who sets out by camel train with her nurse (Deborah) to meet her future husband, Issac. Deborah was a child's nurse and a companion but at times may have been called upon to perform other nursing duties.

Ancient Jews believed that all people should have access to medical care, regardless of their social status. With an emphasis on human brotherhood and social justice, the duties of hospitality to the stranger and relief for widows, orphans, the aged, and the poor were constantly urged as righteous. Visiting the sick was a prominent feature of everyday life and a designated duty. Houses for strangers, called xenodochia, were instituted and later expanded to include the care of the sick. These xenodochia were supported financially through a system of tithing. Whether these institutions had nurses is unknown. They did, however, become predecessors of the modern inn and the modern hospital. Overall, the Hebrews recorded achievement in the practice of hygiene, sanitation, and the systematic and organized prevention of disease.

THE FAR EAST

As the great civilizations of ancient times were developing in the Near East, others were developing on a vast continent that eventually became known as Asia. This region included current-day India, China, and Japan, an area usually distinguished by modern historians as the Far East or Orient. Little evidence of human progress in primitive times is available from this area. It is believed, however, that the stages of development were similar to those experienced by other cultures.

India

India lay in the southern part of the Far Eastern continent. This triangular region was almost completely isolated from the rest of the world by two chains of mountains (Himalayas) along its northern border and waters (Arabian Sea, Bay of Bengal, and Indian Ocean) on its other three borders. It is thought that an advanced civilization existed in the Indus River valley by approximately 3000 BC. Migration from central Asia occurred through the mountain passes on the north by Aryan peoples of Indo-European stock. This group found in India a warm climate, an extremely rich vegetation, and a race darker-skinned than themselves. The difference in skin color may have been the basis for the formation of a caste system that developed gradually and had far-reaching consequences for health and well-being. The immigration continued over a long period, and the descendants, Indo-Aryans, were a vigorous people whose wealth consisted of cattle and amusements included hunting, gambling, and chariot racing. Eventually the native peoples of this area were conquered by the Aryans. An advanced culture developed that had direct access to Persia on the west and indirect contact with China to the east.

Excavated remains indicate that in the first civilization in India (2500–1500 BC) there were large cities and a highly developed culture. Within the carefully planned cities were baths, shops, multiroom buildings, and temples built with burnt brick. An exceptional feature of this pre-Aryan culture was its system of public sanitation. Drainage systems, wells, bathrooms, public baths, and collection chutes for trash were in evidence. Practical arts included cultivation of soil, domestication of animals, and smelting of metals. The script from the writings left by this civilization is yet to be totally deciphered.

The Vedic Age, beginning after 1500 BC, produced the classical Indian civilization and Brahmanism (also known as Hinduism). Agriculture became the principal occupation at this time, although crafts were also practiced. Organized labor appeared in the form of guilds. The territory of the Jumna and Ganges rivers became sacred to the Hindus. India became a home of architectural beauty with a people who were well versed in war and politics, inventors of the decimal system, and discoverers in geometry and trigonometry. A priesthood was established, and the population was divided into tribes ruled by elected chiefs. In time the state replaced the tribes, and kings replaced the chiefs.

India was known as the Land of the Temples. Its temples were masterpieces of artistry and were vitally important to the Hindu people. The idols, however, were usually hideous. Worship was directed to one or more of the prominent deities. Uppermost was the Trimurti, or divine triad of gods: Brahma, the power and spirit of the universe; Vishnu, the preserver of the world; and Shiva, the destroyer and conqueror of death. The other principal deities included Lakshmi, goddess of life, beauty, and good fortune; Soma, personification of the hallucinatory plant used in Aryan rituals; Indra, god of war and weather; Agni, god of sacrifice and fire; Varuna, god of justice and cosmic order; and Dhanvantari, patron god of medicine. The twin Ashvins were also medical gods, patrons of eyesight, who acted as physicians to the gods themselves.

Two philosophical systems greatly influenced the lives of the people of India: Brahmanism and Buddhism. Both were closely connected with strong religious beliefs, and both were pantheistic and nihilistic. Pantheism is the belief that reality is a single being of which everything else is a part. (The deities were parts of the eternal whole because Brahman permeated everything in the universe.) Nihilism is the belief that conditions in the social organization are so poor as to make destruction desirable. It holds that existence is senseless and progress involves destruction for its own sake.

Brahmanism, the religion of the Aryan conquerors, provided religious development during thirty centuries. It revolved about Brahma, the eternal spirit, who permeated everything in the universe. The ideal of perfection rested in absolute unity with Brahma. This was attained by sacrifice, penance, and contemplation. Transmigration of the living soul, the doctrine of reincarnation, was affirmed. A person might be reborn into a lower or higher rank of human being, or even into the form of lower animals after death. Ancestor worship was encouraged, and reverence for animals, especially cows and monkeys, was advocated. Consequently, consumption of products from these animals was forbidden. Inherent in Brahmanism was stratification of the society into four distinct castes: Brahmins (priests and their descendants), Kshatriyas (warriors), Vaishyas (merchants, farmers, and artisans), and Shudras (menial workers).

The religious and moral codes within Brahmanism were written in the Vedas (Vedic, the parent language of Sanskrit, was used), which served as the sacred books or scripture and were the historical documents of India. These doctrines, presented in the form of hymns, prayers, and teachings, were administered by the priestly class. The priests retained a very high position and were responsible for interpretation, enforcement, and preservation of the dogma.

The Vedas, usually dated about 1600 BC, consisted of four books. The Rig-Veda, the Yajur-Veda, and the Sama-Veda were almost entirely religious. In the Rig-Veda, disease was regarded as the result of divine wrath. The Atharva-Veda contained innumerable incantations and charms for the practice of magic; disease, injuries, sanity, health, and fertility were mentioned.

> In India, as in all other countries curative spells and healing mantras (charms) preceded medicine; and the first man of medicine in India was a priest, a Bhisag Atharvan (i.e., magic doctor), who held a superior position to a surgeon in society.
>
> — *Sushruta-Samhita, Introduction, p. xiv*

Supplemental Vedas (Upavedas) were also developed. Of these the Ayur-Veda, or Science of Life, was supposed to have been derived from Brahma himself. It contained eight parts that dealt with subjects such as medicine, surgery, and children's diseases and stressed hygiene and prevention of illness. From these writings various authors made Samhitas or compendiums for which they claimed divine origin. Two of these contributors were regarded as the most influential: Sushruta and Charaka. The dates of origin of these documents vary widely from the fourth century BC to the fifth century AD.

> The surgical treatise (Sushruta-Samhita) is probably the older, though some critics have assigned the two works to the same period, the fourth century BC. The question of date is chiefly important as involving a doubt whether the Hindu medical system is primitive and entirely indigenous, or was influenced by Greece and through Greece by Egypt.
>
> — *Seymer, 1932, p. 9*

Sushruta represented the surgical aspect of Indian medicine; Charaka symbolized the medical aspect. Charaka was believed to have inherited wisdom from a serpent-god with a thousand heads who was the caretaker of all the sciences, especially medicine (Stewart and Austin, 1962). Both authors reveal a highly developed medicine and surgery, which no doubt evolved slowly after the writing of the Vedas and was incidentally influenced by contacts with the cultures of the Near East.

Indian surgery was the most skilled of any ancient culture. Operations such as tonsillectomies, which were unknown to the later Greeks and Romans, were performed in India. Furthermore, Hindu surgeons performed amputations, excised tumors, repaired hernias and harelips, removed bladder stones, couched cataracts (displaced the opacifying lens down and away from the line of vision), reconstructed noses, and delivered by cesarean section. In addition to the procedures related to surgery, about 125 different surgical instruments were described. Hindu physicians drugged their patients with hyoscyamus, henbane, and *Cannabis Indica* and used hypnosis in an attempt to provide anesthesia. Great care was taken in the washing and bandaging of wounds (fifteen principal varieties of bandage were available). The ideal doctor was identified in the following way:

> He should be cleanly in his habits and well shaved, and should not allow his nails to grow. He should wear white garments, put on a pair of shoes, carry a stick and an umbrella in his hands, and walk about with a mild and benignant look as a friend of all created beings. . . . A physician should abjure the company of women, nor should he speak in private to them or joke with them.
>
> — *Bhishagratna, 1907, p. 74*

Many illnesses, such as tuberculosis, typhoid fever, leprosy, hepatitis, neurological disorders, and cholera were described. The epithet "mellitus" (honeylike) was applied to diabetes, and its symptoms were identified as languor, thirst, and foul breath. Variolation was practiced. About fifteen scarifications were made with a needle on the upper arm of a person to be immunized; the area was then covered with cotton dipped in pock material. Transmitters of specific diseases, such as mosquitoes in connection with malaria, were described. It was believed that prevention of disease was more important than the cure. Indian medicine also displayed ideas about pathology, the most notable being that disease might be caused by impurities in the body fluids or humors. This humoral pathology later was emphasized by Greek physicians and ultimately became a basic concept for European medicine.

An interesting portrayal of a team concept of medical care was presented in one Indian document:

> The Physician, the Drugs, the Nurse, and the Patient constitute an aggregate of four. Of what virtues each of these should be possessed, so as to become causes for the cure of the disease, should be known.
>
> *Physician.* Thorough mastery of the scriptures, large experience, cleverness, and purity (of body and mind) are the principal qualities of the physician.
>
> *Drugs.* Abundance of virtue, adaptability to the disease under treatment, the capacity of being used in diverse ways, and undeterioration are attributes of drugs.
>
> *Nurse.* Knowledge of the manner in which drugs should be prepared or com-

pounded for administration, cleverness, devotedness to the patient waited upon, and purity (both of mind and body) are the four qualifications of the attending nurse.

Patient. Memory, obedience to direction, fearlessness, and communicativeness (with respect to all that is experienced internally and done by him during the intervals between visits) are the qualities of the patient.

As in the task of cooking, a vessel, fuel, and fire are the means in the hands of the cook; as field, army, and weapons are means in the victor's hands for achieving victory in battles; even the patient, the nurse, and drugs are the objects that are regarded as the physician's means in the matter of achieving a cure.

Like clay, stick, wheel, threads, in the absence of the potter, failing to produce anything by their combination, the three others, viz., drugs, nurse, and patient cannot work out a cure in the absence of the physician.

— *Kaviratna, n.d., pp. 102–103*

As time passed, the people of India became dissatisfied with the religion of the Vedas. There had long been those who had chosen the life of a recluse to attain a more intimate relationship with the spiritual. Among them was Siddhartha Gautama (560–480 BC?), from the caste of princes, who left home, wife, and child at the age of twenty-nine to find salvation. After wandering and speculation, he announced himself as Buddha, the Enlightened, and offered a new religious philosophy that came to be known as Buddhism. The major premise of Buddhism was based on the idea that perfection consisted of attaining nothingness, which was to be accomplished by severe penances.

"The long period of India's Golden Age was that in which the religion of Buddha prevailed. It was a religion of mercy, compassion, and justice which enjoined humane treatment for animals as well as man" (Stewart and Austin, 1962, p. 24). Buddhism was, however, more of a moral discipline than an organized religion and encouraged the development of social institutions. India's greatest convert to Buddhism was King Asoka (269–237 BC), but he was unsuccessful in instituting its acceptance on a permanent basis. During Asoka's reign the greatest advances in charitable and sanitary work were made. Among his many generous works he established hospitals that are considered to be the first in world history. The exact number of hospitals he developed is not known. According to Shryock (1959), there was difficulty with the Sanskrit word for *hospital,* since it could also be interpreted as *pharmacy* or *dispensary.* However, there is no question that hospitals of some type were built during this period. These hospitals were constructed periodically by government order, serviced by government-paid physicians, and supplied by government stores. Consequently, state medicine had become a reality in India.

The early physicians came from the priestly or Brahmin caste. Later, physicians were drawn from the upper castes, and eventually all practitioners came to be known as Vaidya. High moral standards were expected of those who chose the care of the sick as a life's work. Permission to practice was obtained from the king, a procedure similar to the current licensing system. Appearance, dress, speech, and manners had to be above reproach. Rules for ritual and daily life were dictated by the Laws of Manu, which were compiled between 200 BC and AD 200. These laws have been compared to the Mosaic Law because they include ordinances for regulation of family and personal hygiene and dietary practices. According to the Laws of Manu, physicians could be penalized for improper treatment of patients.

The history of India reveals a more complete description of nursing principles and practice than that of any other ancient civilization. Throughout the historical documents of India frequent references are made to nurses. In most instances these nurses were men; however, in rare cases they were old women. Three main qualities of character—high standards, skill, and trustworthiness—were also required of these attendants. The specific requirements are described in the following passages:

After this should be secured a body of attendants of good behaviour, distinguished for purity or cleanliness of habits, attached to the person for whose service they are engaged, possessed of cleverness and skill, endued with kindness, skilled in every kind of service that a patient may require, endued with general cleverness, competent to cook food and curries, clever in bathing or washing a patient, well conversant in rubbing or pressing the limbs, or raising the patient or assisting him in walking or moving about, well skilled in making or cleaning beds, competent to pound drugs, or ready, patient, and skillful in waiting upon one that is ailing, and never unwilling to do any act that they may be commanded (by the physician or patient) to do.

— *Charaka-Samhita, vol. 1, pp. 168–169*

Nurse. That person alone is fit to nurse or to attend the bedside of a patient who is cool-headed and pleasant in his demeanour, does not speak ill of anybody, is strong and attentive to the requirements of the sick, and strictly and indefatigably follows the instructions of the physician.

— *Sushruta-Samhita, vol. 1, chap. 34, pp. 305–307*

It was apparently the existence of hospitals that created a need for this special group. Although it is certain that nurses were employed in the hospitals of India, it is unclear whether they were viewed as glorified servants or as professional personnel. Women were midwives and in some cases the experts of drug lore. They held a high position in India, and their activities centered about the management of the home. It is assumed that women functioned as nurses when members of their family became ill.

China

Ancient China was cut off from the Mediterranean world by the great range of the Himalaya Mountains. It lay far to the northeast of India and remains somewhat a mystery, since accurate records are not available before the Shang dynasty (c. 1776–1122 BC). The inhabitants of China are believed to have come from central Asia about 3000 BC, settling along the banks of the Yellow River. The land of this region was very fertile. Grain became the staple crop, fruit trees were prevalent, and vegetation was so luxurious that the title of The Flowery Kingdom was conferred upon China.

Information about this early civilization is primarily legendary, yet it emerged in possession of social, religious, and political institutions. China's history became authentic with the appearance of the second Chou dynasty (1122–249 BC), a rule that lasted almost 900 years. Civilization spread south from the Yellow River to the Yangtse River during this time. The people belonged to the Mongoloid race and had great respect for social order. A creative people, they carved in wood and ivory, produced works of art in bronze and lacquer, and used irrigation systems for their fields. Poetry and history were written, although the Chinese writing was slow, complicated, and difficult. It contained symbols that represented objects (pictograms), ideas (ideograms), and sounds (phonograms). Sacred books were also written, and these were comparable to the papyri of Egypt and the Vedas of India.

The Chinese form of government was a patriarchal rule. Since the family was the fundamental unit of the society, the government was concerned with the social group rather than the individual. Local government comprised a group of elders who were representatives of various families making up a particular village. The elders, who met in the local temple to manage the village affairs, were the liaison between the people and the monarch. Shang, the first known dynasty, was followed by the Chou dynasties with a feudal form of government. These were succeeded by the Ch'in in the third century BC, when various feudal states were united into one empire.

鼻衄痘形
一

Selon Courrier, *Infantile Eruption.* Chinese silk, eighteenth century. *(Bibliothèque Nationale, Paris).*

Four social classes were recognized in China: scholars, farmers, artisans, and traders. In reality, however, two classes functioned; these were the officials (mandarins) and the nonofficials. The officials were selected on a talent basis rather than by class, since civil service, an ancient institution in China, opened examinations to all who could qualify.

Three religious systems influenced China: Taoism and Confucianism, which were indigenous, and Buddhism, which was imported from India. "Taoism was characterized by freedom from desire within one's self and an absence of self-determined actions for particular ends in things exterior to one's self" (Frank, 1953, p. 26). It was a religion concerned with obtaining long life and good fortune, often through magical means. The value of charms was emphasized as a method to combat the demons of disease. These charms were written on paper that was burned; the ashes were administered in a liquid such as tea. The study of alchemy arose from the practice of searching for the elixir of life, the transmutation of base metals into gold. Taoism ultimately yielded to Confucianism and Buddhism.

Confucius entered the life of China about 500 BC. He studied the sacred books as a child and later emerged as one of the greatest reformers and teachers the world has ever known. Confucius was a political reformer rather than a religious originator. His political reforms were based on moral principles, and he sought to relieve oppression by returning to ancient customs as a basis for government. Confucius stressed family cohesion, the value of knowledge, right conduct (etiquette), and ancestor worship, which prevented dissections of bodies. (No worship was accorded to female ancestors.) Confucius's philosophy was the negative version of the Golden Rule: What you do not wish done to yourself do not do unto others. On the whole, Confucianism did not promote progress, since it failed to stimulate ambition for better things. Yet some progress was achieved in China. By 200 BC Buddhism became the religion of the land, having been brought from India into the Far East.

The religious practices of China were polytheistic, animistic, and idolatrous. Images of painted wood were adored, and sacrifices were offered to these images because the people believed them to be inhabited by souls. The evil spirits responsible for disease and disaster were frightened off by loud noises. Sacrifice to the gods was an official state function. Only distinguished social groups were permitted to participate in the ceremonies; the people could participate only in those ceremonies for worship of their own ancestors.

Chinese medicine was focused on prevention. Health was considered to be a state of harmony or equilibrium within the individual and the universe. This state was accomplished through the interplay of nature's basic duality: the yang (male principle), which was positive, warm, dry, light, full of life, and the yin (female principle), which was negative, passive, dark, cold, moist, weak, and lifeless. An improper balance of these energies resulted in discomfort and disease. Illness could also be caused by evil spirits and animistic forces.

The works of three legendary emperors provided the basic foundation for Chinese medicine. Fu Hsi (c. 2900 BC) created the *pa kua,* a symbol with yang and yin lines combined in eight separate trigrams. These could represent all yin-yang conditions. Shen Nung (Hung Ti), the Red Emperor, wrote the *Pen Tsao* (*Herbal*), which was the result of his investigations of medicinal herbs. The effects of 365 personally tested drugs were reported. Shen Nung is also thought to have drawn the first charts on acupuncture. Huang Ti (Yu Hsiung), the Yellow Emperor, was credited with writing the great medical compendium *Nei Ching* (*Canon of Medicine*). According to this work, four steps in examination were necessary to determine a diagnosis: look, listen, ask, and feel (observation, auscultation, interrogation, and palpation). All phases of health and illness, including prevention and treatment, were recorded in this canon of medicine.

Medical knowledge in early China included dissection techniques, studies of the circulatory system, massage, the therapeutic use of baths, and the significance of pulse rates. Diagnoses were often made on the basis of a complicated pulse theory in which the pulse of the patient was studied over a period of several hours. Some two hundred types of pulse beat were listed.

> The physician felt the right wrist and then the left. He compared the beats with his own, noting precise time as well as day and season since each hour affected the nature of the pulsations. Each pulse had three distinct divisions, each associated with a specific organ, and each division had a separate quality, of which there were dozens of varieties. Moreover, each division or zone of the pulse had a superficial and deep projection. Thus literally hundreds of possible characteristics were obtainable. In one treatise, *Muo-Ching,* ten volumes were necessary to cover all the intricacies of the pulse.
>
> — *Lyons, 1978, p. 127*

Five methods of treatment were identified in the *Nei Ching:* cure the spirit, nourish the body, give medications, treat the whole body, and use acupuncture and moxibustion. Acupuncture consisted of inserting needles an inch or so into areas along the twelve meridians that traverse the body and using a twisting motion. Moxibustion used the same meridians. However, this treatment used a powdered plant substance (cones of mugwort), which was fashioned into a mound on the patient's skin and burned slowly. This method of counterirritation caused blisters to form on the area.

Smallpox was a widely known disease in China. A more primitive form of variolation than that used in India was performed by the Chinese. Crusts of diseased pustules were ground into a powder and blown into the nostril with a bamboo tube. Surgery was limited to castration of males (eunuchs) seeking advancement at court and to treatment of wounds. The limited development of surgery may have been a result of the belief that mutilation of the body would remain in evidence in life after death. Chinese medicine spread into Korea, Japan, and Tibet, where superstition mixed with these practices.

Little mention is made of hospitals in ancient China, although Halls of Healing are described. These were adjuncts to the temples where the sick prayed for recovery. Berdoe (1893) correlates the absence of hospitals with the duty of the Chinese people to care for their families at home. Even more striking is the lack of reference to nursing in the literature of the ancient Chinese. If there were nurses, they were probably not women, since the woman's position, as defined by Confucius, was inferior. A woman's work was confined to the keeping of the home and the building of families. Her value was greatest when she produced a son. It is also possible that the belief that disease could be caused by evil spirits taking up residence in the patient's body had a distinct impact on care of the sick. The fear that these spirits could enter anyone who touched a sick person would make nursing almost nonexistent.

THE MEDITERRANEAN WORLD

Greece

Ancient Greece was a peninsula that jutted out into the Mediterranean Sea from the southeastern part of Europe. Surrounded by gulfs and ocean, its indented coastline provided good harbors, which led to the establishment of trade. The interior of the country was mountainous; the climate was warm and sunny. This topography led to a particular political organization in which small groups of people settled in the plains and valleys between the mountains. Cities were built within areas of two hundred to three hundred square miles. A location with a commanding view was chosen in each city for use during an attack by enemies. Temples and other buildings were also erected on this site. Eventually government functions were assumed by these cities, which became the ruling authorities in areas with a radius of approximately ten miles. Each area was designated as an independent "city-state" with a king, a council, and an assembly.

Civilization entered Greece through the island of Crete by way of Egypt and Phoenicia and was not unlike that of the peoples of the Near East. Its growth was nourished partly by the inhabitants of the Crete and Aegean islands and the mainland and also by communication with the ancient civilizations of Egypt and Mesopotamia. The Greek people or Hellenes, as the Greeks called themselves, who migrated into the area were of Indo-European stock. They assimilated the preexisting civilization. The Greeks were unlike other ancient peoples because they were keen observers, not experimenters; they were philosophers, not scientists. Their sense of beauty encompassed proportion and spatial relationships, resulting in architecture and temples of the highest artistic caliber. The scattered nation was unified by language, literature, and religious worship. The Panhellenic or Olympic Games, held every four years dating from 776 BC, brought the people together to compete for prizes. In addition, every family aimed to produce participants with healthy bodies.

Recorded Greek history begins with the Homeric Age or Age of Heroes. The writings of Homer, *The Iliad* and *The Odyssey,* became the sacred books of Greece. Through mythology the origins of the peoples were traced and health, illness, and medical practice were discussed. "In the Homeric poems, one gets a glimpse of commonsense remedies and of simple wound surgery, of charms against sickness, and of appeals to this god or that to protect a warrior against injury" (Shryock, 1959, p. 41).

The Greeks had the ancient gods of the earth and the underworld, as well as special healing agents such as snakes and moles. Apollo, the sun god, was the god of health and medicine. Asklepios (in Rome, called Aesculapius), son of Apollo and a human mother, was the chief healer of Greek mythology. His fame may have been created from a mortal of fame and skill, for it is traced to about thirteen centuries before Christ. According to Frank (1953), this

Achilles Bandaging the Wounds of Patroclus, detail from the bowl of Sosias, c. 50 BC. *(Museum of Greek and Roman Antiquities, Antikensammlung, Staatliche Museen zu Berlin-Preussischer Kulturbesitz, 1988.)*

mortal was a Greek physician who was raised to the rank of a god. In addition, two of his sons accompanied the Greek army to the Trojan War. Machaon was a surgeon with "skilled hands to draw out darts and heal sores"; Podalirius was an internist who was "given cunning to find out things impossible and cure that which healed not." Asklepios was represented holding the wand of Mercury, a wayfarer's staff entwined with the sacred serpents of wisdom. The medical caduceus is derived from this portrayal.

The women also shared the work of health conservation in the myth of Asklepios. Epigone, the wife, was revered as "the soothing one." The six daughters included Hygeia, the "goddess of health"; Panacea, the "restorer of health," who personified miraculous all-healing herbs; Aegle, the "light of the sun"; Meditrina, the "preserver of health" (supposedly the ancient forerunner of the public health nurse); and Iaso, who personified the "recovery from illness."

> The whole family of Asklepios has significance for the medical and nursing arts, for if its members were only symbolic, they must have been meant to depict those arts as they existed at that time, and if they were actual persons they combined in their careers all the main lines of specialism that we consider modern.
>
> — *Stewart and Austin, 1962, p. 28*

Above, The Snake Goddess, from the Palace of Knossos, c. 1600 BC. Faience, approx. 34.3 cm high. *(Archaeological Museum, Herakleion, Greece. Photograph Hirmer Verlag, Munich).*

The strong relationship between the snake and the female has its origins in the goddess religions of early history. The snake was the idealization of psychic vision and oracular divination, both of which were traditionally considered to be among women's magical powers. Small Minoan figurines called "snake goddesses" were found in shrines or buried with the dead. These identify Crete as a goddess-worshipping or woman-centered society. Sexuality and the human body were distinguished through images of compelling beauty and power. These goddess figures were usually carved from ivory, banded in gold, and depicted with bell-shaped skirts with tiers or flounces. Snakes were either in their headdresses or around their arms.

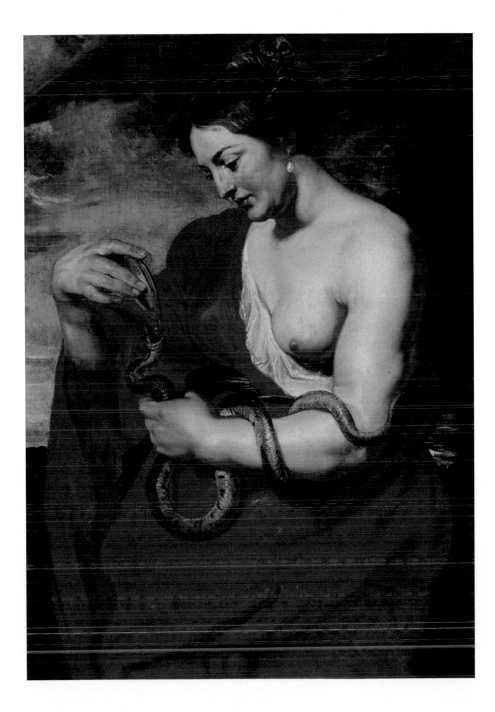

Peter Paul Rubens, *Hygeia, Goddess of Health,* c. 1615. Oil on oak panel, 106.2 × 74.3 cm. *(Gift of Mr. and Mrs. Henry Reichhold. Photograph copyright 1995 The Detroit Institute of Arts, Michigan.)*

The myth of Asklepios became highly complex. Temples were built to him on sites of great natural beauty with pure spring water (often this water had already been noted for its medicinal properties) and refreshing breezes. The buildings, masterpieces of architecture, were exquisitely decorated. Those temples that became famous for cures would emerge as great social and intellectual centers. Theaters, gymnasiums, a stadium, places for worship, a hospital, living quarters for patients, baths, lodgings for visitors and attendants, housing for priests and physicians, and libraries were built nearby and surrounded by gardens and park lands. These health resorts were frequented not only by people who were ill but also by those who enjoyed the beauty and contentment of the surroundings and the brilliance of cultural life and entertainment. The most famous of these centers was Epidauros, situated a few miles from Athens. It accommodated about 500 patients and was serviced by a chief administrator and various grades of attendants, including priestesses.

Upon arrival, patients offered sacrifices of animals to Asklepios and underwent a cleansing or purifying process consisting of a series of baths and a period of abstinence from certain foods and wines. After several days in the outer courts, the patient was admitted to the inner court to participate in religious ceremonies that included elaborate rites and rituals. Finally, the patient was admitted to the abaton to sleep in full sight of a great statue to the god. This incubation or temple sleep would reveal through a dream or hypnotic state the treatment to be administered. Votive tablets were left behind that attested to innumerable cures. Yet maternity patients and the incurably ill were not admitted to the temples for medical assistance.

Two other institutions offered care to the sick: the xenodochium and the iatrion. The xenodochium was similar in function to the Hebrew xenodochium and first provided care for travelers, then for people who were sick

Asklepios and His Daughter Hygeia. (Museo Vaticana, Rome.)

Asklepios became revered as the Greek god of medicine and surgery, a healing god. His daughter Hygeia became the goddess of health and health care. From her name is derived the word *hygiene.* Numerous temples dedicated to Asklepios were erected throughout the Greek empire. Here individuals could come to be healed. The healing process involved a strong belief in Asklepios, techniques that fostered relaxation, and a strong faith.

or injured. In the later centuries of Greek history, it was placed under municipal management and may have been the forerunner of the modern city and county hospital. The iatrion was a facility where ambulatory care was received. It corresponds most closely with the dispensary or outpatient clinics of present-day hospitals.

The cult of Asklepios, which evolved from Greek mythology, provided religious healing and offered a blend of natural and supernatural remedies. Eventually the priests of Asklepios branched into two specialized areas, one strictly medical and the other purely occult. From the medical branch a group of lay physicians developed.

> While the shrines of Aesculapius continued to offer religious healing, lay physicians accumulated factual knowledge about common illnesses and how to handle them. These men moved from one town to another as skilled artisans and learned much from the bedside. They practiced both general medicine and surgery, and the experience of a number of them was finally incorporated in a collection of writings ascribed to Hippocrates. Although there probably was a physician of that name, he did not write all these works; as his name became legendary, it was applied to the whole collection. This became the first general text on medicine and was long viewed as a sort of Bible by the medical profession.
>
> — *Shryock, 1959, pp. 46–47*

As Greek civilization progressed, many changes took place. The healing arts were particularly affected during the Golden Age of Greece between the sixth and fourth centuries before Christ. This was "the birth or age of reason," which culminated in the classical philosophy of Socrates, Plato, Aristotle, and others. These days of the philosopher-scientists were devoted to an attempt to attribute natural rather than supernatural explanations to phenomena. Truth was sought through clear thinking and close observation of physical and social phenomena. This study of nature was eventually called "natural philosophy," the first clear expression of what is now known as science. The results of these scientific and philosophical investigations provided the fundamentals of good living.

Thales (640?–546 BC) was the first of the Greek scientist-philosophers. He made many contributions to navigation, astronomy, mathematics, and geometry but was known best for his explanations of phenomena. Thales did not use religious means to prove the natural processes of the universe; he did not rely on the supernatural. He proposed that the underlying principles of solutions to problems must be found, in addition to the solutions themselves. Socrates and Plato laid the foundation for philosophy and government. It was Aristotle (384–322 BC), however, who had a profound influence on medicine. He was credited with laying the foundation of biology and comparative anatomy. His contributions in the field of both plant and animal biology greatly aided the development of medical thought. In addition, Aristotle dealt with ethical matters in a scientific manner.

Despite the fact that rational medicine had been developing before him and magical medicine persisted long after his time, Hippocrates of Cos (460–370 BC?) was given credit for the establishment of rational or scientific medicine. He belonged to the order of Asklepiades and was believed to have been a direct descendant of Asklepios himself. Hippocrates is considered to have been one of the greatest physicians who ever lived and became known as the Father of Medicine. He taught that disease was not the work of spirits, demons, or deities but the result of the breaking of natural laws. The true art of the physician, therefore, was to assist nature to bring about a cure. The writings attributed to Hippocrates relate to nearly all aspects of medicine—pathology, anatomy, physiology, diagnosis, prognosis, mental illness, gynecology, obstetrics, surgery, therapy, bedside observations, hygiene, and professional ethics. Epilepsy, tuberculosis, malarial fever, ulcers, and other diseases were described. Perhaps the most interesting and significant portions of these

Brygos Painter, *Woman Attending a Man Vomiting,* detail from the interior of a kylix, c. 490 BC. *(Martin V. Wagner Museum der Universität, Würzburg. Photo: K. Oehrlein.)*

writings were the "case histories," which were preserved in the *Epidemics.* These included a compilation of the details of the patient who was ill, the patient's environment, and the complete examination. Even today, these case histories could serve as models for succinct clinical records, since they are comprehensive, concise, and direct.

The practice of hygiene was more than a medical specialty. It was a way of life depicted in part by Hippocrates' discussion of diet, the avoidance of sexual excesses, and the importance of exercise. His emphasis on the role of environment in the spread of disease, as presented in *Airs, Waters and Places,* provided a basic epidemiological text in which the concepts of endemic diseases (those always present) and epidemic diseases (those that broke out at certain periods and involved large numbers of people) were illuminated (Rosen, 1958). Therapy was related to the elements of fire, air, earth, and water. In different combinations these exhibited the four basic qualities of heat, cold, dryness, and moisture. Everything, including the body, was composed of one or more of these elements. This led to the classic "four humors" (blood, phlegm, yellow bile, and black bile) theory of disease. When these humors were in balance, the result was a healthy body; excess or deficiency of one or more caused illness.

The Hippocratic method rested on the following principles (Lyons, 1978):

- Observe all.
- Study the patient rather than the disease.
- Evaluate honestly.
- Assist nature.

These principles were to be combined with the professional spirit, or ethical conduct. The true physician needed to be devoted to his profession and his patients and was to abstain from all that would dishonor one and injure the other.

The literature of the Greeks contains many references to nurses. However, these were primarily children's nurses, wet nurses, and midwives. (Midwives provided most of the obstetrical care; physicians assisted with difficult or abnormal childbirth.) In historical accounts discrepancies exist about who performed the other nursing functions because the activities of a Greek woman were confined to the home unless she was a priestess, a slave, or a harlot. According to Shryock (1959), Greek women could not be admitted to the "mysteries" of any art. Thus, even if the Greeks had nurses, they would probably have been men. Even Hippocrates, the master of medical art, left no direct reference to nurses.

> A most remarkable feature of the ancient medical writings is the scant attention paid to that very important factor in modern treatment—the nurse. Professional nurses were, apparently, unknown, (Note: midwives were common enough) and the general impression that the reader forms is that the physician did not consider the work of the attendant to be of great value. In some cases, doubtless, the household slaves acted as nurses. . . . But the burden of nursing fell chiefly upon the wife. . . . It is clear then that in ordinary cases it was the duty of the wife to nurse the whole household, with the help no doubt of her daughters and maid servants.
>
> — *Jones, 1909, pp. 123–126*

Yet in the Hippocratic writings what we now call nursing is taught in minute detail, and the assistant or attendant is indicated as the co-worker of the physician. Specific directions about poultices, cold sponging, fluid diets, warm baths, light and regular nourishment for heart cases, large amounts of fluid for kidney cases, the use of mouthwashes, and clean, smooth bed linen are given. It is clear from these writings that nursing care existed in ancient Greece. However, what nursing care was actually like is left to the imagination.

Paulus Pontius, *Hippocrates,* early seventeenth century. Engraving after a drawing by Peter Paul Rubens from an ancient marble bust. *(National Library of Medicine, Bethesda, Maryland.)*

Hippocrates as envisioned by a Byzantine artist, c. 1342. Illuminated Greek manuscript 2144, f. 10v. *(Bibliothèque Nationale, Paris)*

Hippocrates became known as the "Father of Medicine." He taught that disease was the result of the breaking of natural laws. He believed that the true art of the physician was to assist Nature to bring about a cure. Although the "Hippocratic Oath" is one of the greatest early documents dealing with medical ethics, most scholars believe that it is not really a part of the true Hippocratic teachings.

Rome

While civilization was progressing in the East and Greece was emerging in the realms of art and thinking, a new power began to form in the West. This occurred in the peninsula we now know as Italy, where an agricultural people known as Latins resided. Italy was separated from Greece by water and divided into two sections by a chain of mountains. The level plains on the western side were initially chosen by the Latins for the location of their homes. This area was occupied in ancient times by various peoples, the oldest of whom were the Etruscans, who had migrated from Asia Minor. The Etruscans achieved a higher degree of culture than other tribes of this area. They were later conquered and absorbed by the Romans.

The Gauls, or Celts, from Western Europe originally occupied the northern part of Italy. The Greeks began to settle in southern Italy about the eighth century BC in an area that became known as Magna Graecia (Greater Greece). Eventually the Romans, who were excellent warriors, conquered and absorbed them all. This Latin tribe had occupied the central and northern portions of Italy. In time, they succeeded in bringing unity to the country under their rule. As a result, the village of Rome passed from a simple farming community to a thriving commercial center.

Legend places the birth of Rome at 753 BC. Located at the mouth of the Tiber River, Rome progressed through the stages of a kingdom, a republic, an empire, and a city. The event of its founding is intertwined with a variety of mythological interpretations. One account is told by Virgil in his great epic poem, *The Aeneid,* which describes the wanderings of Aeneas and his companions in the period from the fall of Troy to the founding of Rome. It is also said that the site of Rome on seven hills "appears to have been the choice of twin brothers, Romulus and Remus, themselves indebted for life to the nour-

Map of the Roman Empire at its greatest extent.

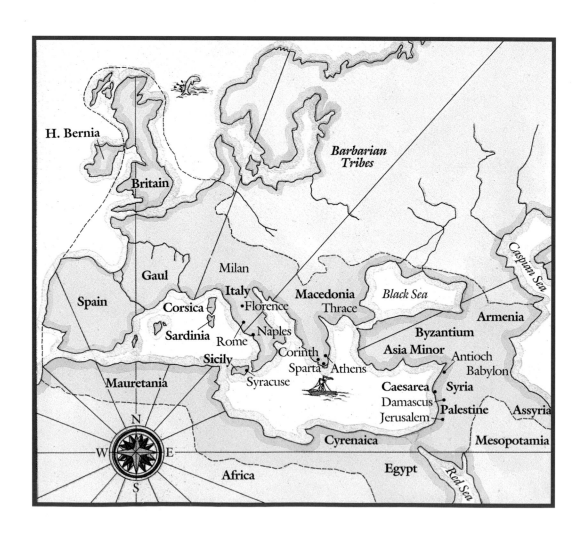

ishment and care given them by a kindly wolf who found them on a mountain top, abandoned by a goddess mother" (Jamieson and Sewall, 1950, p. 74).

The Romans did not develop a religion, a medical system, or an art of their own. These were borrowed from their conquests, from other peoples and nations. From Greece, which was under Roman control by 146 BC, tangible things such as money, textiles, and sailing ships were acquired. Eventually Greek ideas were also absorbed, as well as art and religion. The Greek alphabet was adapted to the Latin tongue.

Early Romans possessed gods whose functions were highly practical. Jupiter guarded the welfare of the city, Juno was the woman's patroness, Mars was the god of war, and Janus was the god of openings or beginnings. Prosperity occurred if one pleased the gods; failure resulted if the wrath of the gods was incurred. During this early period no distinctive gods of healing were identified. However, in a later period gods were borrowed from the Greeks and polytheism prevailed. These gods included Hygeia and Asklepios. It is also said that there was a god or goddess for almost every know physiological function or disease process, for example, Scabies, Angeronia, Fluonia, Uterina, and Febris. Febris became particularly significant to Rome for the power of reducing fevers associated with malaria (Frank, 1953). Yet the ancient Romans were free from the superstition that the sick and insane were possessed by demons.

The Roman population was divided into two classes: the patricians (wealthy or privileged group), who were given civil and legal privileges and whose right to citizenship was hereditary, and the plebeians (poor or lower class), who were denied the right of citizenship. Work was given over to home slaves who were brought from conquered countries. Homes became luxurious, dress elaborate, and social functions extravagant. The demarcation line between the rich and the poor broadened. Internal decay emerged and continued. The Roman Empire lasted about five centuries, from 31 BC to AD 476. The first two centuries were spent in peace and prosperity; the third century was marked by frequent disorder within the empire; the last two centuries were characterized by internal rebellion and external attack. The decline and fall of Rome was unavoidable. The church founded by Jesus Christ was the one institution that remained unshaken during this time.

Before the conquest of Greece, Roman medicine combined folk, magical, and religious practices. After 200 BC the Greek physicians, who were made slaves, did the medical work, and their practices filtered throughout Rome. The most skillful of these were given Roman citizenship during the rule of Julius Caesar. Legend, however, indicates that Greek medicine was introduced to Rome in a year when pestilence was devastating the city (293 BC). Sibylline books were consulted, and the oracle replied that Asklepios be brought from Greece to Rome. A galley was sent and returned with a staff of physicians and attendants. As it came up the Tiber, a sacred serpent sprang out on the little island in the river and established itself there. Since this was a divinely chosen spot, a temple was erected there to Asklepios (Aesculapius).

Several medical practitioners achieved fame during the rise of the Roman Empire: Dioscorides Pedanius, Aretaeus, Asclepiades, and Galen. Dioscorides Pedanius was a Greek physician and a surgeon in the army under Nero. His *De Materia Medica* contained descriptions of more than six hundred preparations from medicinal herbs. He observed these herbs as he accompanied the armies.

Aretaeus refocused the study of medicine on the methods of clinical observation used by Hippocrates. His writings rendered vivid descriptions of such diseases as pneumonia, empyema, epilepsy, tetanus, diphtheria, and a type of diabetes.

Asclepiades of Bithynia was a Greek physician from Asia Minor who assisted with the establishment of Greek medicine in Rome. He repudiated the teachings of Hippocrates, for he believed that the physician, not nature,

Physician Treats a Wounded Soldier, first century AD. Pompeiian fresco. *(The Bettmann Archive, New York.)*

assumed the character of clubs or social centers. Roman cities were cleaner than those of any other ancient civilization. Yet Rome had many epidemics, probably because of a number of factors related to conquests and modernization. For example, tenements were introduced by Rome to assist with the rapid growth of the city.

The Romans were advanced in military medicine and provided excellent care for their soldiers. First aid was rendered on the battlefield, and a field ambulance service was devised. Originally, wounded soldiers were carried to private homes. Later they were cared for in tents or separate buildings and nursed by women and old men of upstanding character. Eventually many military hospitals (*valetudinaria*) were erected, some of which could accommodate two hundred sick or wounded soldiers.

> A few years ago, several of the original military hospitals of about 100 AD were unearthed in the Rhine and Danube valleys. As such border areas had to be constantly defended against barbarians, these buildings probably served as base hospitals for frontier forces. The ground plans reveal long corridors from which opened a series of suites—each of the latter containing two private rooms connected by a small hall. In addition there were central courts for kitchens, dining rooms, pharmacies, and so on. Apparently there were no wards, so it may be assumed that each soldier-patient enjoyed considerable privacy. Many surgical instruments have been found in the ruins, indicating that advanced Roman wound-surgery was here placed at the service of the troops.
>
> — *Shryock, 1959, p. 76*

Facing page, Alma-Tadema, *The Baths of Caracalla,* 1899. Oil on canvas, 152.3 × 95.25 cm. *(Sotheby's, London.)*

Some Roman bathhouses were spectacular achievements, even by modern standards. The Caracalla baths had a temple at each end; one was dedicated to Apollo and the other to Aesculapius, the gods responsible for the nurturing of the mind and the body. Aesthetics was an important aspect of this bath. Outside gardens featured grottoes and nymph's watered by fountains and springs. Shaded porticos displayed masterpieces of sculpture. There were tree-lined promenades for walking. The hypocaust, a room with a cavity beneath the floor where hot air circulated, provided an efficient form of central heating for the baths. Mixed bathing eventually became acceptable, and the baths provided social gathering places where friends could meet and talk, business could be conducted, and entertainment could be enjoyed.

Alma-Tadema, *The Nurse,* 1872. *(Sotheby's, London.)*

A class of orderlies, the *nosocomi,* acted as nurses. Valetudinaria were also established for sick slaves of rich homes or estates, since slaves were considered to be a most valuable commodity. It is probable that slaves functioned as nurses in these institutions.

Roman women were independent and became involved in many activities outside the home. The care of the sick was no doubt undertaken by the mistress and by the male and female slaves of the household. Children's nurses and midwives were still the chief nursing roles for women.

THE FAR WEST

The Americas

The New World, as the Americas were titled by historians, was really an old world in which highly developed cultures had thrived. It may even be that some cultures within the Near East, the Far East, and the Mediterranean had begun and ended before it became known that a rich land lay across the endless sea. It may be that civilization was reached earlier in the Americas than in Egypt. Although the exact date for the habitation of this area is not agreed upon, "it may be assumed with some certainty that highly evolved cultures flourished on the soil of the New World from 2000 to 1000 BC" (Hermann, 1954, p. 188). Some individuals believe it began ten thousand or even twenty thousand years ago.

It is thought that the earliest inhabitants of the American continents came from Central Asia. Access was gained by crossing the Bering Strait into the territory currently known as Alaska. The people (Indians) followed the pattern of other primitive tribes by migrating toward food, water, and acceptable climates. They tended to move in the direction of east and south, and traces

George Catlin, *Chee-Ah-Ka-Tchee, Wife of Not-To-Way* (Iroquois), 1830–39. Canvas, 73.7 × 61 cm. *(Gift of Mrs. Joseph Harrison, Jr. National Museum of American Art, Washington, D.C./Art Resource, New York.)*

of their occupancy have been found as far east as the Atlantic coast. Mexico, Central America, and Peru eventually became the primary sites for their settlements. Hunting and agriculture became a way of life. In addition, the originality of these tribes resulted in the development of various processes such as basket weaving, the tanning of leather with oak bark, and the manufacture of cleaning powder from wood ashes and of glue from fish. The numerous American Indian nations in North and South America eventually decreased, the consequence of tragic events.

Several tribes attained a high degree of civilization: the Mayas, the Incas, the Aztecs, and the Toltecs. Religion, magic, medicine, nursing, and pharmacy were frequently combined in these tribes; these activities were carried out by one individual who was set apart from the rest of the tribe. The medicine men (or shamans and, later, priests) attempted to cure the ills of both mind and body. As in other ancient cultures, it was believed that disease was caused by displeasure of the gods. The sun god in particular was recognized and worshiped by many of these groups.

Health was simply a matter of balance among the person, nature, and the supernatural. Although the systems of healing might vary from tribe to tribe, rituals or ceremonies, prayers, chants, herbal therapy, plans for prevention of disease, and the use of protective devices such as charms and fetishes were an

UNIT 3

Nursing in a Christian World

The care of the sick was only one of many forms of charity undertaken by the Church, but it was always given a place of honor because of the emphasis put on it by the founder of the Christian faith. In the first and second centuries, the visiting of the sick was a part of the duty of all Christians but especially the deacons and deaconesses, who took the poor and homeless members of the group into their own homes and cared for them there. No technical preparation was considered necessary for such service. All that was asked was devotion to the faith, brotherly love, and obedience to the Christian law of hospitality and service. Later, much of this charitable work was centered in hospitals or guest houses requiring full-time staffs. Such institutional workers were chosen, as a rule, from among the widows and virgins and other members of the Church most free from domestic ties. With the rapid growth of the monastic movement, after the sixth century, large numbers of voluntary celibates—men and women—joined religious orders, and the care of the sick, helpless and infirm became in many cases their permanent vocation.

— ISABEL MAITLAND STEWART

Pablo Picasso, *Science and Charity*, 1897. Oil on canvas, 197 × 249 cm. (*Museu Picasso, Barcelona, Spain. Copyright Artist Rights Society (ARS), New York/SPADEM, Paris. Photo: SuperStock, Florida.*)

In this work, a contrast is presented: the detachment of the attending physician with the warmth of a nursing nun as they aid a sick woman. Numerous discussions about this work were evidently held between Picasso and his father. To represent the sick woman, they apparently chose a poor woman who had been begging with her child in her arms. The nun is probably a young boy in disguise, but the habit was possibly lent by Sister Josefa González of the order of St. Vincent. Picasso's father posed as the physician. The title originally decided on for this painting was "The Visit to the Sick Woman." Painted when Picasso was fifteen years old, it shows a doctor taking the pulse of a bedridden woman. A nun with a child in her arm stands on the other side of the bed offering a cup to the sick woman.

69

Nursing in a Christian World

	1	125	250	375	500

Daily Life

1–33 Life of Christ
1–100 Chariot races popular in Roman festivals
64 Persecution of Christians begins
161–181 Marcus Aurelius encourages the establishment of charitable funds to support and feed the poor
164–180 Great plague in the Roman Empire
200 Cotton grown in southwest North America
226–642 Silk weaving industry important in Persia
325 Council of Nicea held
350 Stirrup invented in China

500 Beginning of the Dark Ages
500 Incense introduced into Christian church services
500 Church bells used in France
500–1000 Feudalism and monasticism develop

Science and Technology

14 Pont du Gard Aqueduct built in France
132 First seismograph invented by Chang Heng

400–800 Gold and bronze coins minted in Axum, Ethiopia

The Visual Arts

100–200 Buddha depicted in human form
100–200 Three-dimensional sculptures in China
150 Pyramid of the Sun constructed in Teotihuacan, Mexico
212–217 Baths of Caracalla built in Rome
300 Christian symbols seen on sculpture and tableware

500–600 Coptic art develops

Medicine and Health Care

1–100 Houses of deacons and deaconesses become hospitals called Diakonoia
100–200 Military medicine in Rome well organized
130–201 Galen, regarded as most renowned and influential medical writer
370 Most famous Xenodocheion, the Basilias, founded by St. Basil in Caesarea
390 Fabiola establishes first free Christian hospital in Rome

Nursing

1–500 Rise of religious and social movements leads to systematic development of nursing
1–500 Patients in large numbers cared for by Deaconesses, widows, Roman matrons, and other followers of Christ's precepts
60 Phebe (Phoebe), credited as first visiting nurse and deaconess

300 Parabolani Brotherhood founded
347–404 St. Paula establishes monasteries and a hospital in Bethlehem
410 St. Marcella, considered first nurse educator, dies

end of 6th century St. Dymphna organizes plan for mentally ill and retarded in Belgium
500–600 Monks and nuns serve as nurses
500–600 Nursing and charitable works develop in monasteries under famous abbesses

625	750	875	1000

542 Plague reduces Europe's population by one half
550 Chess game invented in India
570–632 Mohammed, founder of Islam
700 Easter eggs come into use
750 Beds become popular in France and Germany
800–900 Monasteries become centers of alms giving
870 Calibrated candles used to measure time in England
993 First canonization of saints

600 Book printing in China
700 Water wheels used for mill drive
750 Pharmacology and medicine become two separate sciences
850 Salerno University founded
861 New nilometer built to measure height of annual Nile flood
868 Earliest complete woodblock-printed book, *Diamond Sutra*, in China
1000 Vikings sail to Nova Scotia

550 Crucifix developed as an ornament
600 Porcelain produced in China
650 Weaving developed in Byzantine empire
814 Building of Doge's Palace is begun
900 Ethiopian Christian churches decorated with frescoes
900–1000 Great era of Byzantine Art

542 Hôtel Dieu of Lyons established
651 Hôtel Dieu of Paris established
717 Santo Spirito Hospital in Rome established
850–932 Rhazes, one of the greatest Arab physicians
857 Ergotism epidemics in western Europe
900 Founding of medical school at Salerno
936 York Hospital founded by Athelstane
962 Founding of the Hospice of St. Bernard, Switzerland

500–1000 Feudal chivalry brings nursing careers to highborn ladies outside of monasteries
700 Monastic nursing orders flourish

Samuel Bellin, *Christ and the Woman of Samaria*, nineteenth century. Engraving. *(The British Museum, London.)*

the Emperor Constantine proclaimed freedom for the Church. By AD 400 it was probably as dangerous *not to be* a Christian as it had been *to be* one in AD 100. Thus, as the Roman Empire declined, Christianity was bringing Christ into the personal and community life of the people.

THE CHRISTIAN MOTIVE AND NURSING

The history of nursing first becomes continuous with the beginning of Christianity. Pre-Christian records of nursing are fragmentary and scattered; however, records of nursing from the days of the early Christian workers to the present day are continuous. Christ's teachings of love and brotherhood transformed not only society at large but also the development of nursing. "Organized nursing" was a direct response to these teachings and epitomized the concept of pure altruism initiated by the early Christians. The term *altruism* was derived from the Latin *alter,* meaning "other"; hence, altruism means thought for and interest in others. Altruism at this time was not a new idea but an old idea with a new motive:

> Animism had advocated good works as a charm, to prevent misfortune. Judaism urged justice and mercy in order to secure prosperity in this world. Buddhism taught that helpfulness and kindness to others would secure merit in the hereafter. Even in the deteriorated Christianity of the Middle Ages we find the same thing taught, that kindness and service to others stored up merit in heaven.
>
> — *Goodnow, 1942, p. 23*

Pure altruism was disinterested service to humanity, devotion to others without hope of any sort of reward (material or spiritual) but done for the love of God and desire to be like him. From this development of the concept of altruism evolved the care of the sick or disabled as a corporal act of mercy. The Corporal Works of Mercy encompassed basic human needs, recognized the needs of a variety of groups within the society, and reflected the desire for human compassion:

-    To feed the hungry
-    To give water to the thirsty
-    To clothe the naked
-    To visit the imprisoned
-    To shelter the homeless
-    To care for the sick
-    To bury the dead

A spiritual meaning became deeply attached to the care of the sick and the suffering. This flowering of Christian idealism was to forever have a deep and significant impact on the practice of nursing.

The original inspiration of Christians to care for the sick stemmed directly from the teachings of Christ himself. Many instances are cited of Christ's healing the sick and raising the dead by direct intervention and without the use of any medicine or treatment. Faith healing, therefore, was a part of the Christian belief. In addition, those conditions that would promote natural healing were added and eventually supplied the impetus for the establishment of centers for nursing care. Caring for the sick became an activity especially pleasing to God and through which an individual might inherit "eternal life."

Master of Alkmaar, *Seven Acts of Mercy,* 1504. Panel, 101 × 54 cm. *(Rijksmuseum, Amsterdam, Netherlands.)*

The theme of the seven acts is developed by the appearance of Christ as both witness to and recipient of the benefits of the works of mercy and charity. These were acts that a Christian was to carry out to alleviate the suffering of, and bring comfort to, fellow human beings. The Christian reward for performing the acts was the acquisition of a place in heaven. In the specific panel "Visiting the Sick," women attend sick men who are unrelated to them. The hospital ward contains several beds. In the background are a man and woman tending a naked invalid. A scene in the foreground represents caring for the sick, especially those external to the family, as a Christian duty. Here a woman wearing expensive clothing brings a cup into the ward.

SICK & YE VISITED ME

COMMEMORATIVE OF THE ART LOAN EXHIBITION HELD
1878 IN AID OF THE ROYAL INFIRMARY. PRESENTED
BY P CLOUSTON ESQ TREASURER ELECTED 1867

From a chronological point of view, there was a vast difference between nursing in the Christian era and that of the ages that preceded it. A superior type of care was given by those who understood the best medical and surgical techniques of the times. The rich and the powerful who converted to Christianity and engaged in charitable works were socially, culturally, and intellectually endowed. Some were recognized scholars. The educationally prepared included members of the clergy, who for several centuries were the only group that was exposed to any type of formal training. Futhermore, a true integration of services was in evidence because medical and nursing care was seldom separated from other forms of charity for the poor (Sellew and Nuesse, 1946).

Many benefits were derived from the Christian effort. Chief among these were a distinctly humanitarian approach to the care of the sick and the poor and the development of organized nursing services. The positive aspects of nursing's heritage from the Christian teachings are evident and have been specifically identified. Yet this religious thought also handicapped progress in nursing. As nursing became closely identified with religion and religious orders, strict discipline became a way of life. In a sense religion forced nurses to make a strong commitment but a commitment at the expense of money,

Facing page, Adam and Small, designed by Stephen Adam, *Healing of the Sick,* ante-chapel window, 1879. Stained glass. *(Royal Infirmary, Glasgow, Scotland.)*

Charles Allsten Collins, *Convent Thoughts,* 1851. *(Ashmolean Museum, Oxford, England.)*

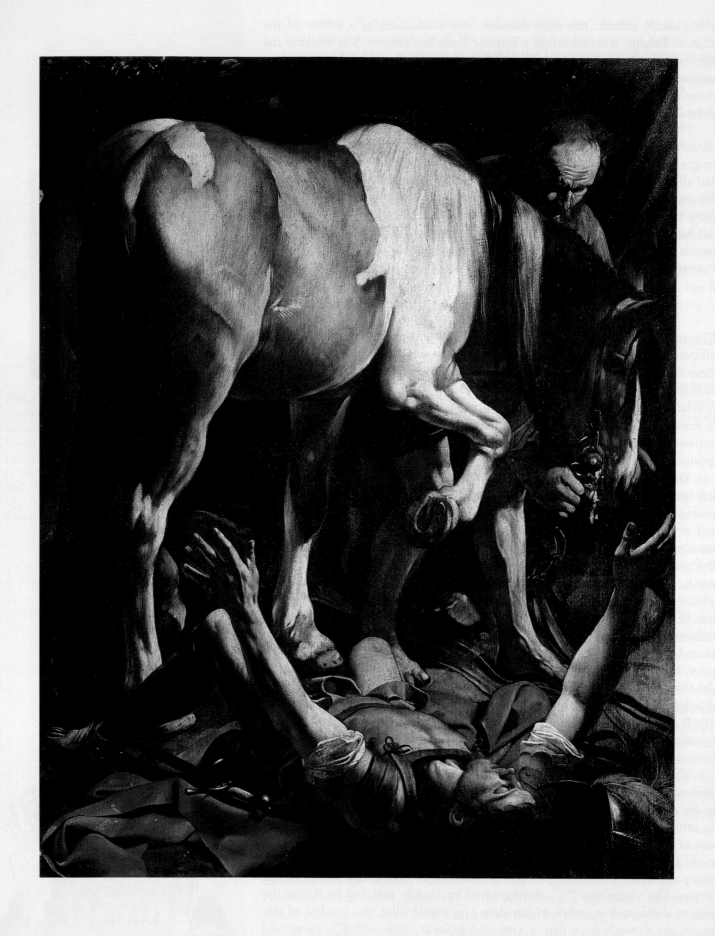

Caravaggio, *Conversion of St. Paul,* c. 1600.
Cerasi Chapel, S. Maria del Popolo,
Rome, Italy. *(SCALA/Art Resource, New
York.)*

Roman Matrons

Deaconesses were rarely mentioned in the Western or Roman Church. Yet illustrious women of Rome devoted themselves to the care of the sick and other charitable works. The noble Roman matrons were active during the fourth and fifth centuries after converting to Christianity. Roman women of the upper classes had, by this time, attained considerable social and legal freedom. They had proven themselves to be successful managers of their wealthy husbands' estates and had participated in public affairs. The names and histories of these matrons, some fifteen in number, have been preserved in the writings of St. Jerome. Their independent positions and great wealth were used to establish community life and to initiate the groundwork for charity and nursing work. The ascetic lives of these women were held in high regard. Three of these matrons, Marcella, Fabiola, and Paula, were particularly significant to continued progress in nursing.

Giovanni Bellini, *Saint Jerome Reading,* c. 1480–1490. Oil on panel, approx. 48.9 × 39.37 cm. *(Samuel H. Kress Collection. Copyright 1995 Board of Trustees, National Gallery of Art, Washington, D.C.)*

Judy Chicago, "Marcella," plate from *The Dinner Party,* 1979. China-painted porcelain, 35.6 cm diameter. *(Copyright Judy Chicago, 1979. Photo copyright Donald Woodman. Through the Flower, Albuquerque, New Mexico.)*

Marcella was known for her dedication to a religious life, her leadership abilities, and her intellect. Her palace became a center for women who aspired to a simpler, more purposeful life. Marcella and her followers ministered to the sick and the needy and established hospitals and the foundation for the great monastic system of Christianity.

The most famous of the Roman matrons was Marcella, who was considered the leader of this group of notable women. She converted her palace, located in a most exclusive part of Rome on the Aventine, into a monastery (the prototype of the later convent), which led to her titles of "Mother of Nuns" and "Founder of Convents in the West." She encouraged other intelligent and spiritually inclined Roman matrons to join her. One of the chief interests of this religious community of women was the care of the sick poor. Marcella was considered to be extremely intelligent and possessed of great virtue and purity. She devoted herself to the study of the Scriptures, and the clergy often consulted with her about scriptural passages. Marcella instructed her followers in the care of the sick, while also devoting her time to charitable works, prayer, and study. She was attacked during the raid on Rome by the Visigoths under Alaric in 410 and died soon after. She is referred to as St. Marcella by some authors (Dolan, Fitzpatrick, and Hermann, 1983; Sellew and Nuesse, 1946); others identify her simply as Marcella (Jamieson and Sewall, 1950; Nutting and Dock, 1937).

One of the most charming, and perhaps the most worldly, of the Roman matrons was Fabiola. A member of the patrician Fabian family, she married, divorced, and remarried, again unhappily. After the death of her second husband and her conversion to Christianity, Fabiola acknowledged her "evil ways" and joined the ranks of penitents. She renounced her earthly pleasures and bestowed her immense fortune on the sick and the poor. The first free Christian hospital in Rome was founded by Fabiola in her own palace in 390. It was described by St. Jerome as a *nosocomium,* a place for the sick as distinguished from objects of charity who were simply poor. Fabiola sought out the poor and the sick in the streets of Rome and cared for them herself. It is said

J.J. Henner, *Fabiola,* nineteenth century. Oil on velvet. *(Author's Collection.)*

that she was particularly skilled with the dressing of wounds and sores that were ugly and repugnant. She has been viewed almost as the patron saint of early nursing, and her idealized portrait is well known. Fabiola not only nursed but shared in the poverty of her patients. Some reports also indicate that she helped to establish a great hospice for pilgrims and strangers at Ostia, a seaport of Rome. Some writers have made the supposition that this hospice was a home for convalescent patients (Haeser, 1857). The entire life and works of Fabiola were related in a famous eulogy by St. Jerome upon her death in 399:

> There she gathered together all the sick from the highways and streets, and herself nursed the unhappy, emaciated victims of hunger and disease. Can I describe here the varied scourges which afflict human beings?—the mutilated, blinded countenances, the partially destroyed limbs, the livid hands, swollen bodies, and wasted extremities? . . . How often have I seen her carrying in her arms these piteous, dirty, and revolting victims of a frightful malady! How often have I seen her wash wounds whose fetid odour prevented every one else from even looking at them! She fed the sick with her own hands, and revived the dying with small and frequent portions of nourishment. I know that many wealthy persons cannot overcome the repugnance caused by such works of charity; . . . I do not judge them, . . . but, if I had a hundred tongues and a clarion voice I could not enumerate the number of patients for whom Fabiola provided solace and care. The poor who were well envied those who were sick.

> — *St. Jerome, Letter to Oceanus (LXXVII)*

Joachim Patinir (active 1515, died before 1524), *St. Jerome in a Rocky Landscape.* Wood, approx. 35.6 × 34.3 cm. *(The National Gallery, London.)*

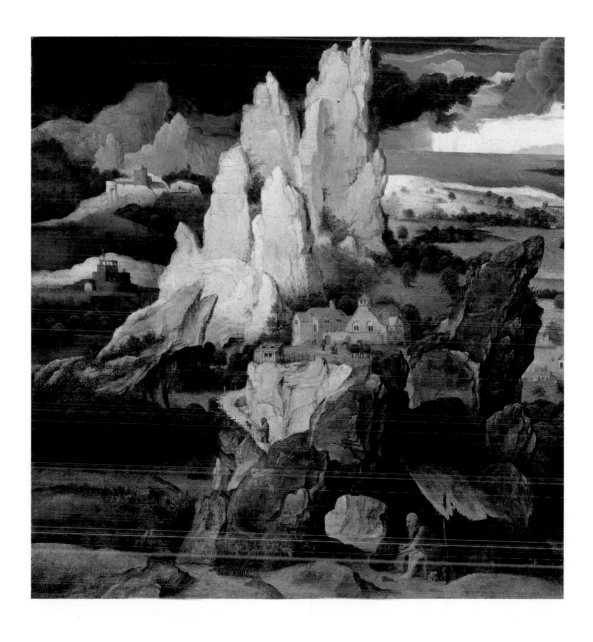

Paula traced her descent to some of the oldest, noblest families, and her husband, Toxotius, was of the Julian family, who claimed descent from Aeneas. Her family was immensely wealthy and owned, among other things, the entire town of Actin. Paula was the wife of a pagan and the mother of five children, four daughters and one son. Her worldly life ended with the death of her husband, when she began to devote herself to strict asceticism. Paula and her daughter Eustochium adopted Christianity, shared in charitable work, and studied with Marcella. Paula was particularly respected for her intellectual ability, which enabled her to develop a relationship with the recognized scholars of the day. This example of colleagueship between the sexes was described by Lord as an important advent of Christianity:

> If to her [Paula] we do not date the first great change in the social relations of man with woman, yet she is the most memorable example that I can find of that exalted sentiment which Christianity called out in the [relationship] of the sexes, and which has done more for the elevation of society than any other sentiment except that of religion itself.

> — *Lord, 1885, p. 63*

Paula was one of the most learned women of this period of history. She studied Hebrew and Greek and assisted St. Jerome with his Latin translations of the Scriptures, known as the Vulgate. In 385 Paula and Eustochium sailed for Palestine. Eventually they settled in Bethlehem, where they attracted a fol-

Francisco de Zurbarán, *St. Jerome With Saint Paula and Saint Eustochium,* c. 1640/1650. Oil on fabric, 235.74 × 173.35 cm. *(Samuel H. Kress Collection, 1952. Copyright 1995 Board of Trustees, National Gallery of Art, Washington, D.C.)*

lowing of devout women and founded a monastery. In addition, Paula built hospices for pilgrims and hospitals for the sick along the road to Bethlehem. The design and construction of the buildings were the plainest, which demonstrated the philosophy that it was better to spend money on the poor than on fine buildings. For approximately twenty years, Paula managed the institutions and personally nursed the weary travelers and the sick. St. Jerome's account of her life emphasized her caring and compassion:

> She was marvellous, debonair, and pietous to them that were sick, and comfort-ed them, and served them right humbly; and give them largely to eat such as they asked; but to herself she was hard in her sickness and scarce. . . . She was often by them that were sick, and she laid the pillows aright and in point; and she rubbed their feet, and boiled water to wash them; and it seemed to her that the less she did to the sick in service, so much the less service did she to God.

It is thought that Paula was the first to train nurses in a systematic way, to teach nursing as a distinct art rather than as a generalized service to the poor. The following description of nurses at work is thought to explain the origin of the tradition of hard manual labor as an expression of good nursing: "They trim lamps, light fires, sweep floors, clean vegetables, put heads of cabbage in the pot to boil, lay table cloths and set tables, hand cups, help to wash dishes, and run to and fro to wait on others" (St. Jerome, Letter to Pammachius).

In the late fourth century in Rome the place in good works was taken by this notable group of women, all friends of St. Jerome. All were Christian

Georges de La Tour, St. Sebastian Nursed by St. Irene, c. 1638. Oil on canvas. 108.6 × 123.8 cm. (Founders Society Purchase, Ralph Harman Booth Bequest Fund. Photograph copyright 1995 The Detroit Institute of Arts, Michigan.)

converts and lived not too many years after Constantine gave freedom to the Church. They were a striking contrast to the decadent, selfish, and apathetic Roman society. Probably no group of women has surpassed them in intellectual powers and commanding characters. Many individuals benefited from their services, including St. Sebastian. Sebastian was company commander in the Praetorian Guards during the reign of Emperor Diocletian (284–305). The public declaration of his faith in Christianity and his affiliation with the Christian Church resulted in his being fastened to a stake and shot by arrows. Later that night, St. Irene, the widow of his martyred friend St. Castulus, found him still alive. She and her associates provided the nursing care that has been documented and portrayed through the years by many artists. Consequently, St. Sebastian became a popular subject of medieval art. The idea that contagious or infectious diseases were shot into the body by invisible arrows fostered the practice of praying to St. Sebastian for prevention or cure.

Men in Nursing

An early organization of men in eastern Rome was the *Parabolani* brotherhood. The name referred literally to those who risked their lives by coming in contact with the sick. The duties of these members of a minor religious order included searching for the needy sick to bring them into hospitals. The members also acted as bodyguards to the bishop and became a burying detail as well. They were forbidden in public places and theaters, perhaps as a way to reduce contagion. It is believed that this group originated during the third century, when the Black Plague depleted the population of the entire Mediterranean area. When this dreaded disease was at its peak in Alexandria, the Parabolani reportedly organized a hospital and traveled throughout the city nursing the sick. These several hundred men and their nursing work were vividly described in *Hypatia,* a novel written by Charles Kingsley (n.d.).

Physicians and Medicine

In the early centuries of Christianity approximately sixteen Christian physicians reached distinction. The majority of them came from Syria, and the group included Aetius of Amida, Paul of Aegineta, and Alexander of Tralles (Frank, 1953). Two of the most prominent ones, St. Cosmas and St. Damian, were twin brothers who were born in Arabia and educated in Syria. They were the youngest of five brothers from a Christian family of some distinction. They became known as the "moneyless ones," since they did not charge for professional services as they traveled to provide services for those in need. It was their hope that this practice would gain converts to Christianity. Although they specialized in both medicine and pharmacy in Asia Minor, St. Cosmas and St. Damian were chosen as the "patrons of the medical profession." They suffered martyrdom in 278 during the reign of Diocletian and soon achieved a following for numerous miraculous cures in life and after death. Their legendary undertakings included the idea of limb transplantation.

Perhaps the best known of physicians of this era was St. Luke, the Evangelist. St. Paul called him the "beloved physician." It has been suggested by several writers that Luke had some type of medical preparation, that he may have studied at the famous school at Tarsus. His writings demonstrate an interest in medical subjects. He traveled extensively and at one point may have been a ship's physician. His several talents included literary and artistic ability.

St. Pantaleon, like Luke, Cosmas, and Damian, practiced free medicine among the sick poor. This, as well as the fact that he was a Christian, created hostility among his pagan friends. Eventually he was put to death and regarded as a healing saint. Later, Pantaleon was associated with the image of the comic in Venetian commedia dell'arte, and his name provided the term *pantaloon* for men's trousers (Petrucelli, 1978).

Ambrosius Francken, *Sts. Cosmas and Damian,* late sixteenth-century. 237 × 89 cm. *(Koninklijk Museum voor Schone Kunsten, Antwerp, Belgium.)*

In the foreground, Saints Cosmas and Damian prepare to transplant the leg of an Islamic Moor onto a recent amputee. These twin traveling physicians, who offered their services without charge to those in need, became known as the "moneyless ones." During the reign of Diocletian and the Christian persecution, they were tortured and beheaded. They received sainthood and were chosen as the patron saints of the medical profession. In the background of this painting appear a cripple, a patient in a sickbed, a physician examining a urine flask, and another surgeon treating a wounded man.

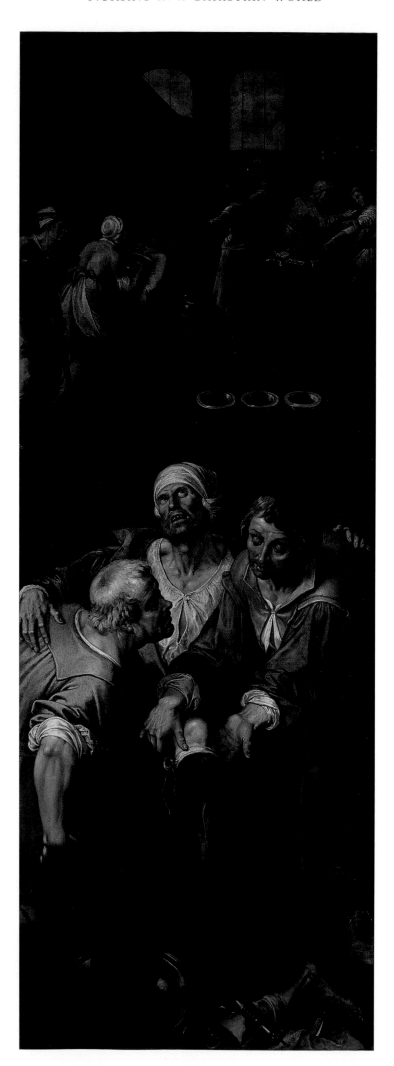

Aetius (502–575), who studied in Alexandria, wrote of treatments for varicose veins, hypertrophied tonsils, hydrophobia, goiter, and aneurysm of the brachial artery (ligation is described). His extensive collection of surgical writings, the *Tetrabiblion,* was first published in 1534 and included some accounts of conditions considered to be the most exact of the time period. Paul (625–690) discussed dietary regimens, pathology, pharmacology, surgery, and medicine; his writings include discussions of cancer, particularly of the uterus and breast. Little is actually known about him, although he, too, studied in Alexandria and was greatly admired for his surgical skills. His *Seven Books,* published in 1528, was a complete, concise synopsis of the medical and surgical literature of the day. Alexander (525–605) wrote of internal medicine and pathology. His excellent powers of observation led to accurate deductions about diseases such as ascites, the origin of epilepsy in the brain, and the detection of an enlarged spleen by palpation. Alexander made a study of diseases of the nervous system and described melancholia as a state of being that could terminate in mania, which he classed as an advanced state of dementia. He traveled extensively and achieved great fame as a skilled physician and an independent scientist. His comprehensive writings on medicine, the *Practica,* also contained magical cures that involved the use of amulets and incantations.

During the period of the Roman Empire and the early centuries of Christianity, medicine experienced a gradual loss of the scientific knowledge that had been attained by the Greeks. This decline was consistent with the deterioration of Roman civilization after the second century. Another contributing factor was the invasion of barbarians into the empire after 400, which helped bring about the disintegration of Roman culture. All of the sciences and medicine were affected; medical knowledge practically disappeared. Of all the Roman institutions, the Church alone survived intact. In addition, the idea that work with the hands was degrading was now applied to medicine.

Hospitals

The development and construction of early Christian hospitals was not left entirely to the charity of individual women. As the Church became freely established, the bishops also assumed responsibility for the expansion of charitable facilities, as well as responsibility for the care of the sick. Consequently, one reads of houses for the sick, for strangers, for the poor, and for the aged that existed in the fourth century. The original rooms in homes for hospitality and the care of the sick were called *diakonia.* The title was indicative of the close association of the nursing care of the sick poor in private homes with the activities of the diaconate. The term *diakonos* later became synonymous with hospital or nursing director.

An expectation of Christianity was that all who needed help would be received. As the congregations grew, it thus became necessary to expand the social services of the Church. As a result, the original diakonia became too small and new rooms, wings, and buildings were added. "Usually it seemed more economical to gather all classes of unfortunates into one institution known as a *xenodocheion,* which was the ancestor of the modern hospital as well as of most other types of charitable institutions" (Shryock, 1959, p. 79). Inns for strangers (hospitality centers); hospitals for the sick, the insane, and lepers; homes for the aged; almshouses; asylums for foundlings, orphans, the maimed, and the deformed; dwellings for nurses and physicians; and offices were included in these institutions. As early as the First Council of Nicaea (325), it was decided that each bishop should establish a xenodocheion. These institutions were administered by deaconesses and visited by widows of the Church. They were financed by Church alms and direct gifts from wealthy Christians. Eventually names for the various special divisions that were found in these charitable institutions arose: *xenodochia,* inns for strangers or travelers; *nosocomia,* wards or rooms for the sick; *brephotrophia,* foundling asylums;

A Medieval Hospital. (Parke-Davis Division of Warner-Lambert Co., Morris Plains, New Jersey.)

orphanotrophia, orphan asylums; *gerontokomia*, homes for the aged; *cherotrophia*, homes for widows; and *ptochotrophia*, almshouses for the poor. According to Nutting and Dock, the evolution of the earliest forms of Christian care of the sick proceeded with the

> diakonia, or rooms in private houses; xenodochia, amplifications of the diakonia; and finally, hospitals; while the forms of the earliest nursing organizations, beginning in the congregation, passed through the diaconate, the widows' sisterhoods, the parabolani, to monks and nuns.
>
> — *Nutting and Dock, 1937 p. 119*

Controversy exists regarding the exact date of the earliest xenodocheion. It is said, for instance, that one was built in Constantinople in the reign of Constantine but also that those built during the time of Julian the Apostate were the earliest. What is certain is that the most famous of these is the one founded by St. Basil the Great in Caesarea (370), often referred to as the "Basilias." St. Basil's institution was almost a "second city" and was as self-sufficient and self-supporting as possible. All individuals who were able to work were given employment in blacksmith shops, in the foundry, in the laundry and the dairy, in shoe and clothing shops, and in the kitchen. Out of gratitude the public officials of the city of Caesarea remitted taxes on the property. This gesture became an important aspect in the development of the precedent whereby properties used for religious or charitable purposes were exempted from taxation.

Three Bed Hospital, fifteenth century manuscript from Ferra: Florence, Laurentian, Gaddian, Ms 24, folio 247 v. Avicenna, *Cannon,* beginning of book IV. *(Biblioteca Medicea Laurenziana, Florence, Italy.)*

The Basilias was an outstanding example of Christian charity that embraced total hospital care—prevention, treatment, and social service. In the hospital were resident physicians, resident nurses, and carriers of the sick (Walsh, 1929). There was an orphanage; a place of hospitality for strangers; an asylum for infants and children; a building for the aged, lepers, and those with contagious diseases; a trade school for the physically impaired; and a hospital that cared for the sick, the crippled, and the poor. In addition, Basil's hospital had a special department for the insane.

The early Christians combined the sacred custom of hospitality with loving service. This resulted in an effective system for the care of the sick and the destitute. Little, however, is known of the specific nursing service that was provided in these hospitals. (Correspondingly, knowledge of medical services is also limited. This perhaps explains why a revival in faith healing occurred.) It is reasonable to assume that deaconesses may have served as nurses. It is also possible that servants did the ordinary labor under the direction of Church authorities. Certainly, no indication is given of any type of formal training for

Following page, Francisco de Herrera, the Elder, *St. Basil Dictating His Doctrine.* Oil on canvas, 242.5 × 194.3 cm. *(Musée du Louvre, Paris. Copyright PHOTO R.M.N.)*

Jean Pucelle, "St. Louis Administers to the Sick," from *The Hours of Jeanne d'Evreux,* French manuscript, fourteenth century, 1325–1328. Text page of the Office of Saint Louis. Illumination, grisaille, and color on vellum, approx. 8.9 × 6.4 cm. *(The Metropolitan Museum of Art, The Cloisters Collection, 1954. Copyright 1991 by The Metropolitan Museum of Art.)*

Jean Pucelle, "St. Louis Feeds a Leprous Monk," from *The Hours of Jeanne d'Evreux,* 1325–1328. Illumination, grisaille, and colors on vellum, approx. 8.9 × 6.4 cm. *(The Metropolitan Museum of Art, Cloisters Collection, 1954. Copyright 1991 by The Metropolitan Museum of Art.)*

the women or men who did participate in the nursing work. Eventually, nursing orders were formed in the Church to serve in the hospitals. The practice of clustering buildings was adopted by monasteries and continued until the twelfth century, when it became customary to separate hospitals from other branches of relief service and build them separately. This intimate connection between the Church and the care of the sick during this period in history is an important factor in an understanding of the organization and functions of the hospital:

> At the outset it will be well to make clear what the hospital was, and what it was not. It was an ecclesiastical, not a medical, institution. It was for care rather than cure; for the relief of the body, when possible, but pre-eminently for the refreshment of the soul . . . . Faith and love were more predominant features in hospital life than were skill and science.
>
> — *Seymer, 1932, p. 36*

THE EARLY MIDDLE AGES (DARK AGES): AD 500–1000

The term *Middle Ages* is used by historians to denote the time between the middle of the fifth century (fall of Rome, 476) and the middle of the fifteenth century (fall of Constantinople, 1453). The thousand-year period that followed the collapse of the Roman Empire is also referred to as the medieval period of history, the division between ancient and modern times. Although this is a useful term because it is fairly well understood, it must be remembered that no period in history has hard and fast boundaries. In addition, this period can be subdivided into the early and later Middle Ages. The early centuries are collectively known as the Dark Ages, a title that clearly demonstrates the prevalent social destruction of the times, the deteriorating world.

During the Dark Ages the domination of society by the Church was practically unchallenged. As the Roman Empire was slowly disintegrating, the Church had been developing into a well integrated and highly organized institution. Its organization followed a pattern similar to that of the Roman government. Each ecclesiastical province paralleled a civil province. Dioceses were formed under bishops, and these corresponded to a Roman governmental unit. Over all was the bishop of Rome, the Pope, who corresponded to the emperor. Finally, when the emperor removed himself to Constantinople in 330, the Pope was left the most powerful figure in the West. The bishops emerged as the natural leaders of the people, and the empire was perpetuated through the Church. All of these events contributed to the evolution of the image of the nurse as a saint. The activity of nursing itself became honored as many royal, noble, and distinguished people engaged in it and regarded it as the work of God. Nursing became a penitential activity used as a means of purgation and purification. It was a work calling for unceasing toil without expectation of earthly reward.

Three large classes of people dominated society in the early Middle Ages. The majority were serfs, who were farmers living under primitive conditions. Above them were the aristocratic and warlike lords. Finally, there was the clergy, both secular and monastic, who were bound by celibacy in order to give undivided devotion to the religious life. Women had again fallen into a subordinate position, but positions in religious orders were open to them as well as to men. It was possible to acquire dignity as a nun.

> There were even joint monasteries of men and women, living in separate houses but ruled over by a woman superior. Certain of the orders, both for men and for women, came to devote themselves to nursing; and it was this trend that brought women into such service for the first time on a large scale. By the modern period, indeed, nursing began to be viewed as primarily a woman's field.
>
> — *Shryock, 1959. p. 89*

The early Middle Ages revealed a crumbling world. Chaos reigned supreme as a result of the impact of the onslaughts of barbarian tribes and extreme moral decay. The middle class disappeared because of exorbitant taxes, widespread epidemics, natural disasters, and wars. Money and cities disappeared along with trade, commerce, and industry. The population declined, crime waves occurred, poverty was abysmal, and torture and imprisonment became prominent as civilization seemed to slip back into semibarbarianism. In essence, the Graeco-Roman culture stumbled to a halt.

"The fate of civilization rested upon health protection, a different form of government, the education of thousands of barbarians to civilized standards, and many changes in Roman outlook and attitudes" (Jamieson and Sewall, 1950, p. 128). Medieval life became increasingly dangerous and necessitated the formation of protective groups by the populace. The people had lost their sense of security and gathered together in search of safety. This phenomenon was characterized by three great movements that arose during this early period of the Middle Ages: feudalism, monasticism, and Islamism. These movements developed simultaneously and were thought to be possible solutions to the chaos of the time.

Feudalism

Feudalism was a new system of land tenure with complex social arrangements in which self-sustaining groups prepared themselves to resist attacks from bands of fighting men sworn to uphold the might of their leaders. It involved cooperative farming units, isolated from each other and governed by individuals known as knights, counts, earls, barons, or lords. Feudalism was a type of patriarchal rule that provided men with homes for their families, food, and bodily protection. In return for these services, the tenants worked the land as farmers and became soldiers in the case of war. These serfs could not be sold as slaves. Political, economic, and social life were based on the holding of land. The typical edifice was the rural manor or estate owned by the lord. It was usually set high in an inaccessible location, and massive turreted walls enclosed the manor, which was also encircled by a moat.

"Midwife Attending Childbearing Woman Seated on Obstetrical Stool," from Jacobus Rueff's *Ein Schoen Lustig Trost-buechle Von Den Empfengknussen Und Geburten Der Menschen.* Zurich, 1554. Engraving. *(The Wellcome Institute for the History of Medicine, London.)*

In ancient art only two types of scenes illustrate women caring for the health of others: childbirth and the bathing of infants. During childbirth, the midwife functioned while sitting or kneeling in front of the woman. Rueff's *Trostbuechle* was a sixteenth-century book of instruction for midwives.

Feudalism acted as a cohesive force in the new society and demanded a strong bond of loyalty between lord and tenant. It offered a temporary solution to the land problem and provided an armed force for Europe against Frankish and Islamic invasions. Feudalism did, however, have drawbacks that eventually led to many abuses within the society. Although protection was indeed provided, constant warfare prevented progress. In addition, government consisted of numerous insignificant principalities that were united merely by fidelity of small lords to greater ones. Only the Church rose above this confusion through continued systematic organization.

Most women were forced to marry young, often without their consent. Their chief value to society was their breeding power and the ability to manage a home. The lord's wife, the lady of the manor, was faced with a difficult life. She was responsible for the supervision of the entire establishment, for bearing and caring for children, for riding and hunting, for whatever needed to be done. She was frequently called upon to nurse family guests or villagers. The lady was in charge of the care of the sick of the manor and was a combination of doctor and nurse. She applied first aid, faced surgical emergencies, and had an extensive knowledge of home remedies for all types of illnesses. Empirical medicine was almost entirely in the hands of such women. The number of doctors was small, and only a few of them were located in the manors.

> The lady was thus obliged not only to be housewife in her own capacity, but also amateur soldier and man of the house in her husband's absence and amateur physician when no skilled doctor could be had. She was supposed to be manager of the household and know how to choose and treat servants, to air and mend and keep moths out of clothes and furs, to know the best recipes for catching flies and other "familiar beasts to man," and for keeping bedrooms free of mosquitoes and barns of rats. There is even an injunction to his [the lord's wife] "If one of your servants fall ill, do you yourself lay aside all other cares, very lovingly and charitably care for him or her."
>
> — *Walsh, 1929, p. 35*

Monasticism

The idea of finding the ineffable love of God by renouncing the world found a practical outlet in monasticism. The dangers of medieval life led many men and women who were spiritually minded to the monasteries to escape worldly chaos. Others probably entered the monasteries to obtain security and protection. From the efforts of St. Basil in the fourth century, the monastic movement spread to the West and assumed prominence in the social structure of the early Middle Ages. Through the fifth century the movement spread slowly because the majority of monasteries were weak, poor, and disorganized. The monks tended to be idle and dissolute, often wandering from one monastery to another in search of the easiest path. By the sixth century, however, monasticism provided great practical and spiritual value to concerned individuals and to society at large.

The basic concept of monasticism was withdrawal from society for the sanctification of one's soul. Ascetism was also a marked feature of this religious life, particularly in the earlier periods. All degrees of self-mortification, self-denial, and strict discipline were observed. The monks and nuns were governed by a rule—the constitutions, bylaws, and directives by which they were to live. Four rules were recognized by the Church for the government of monastic orders, those of Basil, Augustine, Benedict, and Francis. Monasteries were not established to care for orphans, to educate children, or even to nurse the sick. These were secondary works that arose serendipitously and were done well by the monks and nuns who performed them; they were not an essential part of their calling.

The credit for the organization of many of these institutions is given to St. Benedict of Nursia (480–543), who founded the order of Benedictines in the sixth century. St. Benedict began life as a hermit who practiced the most excessive and excruciating asceticism, which led to his ultimate fame. His followers were formed into twelve communities of twelve monks. St. Benedict established the most influential monastery in western Christendom at Monte Cassino. This monastery became a Nazi stronghold during World War II and was bombed by the Allied forces. About the year 529, St. Benedict composed his rule, the Benedictine Rule, which had a great influence on Western civilization:

> Before all things and above all things care must be taken of the sick so that they may be served in the very deed as Christ Himself; for He has said: "I was sick and ye visited me" and "As long as ye did it to one of these my least brethren, ye did it to me." But let the sick themselves consider that they are served for the honor of God, and not grieve their brethren who serve them by their importunity. Yet must they be patiently borne with, because from such as these is gained more abundant reward. Therefore the Abbot shall take the greatest care that they suffer no neglect.

The success of the Benedictine Rule lay in its moderation, an adaptation of monastic tradition to Western conditions. It helped to bring stability and organization out of chaos, to bring calm out of panic. The rule provided for reasonable and moderate conditions, which included adequate sleep, rest, diet, and clothing and a balance of study, prayer, and manual labor both indoors and out. Members, after a year's probation, vowed to never return to the world, to render complete and unquestioning obedience to their leader, and to totally deny themselves through humility and service. It was, therefore, possible for persons of ordinary spiritual gifts to follow the rule. Communities were able to retain monks, to be physically, spiritually, and socially healthy and, most important, to be effective.

The Benedictine monasteries became centers of influence, learning, and culture. The monks revived agriculture through labor in the fields, orchards, and vineyards. They improved the plow and invented the windmill, the

Map of the centers of hospital, medicine, and nursing activity, 5 BC–5 AD.

waterwheel, and the horse collar. They not only labored for souls but tilled the soil and made barren lands bountiful. The excess food produced was used to feed the poor. The monks increased the available knowledge in many ways. They were scholars, librarians, and teachers and opened schools so that all, not only their own members, could read and write. They laboriously copied, clarified, and illustrated precious manuscripts. They used their knowledge of medicine and herbs to care for the sick. The monasteries offered hospitality and shelter to the homeless and refuge to the persecuted.

> The work of the Benedictine monasteries manifested itself in several directions: in the conversion of the Teutons, in civilizing northwestern Europe, and in extending the works of education: literature, arts, sciences, libraries. It is to the monasteries that we are indebted today for practically everything extant in ancient secular and religious literature. The monks were not only the official copyists of manuscripts, they were also the official chroniclers of the history of their times.
>
> — *Frank, 1953, p. 84*

Nursing of the sick eventually became a chief function and duty of the community life. This command was stated in the rule: "Before all things and above all things care must be taken of the sick." Every monastery provided an *infirmarium* for its members and a *hospitalarius* just inside or outside the gates for the needy of the community. These were at first hospices rather than hospitals, since they were refuges for the poor, devoted more to shelter and comfort than to cure. More affluent monasteries later sought to divide the sick from the poor and to offer more than food and shelter to those who needed help. As time elapsed, it was not only the sick poor who requested assistance. Monks were called from their monasteries to the courts of kings and nobles and to the homes of the wealthy. From the original refuges city hospitals grew and became the responsibility of a monastic order. In most instances the nursing in these institutions was done by a monastic sisterhood.

Information about the nursing personnel of these earliest monastic hospitals is scanty. It is possible that deaconesses were still active as nurses. In some

After Abraham Bosse, *Interior Scene With Woman Being Phlebotemised by a Barber Surgeon,* c. 1635. Engraving. *(National Library of Medicine, Bethesda, Maryland.)*

cases religious societies were instituted to meet the needs of specific situations. It was also the custom for the monks and nuns of related orders to serve the hospitals. Monastic orders for women had developed concurrently with those for men and followed the same pattern. Monks did nursing in the men's wards and nuns in the women's wards, an arrangement that became common toward the middle of the thirteenth century. In some cases the nuns were in charge of an entire hospital and the monks of the same order acted as priests. It is doubtful, however, that all the nursing work was done by the nuns and priests, since they had many lay attendants and perhaps volunteers.

Little is known about the actual care given the sick during the Dark Ages. Secular medicine was almost completely extinguished, and there was little impetus toward advancement in the science and art of nursing or of medicine. In fact, little distinction was made between medicine and nursing. The monks and the nuns practiced medicine as well as nursing and for long periods seemed to have been the only practitioners. Medical historians report that the medical practice was almost entirely confined to the members of these monastic orders. Considerable folk and drug lore, mysticism, religious faith, and, at times, superstition crept into the care of the sick. Bloodletting, diet, and baths were common treatments of the day, along with the application of cups and leeches and the use of blisters, cautery, scarification, and enemas. "The main advancement in nursing during this period probably came through the internal organization and operation of monastic institutions and the discipline and training of large groups of sisters and brothers in their cooperative undertakings" (Stewart and Austin, 1962, p. 50). The nursing of the times was done partly by monks and nuns and partly by servants. It is difficult, however, to determine the division of labor between the two and whether either received much formal training.

Monastic Nurses

Monastic houses for women grew in number in the sixth and seventh centuries. Many of the women who entered these houses were wealthy and had great influence in the community. The two primary reasons given for women's entry into these orders were the prevailing need for protection and the opportunity to follow the occupational career of one's choice. The women in these monasteries were sheltered by a rule, granted by the Church, that afforded freedom and safety to pursue intellectual studies or practical interests. Many famous women of the early Middle Ages were connected to the monastic life. They included Hrotswitha, who knew the Latin classics and wrote dramas; Lisba, Walburga, and Berthgythe, who went from Ireland and England to evangelize Germany; and Hildegarde, whose medical knowledge and political insight were remarkable. Other women carried on hospital nursing and medical work.

Large twin communities, or double monasteries, of men and women were also a feature of early monastic life. These were under the direct control of an abbess, who held a position of great importance. The two related houses, one of monks, the other of nuns, were usually kept rigidly apart. The opposite system of the rule of women's orders by an abbot met with failure; the groups did not flourish or survive (Tuker and Malleson, 1900). A sense of joint ownership united the members of these religious settlements and resulted in the emergence of centers of culture and of art. Famous abbesses who ruled the twin communities were Radegunde at Poitiers; Hilda at Whitby in England, who had some of the great bishops as her scholars and taught Caed mon, the first English poet; and Hersende at Frontevrault, who ruled a vast establishment of three thousand members. Each abbess administered the property of the monastery and maintained discipline. The monks and the nuns swore obedience to her.

The most famous double establishment was founded and ruled by St. Radegunde (519–587) at Poitiers in 559. Radegunde, the daughter of a Thuringian king and a descendant of Theodoric, experienced numerous tragedies in her young life. Her father was murdered by her uncle; she was captured and forced to marry Clotaire, the Frankish king of Neustria, becoming one of his six wives; and she fled to Noyan after her husband murdered her brother. Eventually Radegunde made her way to Poitiers, where she took refuge in the Christian Church. She founded the Holy Cross Monastery, a religious settlement of about two hundred nuns.

Scripture reading, the study of ancient literature, the transcription of manuscripts, and the performance of dramas (mystery plays of the Middle Ages) were important activities of this community. The care of the sick, however, was the chief function. Radegunde nursed the patients herself in the hospital she established. She was particularly sensitive to the lepers, who were social outcasts, and was seen giving a kiss to their diseased bodies. There is no indication that physicians were connected with this hospital. Nursing care seems to have been the key to the restoration of health. Baths were built at the instigation of Radegunde. This was particularly significant because Christian monasticism had destroyed the cult of the Roman bath. Stimulation of the skin was condemned as a provocative sexual desire in an age of asceticism. In a sense Radegunde carried on the forgotten tradition of the Baths of Caracalla (Robinson, 1946).

The monastic ideal of humility led to the use of plain, coarse materials for clothing. This ideal was perpetuated by the poverty of many of the earliest convents. Yet abbesses and nuns of royal birth wore beautiful clothing, as depicted by the following description:

> A vest of fine linen of a violet colour is worn, above it a scarlet tunic with a hood, sleeves striped with silk and trimmed with red fur; the locks on the forehead and temples are curled with a crisping iron, the dark head-veil is given up for white and coloured head-dresses which, with bows of ribbon sewn on, reach down to the ground; the nails, like those of a falcon or sparrow-hawk, are pared to resemble talons.

> — *Putnam, 1921, p. 85*

Criticism of this costume as incongruous with monasticism paved the way for a clothing reform that ended in uniformity. A distinctive dress for religious women became a custom. The veil as part of convent dress symbolized humility, obedience, and service. Regulations were developed that governed the use of the veils. They came to be a part of the prescribed habit and were always white during the probationary period of the novice. Various forms of the veil were worn by women to distinguish social position. The cap of the modern nurse was a modification of the religious veil and has been associated with humility and the rendering of service to mankind.

St. Brigid (452–523) introduced female monasteries into Ireland as early as the fifth century. She was the daughter of an Ulster prince and a disciple of St. Patrick. Brigid became a famous abbess in Ireland at Kildare and was respected as a scholar, educator, counselor, and an expert in the healing arts. References are made to the miracles of Brigid, who was also known for her healing of the lepers and her care of the sick. She was labeled "the patroness of healing." The monastery at Kildare became a center for culture, the arts, learning, and spirituality.

St. Scholastica, the twin sister of St. Benedict, founded a Benedictine community for women. This order was established near Monte Cassino, and Scholastica became its abbess.

Islamism

During the early centuries of the Christian era and into part of the Middle Ages, Arab kingdoms extended from Spain, through northern Africa, and into western Asia. The Arab influence was felt as far away as India and China. The conquests of the Arab people exposed them to a variety of native cultures, and they developed a certain tolerance for different beliefs and ways of living. They learned from the achievements of the Egyptians and the Greeks. They built universities where experimental research and scientific studies in astronomy, mathematics, and chemistry were conducted.

Muhammad (570–632) was born at Mecca, the religious and commercial center of Arabia. His tribe was one of the most influential and guarded the sacred Kaaba, the idolatrous shrine where heathen Arabs made an annual religious pilgrimage. He was considered to be the first and only prophet of a new world religion: "There is no God but Allah, and Muhammad is his prophet." At Muhammad's command primitive gods and native animism were abandoned. Submission was the core of the religion and the basic ideal that led to the name of *Islam* ("surrender to the will of Allah"). The followers of the monotheistic religion were called Muslims. The teachings of Muhammad were written down and incorporated in the *Koran*. Both the civil and religious lives of Muslims were directed by the tenets of this new religion. Muhammadanism has been called a "religion of the sword," since the followers of Islam were inspired by the creed to spread their conquests throughout the Mediterranean and to threaten the gates of Europe.

Medicine was an interest of the Arabs, and they strongly encouraged its study. They translated many Hellenic works into Arabic, particularly those related to medicine and including the works of Hippocrates and Galen. The Arabs studied hygiene and developed an extensive materia medica. Their belief in the uncleanliness of the dead forbade dissection. Thus knowledge of anatomy and physiology was hampered. Surgery, however, was practiced, and the Muslims are credited with the use of catgut for sutures. Physicians were held in high esteem and were required to pass qualifying examinations.

The Arabs built large, well-constructed hospitals and introduced new methods of caring for the sick. The hospital at Cairo had chief physicians who held clinics for medical students. Some of the unusual features of this hospital included classified wards, male and female nurses, streams of running water in some of the wards, and fever wards cooled by fountains.

> The great Al-Mansur hospital of Cairo was a huge triangular structure with fountains playing in the four courtyards, separate wards for important diseases, wards for women and convalescents, lecture rooms, an extensive library, out-patient clinics, diet kitchens, an orphan asylum and a chapel. It employed male

and female nurses, had an income of about $100,000, and disbursed a suitable sum to each convalescent on his departure, so that he might not have to go to work at once. The patients were nourished upon a rich and attractive diet, and the sleepless were provided with soft music or, as in the Arabian Nights, with accomplished tellers of tales.

— Garrison, 1913, pp. 92–93

Alexandria and Damascus also had well-equipped hospitals under the control of expert physicians. The one at Damascus gave free treatment and drugs for more than three centuries. The hospital at Baghdad employed sixty salaried physicians on its staff, probably the earliest instance of a paid staff. A system of care of the patient incorporated spiritual and mental aspects as well as attention to the body. Yet the care of a woman during childbirth and in the case of gynecological disease remained in the hands of untaught midwives.

Among the many outstanding physicians, three in particular are remembered: Razes, Avicenna, and Maimonides. Rhazes (Razi-abu-Bakr Muhammad ibn-Zakariya al-Razi, 850–932) was one of the greatest of the Arab physicians. He was especially known for his writings on measles and smallpox and contributed material to an encyclopedia of medicine. Rhazes was respected for his clinical descriptions of illness, his observations, and his pragmatic approach to treatment.

Avicenna (abu-Ali al-Husayn ibn-adallah ibn-Sina, 980–1037) was considered to be both a philosopher and a scientist. He received his medical education in Baghdad and eventually was made the physician-in-chief of its largest hospital. Although he may have practiced medicine, his principal contribution in this area was his writings. The *Canon of Medicine,* in use for centuries after his death, was considered one of the most important textbooks in the field of medical education. Until the middle of the seventeenth century, medical curricula of the Christian universities were based on his writings.

Maimonides (Rabbi Moses ben Maimon, 1135–1204) was the most famous Jewish physician in Arab medicine. He was born in Muslim-controlled Cordova, Spain, but fled with other Jews to Fez in Morocco when nonbelievers began to be harassed. Later he went to Palestine and then to Cairo, where he entered medicine for financial reasons. He finally became court physician to the sultan Saladin. Maimonides aimed at practical therapeutics and gave advice on such things as hygiene, poisons, diet, and first aid. However, he was basically a philosopher who attempted to reconcile scientific reasoning and religious faith. He is remembered specifically for codifying the Talmud. Although attributed by some with composing the Morning Prayer of the Physician, Maimonides probably was not the author (Lyons, 1978). This section of the prayer is often quoted:

> O God, let my mind be ever clear and enlightened. By the bedside of the patient let no alien thought deflect it. Let everything that experience and scholarship have taught it be present in it and hinder it not in its tranquil work. For great and noble are those scientific judgments that serve the purpose of preserving the health and lives of Thy creatures.
>
> Keep far from me the delusion that I can accomplish all things. Give me the strength, the will, and the opportunity to amplify my knowledge more and more. Today I can disclose things in my knowledge which yesterday I would not yet have dreamt of, for the Art is great, but the human mind presses on untiringly.
>
> In the patient let me ever see only the man. Thou, All- Bountiful One, hast chosen me to watch over the life and death of Thy creatures. I prepare myself now for my calling. Stand Thou by me in this great task, so that it may prosper. For without Thine aid man prospers not even in the smallest things.
>
> *— Morning Prayer of the Physician*

School of Salerno

The earliest universities were established at Salerno, Bologna, Paris, and Oxford. The circumstances of the founding of each remain obscure. Their growth, however, was gradual. Salerno began as a medical center and served a vital role in the transition from monastic to lay medicine. The date of its founding and its origins are unclear. Some speculate that the Benedictines had a monastery and a hospital there about 820. Legend states that the school was started by four physicians; one Jew, Elinus; one Greek, Pontius; one Latin, Magister Salernus; and, one Arab, Adala. Until the twelfth century it prevailed as the leading medical institution in western Europe under secular authority.

Salerno became an important center of medical learning and assisted with the revival of medicine in Europe. It was open to female students, and women physicians were on the faculty. Trotula and Abella were the two most famous women of this school. Trotula was supposedly the author of an obstetrical and gynecological treatise entitled *Trotulae Curandarum Aegritudinum Muliebrum* (*Trotula on the Cure of Diseases of Women*). She was also the head of the department of diseases of women. Throughout the early Middle Ages, however, midwifery was the province of women, and other medical concerns were generally forbidden to them. Women physicians usually specialized in diseases of women and children, even though they were licensed for general practice.

Standard requirements of the school of Salerno included three years of premedicine at the college level in the study of logic, philosophy, and literature, five years of medicine and surgery, and one year's practice with a reputable physician. A law was enacted about 1140 to prohibit anyone from practicing medicine without a license. *Regimen Sanitatis Salernitanum* or *Flos Medicinae* was the most famous work of the Salernitan school. This Latin poem, consisting of rational dietetic and hygienic precepts, underwent many versions, more than three hundred editions, and numerous translations. It appeared in the form of verse so that it could be easily memorized:

> If thou to health and vigor wouldst attain,
> Shun weighty cares—all anger deem profane,
> From heavy suppers and much wine abstain,
> Nor trivial count it, after pompous fare,
> To rise from the table and to take the air.
> Shun idle, noonday slumber, nor delay,
> The urgent calls of nature obey.

> — *Portion of a verse.*

Medieval Hospitals

Three famous medieval hospitals, the Hôtel Dieu of Lyons, the Hôtel Dieu of Paris, and the Santo Spirito Hospital of Rome, were built outside monastic walls and are still in existence. The most complete records dealing with the nursing arrangements are available for the Hôtels Dieu of Lyons and of Paris. The name *Hôtel Dieu,* meaning "God's house," was generally used to indicate the principal hospital in a French town or city (Nutting and Dock, 1937). The original hospitals were established as xenodochia or almshouses and attended to the needy and infirm as well as to the sick.

The Hôtel Dieu of Lyons was founded in 542 at the request of Sacerdos, the archbishop of Lyons. It was originated on the almshouse plan and was managed by lay groups. Including other charitable works besides nursing, it was designed to shelter pilgrims, orphans, the poor, the infirm, and the sick. Its earliest nurses were laywomen who were recruited from penitents (fallen women) and widows. Eventually, men who were originally called *servants,* and later *brothers,* assisted with the nursing work. This particular hospital provided a striking contrast to other institutions of the time in that it was free from clerical control.

The Hôtel Dieu of Paris dates from 650 or 651. It was founded by Bishop Landry (Landericus), whose statue stands in its courtyard. This "house of God" was built with an open door for all who suffered. Also patterned after the almshouse, it was governed by a lay administration. The Hôtel Dieu began as a small hospital and grew to immense proportions. The original group of laywomen who cared for the sick were organized into a religious body by Pope Innocent IV. They became known as the Augustinian Sisters, since they adopted the Rule of St. Augustine. Brothers, too, belonged to this strict order. These sisters were responsible to the clergy and for all practical purposes were about the same as cloistered nuns. They are considered to be the oldest purely nursing order of sisters in existence. The importance of the Hôtel Dieu of Paris is noted in the following description:

> No other ancient hospital has bequeathed to posterity a nursing history so extensive or one that has thrown so much light on internal hospital management. For the publication of these interesting records we have mainly to thank the unremitting and bitter contest which for centuries was carried on by the clerical and civil powers over the administration of the important and extensive institution. In this, as in every similar contest, the nursing service was the chief storm centre, and to gain control of the nursing staff the main point of vantage sought. The story of this struggle points anew to the elemental importance of the nursing factor in the composition of hospitals, and many useful lessons may be taken therefrom.
>
> — *Nutting and Dock, 1937, p. 294.*

Both the brothers and the sisters were assigned specific activities that fell into the categories of exterior work, hospital administration, care of the sick, and religious services. Some nursing was done by the brothers in the general wards, but in the women's wards only sisters did the nursing care. The Augustinians went through three stages of training. Their nursing role included the admission and discharge of patients, responsibility for the kitchens and the laundry (all the washing was done on the banks of the nearby Seine), and the burying of the dead. In addition, religious rites were an essential part of the hospital routine, with services conducted for both patients and staff.

The Santo Spirito Hospital in Rome, established in 717 by order of the Pope, was probably the largest of the medieval hospitals. It was built for the primary purpose of care for the sick. By 1500 it possessed a main hall that contained nearly one thousand beds. Several distinct wards were included for

A nursing scene is portrayed on a page of a Parisian manuscript. Illustrated are the various vows of the sisters. Groups of nuns stand with figures representing the four Virtues as the nuns gather in front of the sick in a ward. The manuscript by Jehan Henry was a spiritual guide for the Augustinian nuns who nursed at the Hôtel Dieu.

"Nuns at Work on a Ward at the Hôtel Dieu, Paris," c. 1650. Wood engraving. From Casimir Tollet's *Les Edifices Hospitaliers*, 1892. *(National Library of Medicine, Bethesda, Maryland.)*

Interior Scene at the Ospedale de Santo Spirito, Rome, c. 1840. Several monks and a nun tend the patients in the immense ward at Santo Spirito. Lithograph. *(National Library of Medicine, Bethesda, Maryland.)*

men, women, and convalescents. As the revival of a lay medical profession in the later medieval period brought physicians into the hospitals, Santo Spirito encouraged this connection. It is said that more than one hundred physicians and surgeons were eventually in attendance at this hospital. This institution became a well-known prototype for the development of other medieval hospitals.

U N I T 4

Nursing in a Changing World

Aristocratic and Military Influences

The most spectacular product of the feudal system was the Crusader, a man who was supposed to combine a lofty spirit devoted to the service of God with a fierce, belligerent temper, ready to fight the infidel wherever he was to be found, that the holy ground upon which Christ trod might again belong to his followers. He carried the principles and the glory of knighthood to their fullest as he traveled over the continent of Europe and throughout the Mediterranean basin. When he traveled in the Near East, he learned much from the enemy; the idea of the organized hospital was originally borrowed from the Arabs. The natural places for the establishment of hospitals were the outposts, particularly Jerusalem itself, where those wounded in battle sought refuge while they recovered. The hospital had to be staffed by physicians and nurses who were members of the regular orders. The nurses went to battle and then retired to attend the sick. They were called "knight hospitalers."

— GERALD JOSEPH GRIFFIN AND JOANNE KING GRIFFIN

Giovanni Bellini, *St. Francis in the Desert*, c. 1485. Panel, 124.5 × 142 cm. *(Copyright The Frick Collection, New York.)*

With St. Francis came the emergence of the nun from her cloister and her close association with nursing in hospitals. St. Francis stressed the need for care for the homeless and the poor sick of the towns as a matter of Christian duty. Nursing care of the sick expanded beyond hospital walls.

Nursing in a Changing World

| 1000 | 1050 | 1100 | 1150 | 1200 | 1250 |

DAILY LIFE

1066 First record of comet, later called Halley's

1094 First record of gondolas in Venice

1096 First Crusade occurs

1151 First fire and plague insurance in Iceland

1180 Glass windows appear in England

1200 Engagement rings become fashionable

1215 Magna Carta signed

1230 Leprosy introduced into Europe by Crusaders

SCIENCE AND TECHNOLOGY

1041–1048 Earliest movable type for printing invented in China

1044 Exact formula for gunpowder published

1090 Chinese develop first water-driven mechanical clock

1100s Magnetic compass invented in China

1180 Windmill with vertical sails invented in Europe

1233 Coal mined in Newcastle, England

THE VISUAL ARTS

1000 Artistic revival in Italy with frescoes and mosaics

1000–1100 Illustrated books in Iran

1050 English monks excel in embroidery

1078 Tower of London built

1100 Appearance of Gothic architecture

1174 Leaning Tower of Pisa built

MEDICINE AND HEALTH CARE

c. 1098–1179 St. Hildegarde considered leading medical authority

1100 Barber-Surgeons form guilds

1101 St. Giles' Hospital built for the care of lepers

1123 St. Bartholomew's Hospital founded in London

1200 Alcohol used for medical purposes

1213 St. Thomas' Hospital founded in London

1247 Bethlehem Hospital founded in England

NURSING

1000–1500 Midwives, not physicians, deliver infants

1000–1500 Rich period of nursing saints and mystics

1095 Antonines founded and devoted to sufferers of "St. Anthony's Fire"

1096–1272 Military nursing orders (Knights Hospitallers) carry chief burden of nursing

c. 1100 The Benguines movement begins

1170–1221 St. Dominic establishes Order of Preachers and other orders involved with nursing

1182–1226 St. Francis of Assisi establishes three religious orders involved with nursing

1194–1253 St. Clare of Assisi, abbess of Poor Clares

1207–1231 St. Elizabeth of Hungary, patron saint of nursing

1244 Misericordia functions primarily as volunteer ambulance society

1300	1350	1400	1450	1500	1550	1600

1290 Spectacles come into use

1348 Worst occurrence of Black Death
devastates Europe

1464 Royal mail service begins in France

1492 Columbus lands in America

1495 Syphilis epidemic spreads throughout Europe

1500 Black lead pencils used

1509 African slave trade begins

1517 Coffee drinking begins in Europe

1532 Sugar cane cultivated in Brazil

1547 Moscow
destroyed by fire

1596
Water
closets
installed in
England

1337 Attempt made at scientific
weather forecasting

1452 Metal plates used for printing

1480 Leonardo da Vinci develops the parachute

1492 First terrestrial globe constructed

1440–1513 Bihizad, most famous artist for
illuminated manuscripts

1450 Florence becomes center of Renaissance

1452–1519 Leonardo da Vinci, Italian artist and universal genius

1471–1528 Albrecht Dürer, German artist

1475–1564 Michelangelo Buonarroti, Italian sculptor

1477–1576 Titian, Italian artist

1483–1520 Raphael, Italian painter

1300 Urine examination used in
medicine as means of diagnosis

1350 Fallopio discovers "fallopian tubes"

1400 Rise of municipal hospitals

1451 Ospedale Santa Maria
degli Innocenti built
as asylum for abandoned
children in Italy

1500 Civil authorities take over all
hospitals in Protestant countries

1510–1590 Ambroise Paré, French surgeon

1514–1564 Andreas Vesalius, founder
of modern anatomy

1557 Influenza epidemic
spreads over all
Europe

1347–1381 St. Catherine of Siena, hospital and visiting nurse

1348 Alexian Brothers form to care for bubonic plague victims

1400 Great extension of nursing by secular orders occurs

*T*he roots of a movement toward the creation of religious orders of men and women with the primary motivation of nursing the sick began to occur in the late Middle Ages. This was accompanied by a marked tendency toward the secularization and commercialization of nursing.

THE LATE MIDDLE AGES: AD 1000–1500

Numerous interacting forces were activated in the period known as the late Middle Ages, the end of the Dark Ages. As a result of these forces, society would never be the same again. By this time many barbarian tribes had settled somewhere in Europe, staked claims to lands, and often been Christianized and civilized. It was a period in history characterized by mobility of the population and eventually the detachment of individuals from protective units. It was a time in which surprising progress was made, not only in the arts and writing (greatly aided by the invention of printing) but also in architecture and the healing arts. In some ways it was marked by a spirit of optimism and enthusiasm that would become shattered nearly five centuries later by war, plagues, famine, and instability.

Trade promoted the development of inland cities and a middle class of merchants, bankers, shop owners, and shopkeepers; craftsmen arose and became as wealthy and powerful as the land barons. New inventions in crafts and trades occurred in relation to these changes. Learning was revived, and university education became a privilege of the middle class. This middle class grew as social forces freed the serfs from their manor duties and set them adrift into the cities to seek paid employment. The protection that the castle or monastery walls had previously offered was secured by the building of town walls. The gates in the walls were secured at sundown; the bridge was raised in those cities surrounded by moats. In many instances the walled cities were overpopulated. There were limited, if any, facilities for sanitation and for the provision of pure water and food. Slums became hotbeds of disease, crime, violence, and death.

A new spirit challenged the domination of the Catholic Church, which remained the chief influence over the people. This spirit was characterized by an emerging interest in the things of this earth and the life of the present rather than a focus on life after death with its emphasis on the soul. The Church had grown rich and powerful, and this caused criticism of the priesthood and monastic orders as well as the Church itself. Wealth, laxity, and greed failed to exemplify the teachings of Christ. Unrest occurred as the middle class grew more independent, knowledgeable, and sophisticated. Various reform movements, which included new patterns of religious thought and action, tended to divert the unrest, at least for a time. Eventually a new interpretation of the doctrine of the Church was demanded. Individuals such as Peter Abelard (1079–1142) broke from the rigid Augustinian doctrine of predestination. In the Augustinian doctrine the life of the body was held to be of little importance except as an opportunity for the soul to find unity with God. This unity could be achieved through suppressing physical desires and appetites, having faith in Christ, and obeying the commands of Christ. Life in this world was a journey between life and death. Each person would struggle with the forces of good and evil and would be rewarded in the next world on the basis of success. Reason and logical analysis as the means to truth began to be advocated as an alternative. The writings of St. Thomas Aquinas (1225–1274) became a part of this new ideology and the basis of Catholic doctrine for many centuries thereafter. Aquinas, also known as the "angelic doctor," incorporated his interpretation of the whole doctrine of Catholicism in *Summa Theologica*.

A resurgence in religious fervor demonstrated itself in reforms of the monasteries and priesthood, crusades against the heretics of the Near East, and an increase in pilgrimages to the Holy Land. Nursing was affected by these events because crowded living conditions and the resulting increase in the spread of disease created a need for the establishment of new and different types of orders to care for the sick. The redistribution of the population and urban growth brought nursing out of the institutions and back into the home. Those individuals who were drawn to nursing continued to be of high intellectual and social backgrounds. Great numbers of men became nurses, and the military ideal of discipline and order entered nursing. This era was rich in nursing saints, several of whom were widely acclaimed and highly honored.

Among the momentous forces and developments of this period that in one way or another influenced health practices generally and nursing in particular were the Crusades, the military nursing orders, the institution of chivalry, the guilds, the further development of hospitals and medicine, the decline of monasticism, the rise of the mendicant orders and the devastation of Europe by the great plague. None of these factors in what was a changing world can be considered in isolation from the rest.

— Frank, 1953, p. 96

Domenichino, *St. Cecilia Distributing Alms to the Poor,* c. 1615–1617. Fresco. *(San Luigi dei Francisi, Rome. SCALA/Art Resource, New York.)*

Guilds

According to many historians, references to guilds are thought to have first been made in England. Guilds were initially mentioned in the eighth century. In England they were primarily religious and played an important role in English social life as charitable institutions. These social organizations demonstrated a localized system of control that involved self-regulation by the members.

The earliest guilds were specifically religious and social in orientation, an attempt to balance the spiritual and temporal needs of the members. They were often named for a saint whose patronage they sought. Activities included the building of chapels, the founding of schools, and the presentation of mystery plays. Eventually hospitals were maintained and social insurance (distress assistance for sickness, poverty, and death) was provided through dues paid by the members. Other types of guilds also developed. These included the peace guilds for the maintenance of justice in the town and merchant guilds for the purpose of carrying on trade. Frequently the law of the guild became the law of the town, as exemplified in London in the tenth century.

The first associations of workers arose in the form of guilds and were extremely important in the late Middle Ages. These were usually known as craft guilds, which divided workers into three levels of vocational training: the *apprentice,* who remained under the direction of a master craftsman for three to ten years; the *journeymen* or *craftsmen,* who hired their services to another, and the *master craftsmen,* who were required to make an original contribution to the craft, pass an examination, and be economically stable in order to achieve this status. The craft guilds were the vocational training schools of the era. Under an apprenticeship method learners worked with an expert, were motivated to become masters, and recognized the value of their craft. These guilds were also the labor organizations of the day and as such protected and improved the status of the members. Wage scales and prices were fixed, hygienic working conditions were demanded, reasonable hours of labor were established, and quality in the work of the crafts was demanded.

Men in the same crafts and professions thus banded together to promote high standards. Ultimately physician guilds were established and fostered the separation of surgeons from medical practitioners. This was necessary because of the inclination to draw individuals together according to the similarity of their tools and materials rather than a consideration of their purposes. For example, surgeons' guilds admitted barbers who were able to perform such services as routine bleeding; physicians were joined with apothecaries and artists because of their common use of powders.

In general, the guild system provided an element of stability to the larger social order. It was a viable method of regulating economic life and providing for the discharge of personal responsibility to the community as a whole. It was a system whereby the consumer and the worker could be protected and a quality product could be ensured. In addition, the medieval apprenticeship system survived and affected the development of some types of workers throughout various periods in history. The apprenticeship form of nursing prevalent in the United States until the 1940s was probably influenced by the pattern of the craft guilds. This type of system did not foster a bona fide educational process; rather, it encouraged a strong aspect of service, which impeded the progression of nursing for many decades.

The Crusades

The Crusades have been identified as the "supreme folly of the Middle Ages" in one source (Nutting and Dock, 1937). This statement, however, is in direct opposition to the idea that throughout history people have regarded certain places, events, and objects as sacred and have journeyed long distances to revere them. From the fourth century, people had made pilgrimages to shrines and to the Holy Land. By the eleventh century, both the number and size of these pilgrimages had greatly increased, until some were made up of thousands of individuals. There are records of 6 pilgrimages in the eighth century, 12 in the ninth century, 16 in the tenth century, and 117 in the eleventh century.

Pilgrim travels to Palestine started soon after the Crucifixion. Initially these journeys were made by the inhabitants of the Holy Land itself but eventually included inhabitants of distant lands. By the late eleventh century, however, a series of military and political changes took place in the Middle East, and the Seljuk Turks, who had embraced Islam, captured Jerusalem. Mosques were erected in the Holy City of Jerusalem, and Christians who had been making pilgrimages there were persecuted. Therefore a united effort to stop the actions of the Turks was launched in the form of military expeditions known as *Crusades*. Hundreds of thousands of men answered the call of Pope Urban II to initiate this movement:

> Come forward to the defense of Christ. O ye who have carried on feuds, come to the war against the infidels. O ye who have been thieves, become soldiers. Fight a just war. Labor for everlasting reward, ye who were hirelings, serving for a few solidi.
>
> And more—whosoever shall offer himself to go upon this journey and shall make his vow to go, shall wear the sign of the cross on his head or breast.
>
> — *Lamb, 1930, pp. 39–41*

Each Crusader was identified as a soldier of Christ by a red cross on his head or breast. The first expedition of these crossbearers began in 1096.

Numerous Crusades occurred between 1096 and 1291. (The dates may vary somewhat according to the reference used.) They are generally divided into four major expeditions and four minor ones.

The major expeditions included the First Crusade (1096–1099), led by knights of France and the Normans; the Second Crusade (1147–1149), under the direction of the kings of France and Germany; the Third Crusade (1189–1192), led by the kings of France, England, and Germany; and the Fourth Crusade (1202–1204), led by French nobles and the doge of Venice.

The minor Crusades took place from 1216 to 1220, 1228 to 1229, 1248 to 1254, and 1270 to 1272. Jerusalem was captured during the First Crusade but was lost once again to the Turks in 1187. It was never regained by the Western world until the First World War.

Innumerable fanatical efforts also occurred, including the Peasants' Crusade and the Children's Crusade. The former resulted from the preaching of such men as Peter the Hermit and was the first stirring of the serfs against

The *Crac des Chevaliers,* a famous stronghold of the Hospitallers in the eleventh century. (*The Bettmann Archive, New York.*)

O. Cennl, *The Knights of Malta Entering Jerusalem,* 1908. Drawing. *(The Bettmann Archive, New York.)*

their lot. The latter was organized with the idea that Jerusalem would fall to a band of children so young as to be pure of heart. All the children, who were under twelve years of age, eventually fell ill or were captured and made slaves.

The Crusades were extensive expeditions to conquer the Holy Land, which had been in the hands of the Muhammadans for several centuries. Among the participants were members of the clergy, adventurers, pious individuals, and others who sought an opportunity to satisfy a variety of motives. The Crusades, indeed, represented many things to many people: aristocratic and military ideals in social life, political ambition, economic gain, the desire for adventure, and the extension of Christianity by means of war, a holy war.

These enterprises extended over a long period and increased the need for hospitals along the Crusader and pilgrim routes and in Syria and Palestine. An acute demand arose for hospitals and for providers of health care because of the effects of the war, which became more and more deadly as disease was carried wherever armies were sent.

> That the Crusades were turned back by epidemics much more effectively than they were by the armed power of the Saracens can hardly be questioned. The history of the Crusades reads like the chronicle of a series of diseases, with scurvy as potent as infections. In 1098, a Christian army of 300,000 men besieged Antioch. Disease and famine killed so many and in such a short time that the dead could not be buried. The cavalry were rendered useless within a few months by the death of 5000 of their 7000 horses. Nevertheless, the city was captured, after a nine months' siege. On the march to Jerusalem, the hosts were accompanied by an enemy more potent than the heathen. When Jerusalem was taken, in 1099, only 60,000 of the original 300,000 were left, and these, by 1101, had melted to 20,000.
>
> The story of the second Crusade, led by Louis VII of France, is sadly similar. Of half a million men, only a handful—most of them without horses—managed to get back to Antioch, and few returned to Europe.
>
> — *Zinsser, 1934, p. 155*

The response to these identified needs resulted in the development of military nursing orders, knighthood, additional hospitals, mendicant orders, and the rise of several great nursing saints. In addition, with the advent of the military order a harsher element entered nursing. Emphasis was now placed on rank, deference to superior officers, and the vow of unquestioning obedience. All of these would profoundly affect the progress of nursing and nursing education for many years.

Military Nursing Orders

The military nursing orders were an outcome of the Crusades to the Holy Land. They were a special type of nursing order that appeared in the military brotherhoods. These orders combined the attributes of religion and chivalry, as well as militarism and charity, in their dedicated services. The chronicles and histories of this period contain little information about how the knights cared for the sick and the wounded because the primary emphasis in these documents was on the military aspects of the pilgrimages. However, they do indicate that great hospitals were built and equipped and that knights nursed patients (Austin, 1957). So great was the influence of these orders on nursing that Nutting and Dock devoted an entire chapter of the *History of Nursing* to the origin and development of them. There is no doubt that the religious zeal that called forth groups of knights to care for the wounded and the sick was important to the organization and structure of European hospitals and to the pattern of nursing service that was established and standardized by them. The majority of what was written about these orders is good; the members were benevolent, brave, and charitable. Yet the accumulation of vast riches and large land holdings proved to be the eventual downfall of the orders. Soon after the Holy Wars ended, devotion to the calling of nursing diminished, works of mercy dwindled, and warfare against unbelievers became the sole focus. "The pride of riches and power, with the gradual abandonment of the humbler humanitarian duties for a spiritual dominance, had made the once peerless order of serving brothers a menace to the secular power" (Nutting and Dock, 1937, p. 206).

Great orders were formed, all called by the name *hospitallers*. The membership of these orders consisted of three classes—knights, priests, and serving brothers. The knights were men of patrician birth who bore arms, protected pilgrims, and fought in the Crusades. When they were not engaged in battle, they helped to nurse the sick. The priests attended to the religious duties in churches, camps, and hospitals. The serving brothers (*serjeus* or half-knights) were primarily responsible for weary travelers and the care of the sick. Three of these nursing orders stand out as being the most famous and the most important in history: the Knights Hospitallers of St. John of Jerusalem, the Teutonic Knights (der Deutsche Order), and the Knights of St. Lazarus. Both the Hospitallers and the Teutonic Knights formed women's orders that were subordinated to the men's communities, as was often the case. Frequent references are also made to the Knights Templars or Red Cross Knights, although this group was always purely military.

Knights Hospitallers of St. John of Jerusalem. Rich merchants of Amalfi, Italy, established two hospitals (one for each sex) in Jerusalem about 1050. These were placed under the protection of St. John the Almoner (neither the Evangelist nor the Baptist but a Cypriot) and St. Mary Magdalene. These hospitals originally tended any individual who was sick, including the pilgrims and the insane, but they became crowded with wounded and dying Crusaders during the siege of Antioch and the battle for Jerusalem. Many Crusaders of noble birth laid aside their arms to help with the work of tending the sick in the Hospital of St. John. Thus was born the order of the Knights Hospitallers of St. John of Jerusalem.

Fr. Alberto Arringhieri, *'In the Convent' a Knight of Rhodes. (The Bettmann Archive, New York.)*

From the fifteenth century painting by Pintoricchio in the Siena Cathedral.

Following pages, John Singleton Copley, *The Red Cross Knight,* 1793. Oil on canvas, approx. 213.4 × 273 cm. *(Gift of Mrs. Gordon Dexter. Copyright 1995 Board of Trustees, National Gallery of Art, Washington, D.C.)*

The first duty of knights, or men-at-arms, was to fight; those who were expected to serve in the hospital wards when not engaged in battle wore a white cross on their habits. Frequent references are also made to the Red Cross Knights (Knights Templars), although this group was always purely military.

Decaisne, *The Institution of the Hospitallers as a Military Order. (Museum and Library of the Order of St. John, London. By permission from the Musée Nationale du Château de Versailles.)*

The nuns of St. John of Jerusalem Order distinguished themselves as nurses in the Hospital of St. John of Jerusalem during the Crusades. *(The Bettmann Archive, New York.)*

Until 1099, when Godfrey was made King of Palestine, the order was secular and was directed by Peter Gerard, who was considered to be a pious and saintly man. Gerard developed a code of rules; major decisions were voted upon in adherence to a democratic constitution. A female branch of the order, the Hospitaller Dames of the Order of St. John of Jerusalem, served the Hospital of St. Mary Magdalene. The women met at first on terms of equality with the knights; both nursed, ate, and worshiped together. Eventually the men and women formed a religious fraternity and dedicated themselves as servants of the poor and of Christ to function under the rule of St. Augustine. Segregation became total, and the sisters were subordinated to the brothers. Solemn vows of poverty, chastity, and obedience were taken, and a black robe with a white linen (Maltese) cross embroidered on the left breast was donned. (Later the Knights of St. John were differentiated from other hospitallers by a white cross on a red background.) The order became extremely wealthy through gifts of grateful benefactors, which enabled the building of additional hospitals, hostels, and hospices. Rules were drawn up for hospital management, and they were followed by the best city hospitals or *Maisons-Dieu* of Europe for many centuries.

The career of this order was one of distinction in nursing until the expulsion of the Christians from Palestine. Nursing was gradually neglected as the Sisters of St. John disappeared temporarily and the men's order fled to Cyprus and then to the island of Rhodes, where they remained for approximately two hundred years. With the conquest of Rhodes by the Turks the care of the sick became a secondary objective. In 1522 the Knights were forced out of Rhodes and were without a headquarters until Emperor Charles V granted them the isles of Malta, Goza, and Tripolis in 1530. Finally the Knights were turned out of Malta by Napoleon in 1798. The name of the order changed

122

Knight Hospitallers, 1588. Engraving. From Verdala, *Statues of the Order of St. John.* *(Courtesy of the Museum and Library of the Order of St. John, London.)*

123

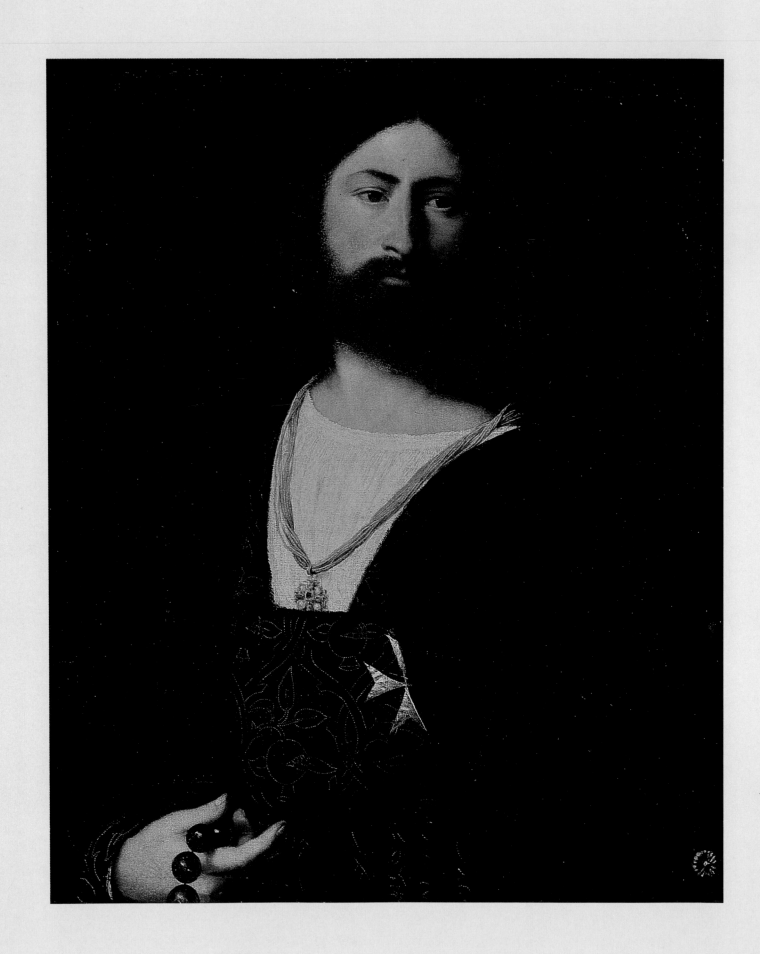

as its geographical location shifted. The members were successively known as the Knights of St. John of Jerusalem, the Knights of Rhodes, and the Knights of Malta. The significance of this organization in nursing history is great:

> First and foremost, the glamour shed on its activities by what we may call the "Crusading spirit" gave to it such a position that membership was sought after by the flower of knighthood of the day and the prestige thus received caused it to influence and stimulate all subsequent hospital organization.
>
> Secondly, as the Knights were always very rich they could equip and conduct their hospitals far better than any other community of that period.
>
> — *Seymer, 1932, p. 38*

The most important and the largest of the many hospitals of the order was established in 1575 at the seaport town of Valetta in Malta. In its early days this hospital was a model for all of Europe, but by the time of John Howard's

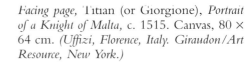

Facing page, Titian (or Giorgione), Portrait of a Knight of Malta, c. 1515. Canvas, 80 × 64 cm. (Uffizi, Florence, Italy. Giraudon/Art Resource, New York.)

The Knights of St. John of Jerusalem became known as the Knights of Malta when Emperor Charles V granted them the Isles of Malta, Gozo, and Tripolis in 1530. The Knights of Malta are famous as the only military order that cared for insane patients.

Great Ward of the Hospital of the Knights of St. John in Valetta, c. 1650. Engraving. Printed in Augsburg, Germany. (Courtesy of the Museum and Library of the Order of St. John, London.)

This illustration depicts knights attending the sick, who are in beds with mosquito curtains. In the foreground is a funeral ceremony.

visit in 1786 it had fallen into a deteriorated state. The hospital, which remains a magnificent monument of architecture, initially accommodated somewhat less than a thousand patients. A well-defined organizational structure provided for department heads, nursing, almsgiving, distribution of food to the poor, mending of clothing, and foundling care. Acute cases and cases of hemorrhage, lithotomy, and insanity were isolated. Visitors to the hospital frequently remarked about its cleanliness and expressed their surprise that the Knights actually attended the patients. Chaplains attended spiritual needs; paid physicians assisted knights in anatomy and the care of disease.

> A peculiar interest attaches itself to this institution because of the remarkable splendour of its equipment and service. They were unrivaled in their day, and indeed, with all the improvements in hospital service which modern progress has brought, we would find it hard to better some of these old regulations of 1533. In reading them over one is struck with the careful arrangements made for the division of labour, and the proper conduct of the work.
>
> — *Nutting and Dock, 1937, p. 196*

The Knights of St. John were finally suppressed but later continued their activities in a modified form. Branches were developed in several countries, including England and the United States. Continuing a semimilitary tradition, the Hospitallers functioned as units in Europe, supplying ambulance and other medical services during times of war. "But their original functions have been largely taken over and expanded during the last century by the International Red Cross" (Shryock, 1959, p. 109). The order lives in the St. John's guilds and ambulance corps and societies that provide first aid to the injured. The hospital buildings established by the Knights of St. John can still be seen on Rhodes and Malta.

The Maltese cross, once worn by the Knights of St. John, survived the Crusades period and became a part of the insignia of many groups caring for the sick. It was on the banner of the United States Cadet Nurse Corps and was worn on the shoulders of the nurse's uniform. The eight points of the cross signify the beatitudes that knights were expected to exemplify in the works of charity in their daily lives:

- Spiritual joy
- To live without malice
- To weep over thy sins
- To humble thyself to those who injure thee
- To love justice
- To be merciful
- To be sincere and pure of heart
- To suffer persecution

The Teutonic Knights. The German order of Knights Hospitallers formed in 1191 was called the Deutsche Orden, or Teutonic Knights. German pilgrims during the Third Crusade set up a temporary hospital beside the walls of the Acre, engaged religious knights for defense, and originated this group. The Teutonics followed the hospital rules of the Knights of St. John and the military structure of the Templars. The first members were from noble families. They took the usual vows of poverty, chastity, and obedience but added a fourth vow that required them to care for the sick and defend the faith. They, too, were divided into three classes—warriors, nurses, and spiritual brothers. The Teutonic Knights had from the very beginning both nursing and military duties. They were distinguished by a black habit over which was worn a white cloak with a black cross embroidered in gold on the shoulder.

A women's order was founded in Germany to specifically perform hospital work. The women were not, however, admitted to full membership and were called *consorores* (lay sisters). They took vows but lived outside the monastic precincts. Their nursing duties were perhaps regarded as menial,

The Monaco 1961 stamp was issued to honor the Sovereign Order of the Knights of Malta (Knights Hospitallers). The Knights Hospitallers traces its origin back to the eleventh century; the Knights of Malta, back to 1530. The hospital at Malta was the equal of any other in Europe. In 1926 an association was established in the United States devoted to the care of the sick and wounded. The stamp depicts a medieval town and a leper beneath the Maltese Cross. *(Courtesy of Howard B. Hurley.)*

since the Rule of 1280 says that women are to be admitted "because services to cattle and to sick persons in hospital are better performed by the female sex."

The Teutonic Knights became powerful in Germany, and many hospitals were given over into their hands. From different princes they received rich possessions in various countries, particularly in Sicily. According to reference material, their history is similar to that of the Knights of St. John but their nursing service was not as effective. By the fourteenth century they had fulfilled their destiny.

The Knights of St. Lazarus. According to some historians, the Knights of St. Lazarus were the oldest of all the orders of hospitallers. It is speculated that this order originated from the hospital built by St. Basil at Cesarea, which kept a separate house for lepers. Attempts have also been made to trace it back to the days of Christ's raising of Lazarus, the brother of Mary and Martha. Whatever the origins of this order, the fact remains that leprosy, which had always been a problem in society, became its special cause. Lepers had been excluded from society and confined to institutions called *lazarettos* in honor of the leper spoken of in the parable of the rich man. Those who were not confined to institutions were obliged to wear a distinctive dress and carry a wooden clapper to warn of their approach; they were isolated and considered to be incurables. At this time the term *leprosy* was also applied to syphilis and many chronic skin diseases.

The members of the Knights of St. Lazarus were not only knights who participated in the wars of the Crusades but also those who had been stricken with leprosy, which was endemic in the Near East. Initially the order was a purely nursing order, but by the thirteenth century it added armed combatants to membership. This action created two categories of knights, the warriors and the hospitallers, who were headed by a grand master of a noble family who was himself a leper. This rule was in effect until 1253, when permission was given by Pope Innocent IV to elect a nonleper to this office. With the addition of the warring aspect, care of the lepers became secondary and the order became purely military. Decay and deterioration set in until Pope Innocent VIII suppressed it in the fifteenth century. The order ceased to exist by 1830.

Details of the work of the order is obscure. There is little information regarding what real service was rendered to the sick poor or to the lepers. After the Crusades, however, the incidence of leprosy began to decrease and the need for the special work of the order diminished. As with the other hospitallers, the Knights of St. Lazarus received lavish gifts and rich possessions. According to Nutting and Dock (1937), there were also sisters of the order. Yet few sources mention the existence of a female branch.

The first Knights of St. Lazarus varied both their habit and their cross in different countries. The color of the original cross is unknown, but its form was distinguished by four arms of equal length, somewhat flared at the ends. The French cross was an eight-armed golden and green or purple-red cross with tiny golden lilies in the corners. The Italian cross was white and green. The emblem of the order of St. Lazarus was adopted by the German Nurses' Association.

Rise of Mendicant Orders

Social groupings for nursing and neighborhood work occurred with the rapid spread of sickness and disease and the fear associated with the plagues. Religious fervor escalated and led to the development of types of care different from that required when monasteries were the focal points of the communities. Emphasis began to be placed upon the great reward that could be achieved through total withdrawal from the world. Religious missionary

A German Templar Knight. (The Bettmann Archive, New York.)

The Knights of St. Lazarus were prominent in hospital work during the Middle Ages. (The Bettmann Archive, New York.)

bodies thus arose and pledged themselves to literal poverty. These groups exemplified the democratic and secular tendencies that developed along with the military orders. Extension of Christianity, however, in this case would transpire through peaceful means. Many devout individuals took part in this movement.

Success in this endeavor meant taking religion and nursing out among the people. The mendicant orders were founded to accomplish this goal. The members lived as part of the world, owned no property, gave their possessions to the poor, and followed the teachings of Christ. They depended on begging for sustenance, a practice that earned them the name of *mendicants.* The personification of this approach was St. Francis of Assisi (1182–1226), who instituted three religious orders. The first order, Friars Minor (Little Brothers), was for friars; the second, called Poor Clares, was for nuns; the third order, Tertiaries, was for lay men and women who wished to continue to lead secular lives. (St. Dominic also founded three orders and patterned them after these.) The members lived outside the monastery walls and were guided by an order or rule. Care of the sick as well as the poor, the needy, and the outcast became a primary duty. The Franciscans, the Dominicans, the Carmelites, and the Oblates of St. Benedict became the most famous of these third orders.

St. Francis of Assisi.   St. Francis became one of the best-known and best-loved saints in history. Born to a life of wealth and ease as the son of a cloth merchant in Assisi, he spent his youth as an exuberant, carefree cavalier. His style of living changed after Francis suffered from a serious illness in his early twenties. Even before the illness, however, he looked with aversion upon the miseries that were prevalent in the society and was particularly affected by the plight of the lepers. A variety of circumstances, particularly his giving of great amounts of alms to the poor, led to Francis's being disinherited by his father. Rejected by his family, Francis set out alone, barefooted and clothed with a rough brown tunic tied at the waist with a heavy white rope, to travel the countryside. Appalled by the sufferings of the poor and the sick, he devoted his life to their ministrations. Most important, he provided a necessary example of consideration of human beings as individuals:

> What distinguishes this very genuine democrat from any mere demagogue is that he never either deceived or was deceived by the illusion of mass-suggestion. . . . To him a man was always a man and did not disappear in a dense crowd any more than in a desert. He honored all men; that is, he not only loved but respected them all. What gave him his extraordinary personal power was this; that from the Pope to the beggar, from the sultan of Syria in his pavillion to the ragged robbers crawling out of the wood, there was never a man who looked into those brown burning eyes without being certain that Francis Bernardone was really interested in *him;* in his own inner life from the cradle to the grave; that he himself was being valued and taken seriously, and not merely added to the spoils of some social policy or the names in some clerical document.
>
> — *Chesterton, 1924, pp. 141–142*

St. Francis became known for his great compassion and capacity for love. He became the champion of lepers and urged his followers to go to leper hospitals. He frequently visited the leper houses where the lepers were always waiting for him, knowing that he brought not only alms but also love. Initially St. Francis became the jest of the town because the people could not understand his close association with the lepers. Adults and children flung mud at him and shouted "Pazzo! Pazzo!" According to Robinson (1946), the pale, gaunt appearance and cadaverous face with the burning eyes probably did make him look like a madman. Francis's work for these sufferers eventually influenced and inspired others to improve their conditions.

Slowly, disciples began to gather around and follow Francis of Assisi. When they numbered twelve, they went to Rome to seek permission of Pope

Innocent III to preach and follow an ascetic life. With papal sanction the Franciscans, or the Order of Friars Minor (Brothers Minor), grew rapidly. The habit of the Franciscans was the same rough tunic with rope girdle that St. Francis himself had worn. The shade of the garment might be brownish or grayish, and the wearers were called Gray Friars. Poverty and humility were emphasized in the Franciscan order; begging was done for the members themselves and for the poor.

St. Francis ultimately became a victim of a barbaric medical practice. His vision began to fail and it was believed that he would become blind. His eyes were cauterized with a red-hot iron, a treatment conducted without the benefit of any type of medicine or herbs that would allay or prevent discomfort. He died in 1226, aware that his order was departing from his original concept of complete poverty and simplicity. Leadership passed into other hands and a new rule was established. The structure of the order became more elaborate and properties were acquired. Some of the brothers had even established themselves in universities before the death of St. Francis, despite his great opposition to scholarship. Both Francis and Clare were canonized, and the bodies of these two saints repose in their native Assisi. The feast of St. Francis of Assisi is kept on October 4. His prayer has guided numerous individuals in contemporary society as it guided him:

> Lord, make me an instrument of your peace.
> Where there is hatred, let me sow love.
> Where there is injury, pardon.
> Where there is doubt, faith.
> Where there is despair, hope.
> Where there is darkness, light.
> Where there is sadness, joy.
> O Divine Master, grant that I may not so much seek
> To be consoled as to console,
> To be understood as to understand,
> To be loved as to love,
> For it is in giving that we receive,
> It is in pardoning that we are pardoned,
> It is in dying that we are born to eternal life.

While the Franciscans were achieving success, St. Dominic (1170–1221) established the Order of Preachers, the Dominicans. A member of a noble family of Guzman of the village of Castile, Dominic had given up his plan of becoming a monk in a monastery in order to have closer contact with the rich and the poor who needed spiritual assistance. He set forth to restore to the Church those who had fallen away and to convert others. Both men and women gathered about him, and this led to the development of the Dominicans. The followers were sent abroad as traveling preachers in an effort to make Christianity the one religion. The order practiced both individual and corporate poverty. The Dominican robe was made of white wool and topped by a black cape with a hood. The hood could be pulled over the head for warmth. This cape led to the title of Black Friars.

Eminent scholars arose from the Franciscans and the Dominicans. Many of them taught at great universities such as Padua, Cologne, Vienna, Prague, and Paris. Among them were the Dominican Albertus Magnus; the Franciscan Roger Bacon, who stressed the value of observation, experimentation, and inductive reasoning, which assisted with the development of experimental science; and the Dominican St. Thomas Aquinas, who studied under the Benedictines at Monte Cassino and completed the *Summa Theologica,* his greatest work.

St. Clare of Assisi. The life of St. Clare of Assisi (1194–1253) was closely interwoven with that of St. Francis. Clare, a beautiful daughter of a knightly family of the Sciffi, at the age of sixteen heard St. Francis preach in

Lippo Vanni, *Madonna and Child With Donors St. Dominic and St. Elizabeth of Hungary,* late fourteenth century. Tempera-agesso on panel, 171.5 × 201 cm. *(Samuel H. Kress Collection. The Lowe Art Museum, University of Miami, Coral Gables, Florida.)*

the churches of Assisi. She became convinced that his way of life, extreme poverty, was what the Lord wished for her. She believed that the adoption of this type of life would provide her with contentment, peace, and joy. Clare remained in the household of her father until the age of eighteen, then ran away to the chapel of the Franciscans where she exchanged her expensive dress and jewels for a rough woolen robe. Francis cut off her long hair and received her vows of poverty, chastity, and obedience. Clare lived in a Bene-dictine convent for a brief period until a special convent was established for her. Other women who wished to share this simple life joined her. Thus began the second order of St. Francis, more commonly referred to as the order of Poor Clares (Clarisses), with Clare as its abbess. A short time later Clare was followed by her younger sister Agnes.

It is said that the Poor Clares cared principally for lepers, whom they housed in small mud and wattle huts around their convent in San Damiano. Accounts vary, however, about the actual services they provided. One author (Austin, 1957) suggests: "It would probably be a mistake to ascribe to the Poor Ladies any widespread activity in the care of the sick. Their chief pre-occupation seems to have been with the contemplative life" (p. 67). Austin adds that "the Rule of 1253 indicates that the Poor Clares cared for their own members, but whether their care extended to the surrounding community is uncertain" (p. 69). Other authors (Jamieson and Sewall, 1950; Nutting and Dock, 1937; Robinson, 1946; Shryock, 1959) discuss the nursing activities of this order of Franciscan nuns.

Bartolomé Esteban Murillo, *St. Elizabeth Bathing People Afflicted With Ringworm,* c. 1670–1674. Canvas. *(Hospital de la Caridad, Sevilla, Spain.)*

St. Elizabeth, along with many healing saints, is portrayed in fifteenth and sixteenth century art. However, in contrast to the other saints, she is shown performing some of the Seven Works of Mercy—visiting or nursing the sick, giving bread to the hungry, and giving her jewels to the poor.

Clare outlived St. Francis by more than twenty-five years. After her death the order experienced many changes. It has been known at different times and in different countries by a variety of names: Order of Poor Ladies, Clarisses, Minoresses, and Poor Clares. It eventually became a strictly cloistered order whose members functioned under the most austere conditions. Professed sisters living under rule did not go outside their walls; nor were they in contact with the outside world until after the Protestant Revolt. Since its original founding, the Poor Clares, and numerous sisterhoods that have adopted Franciscan rule, have founded many hospitals and other institutions for the sick.

Tertiaries: Third Orders of St. Francis and St. Dominic. The Tertiaries, or Third Orders, were founded for the laity of both sexes who wished to continue their ordinary lives in the world. They were to practice charity and devotion to God in a manner similar to that of the religious orders. Several communities of tertiaries lived almost the same life as the religious without being cloistered. These orders attracted thousands of people of all classes and were a powerful force for a number of years. Some were later formed into communities (convents arose in different countries) that often undertook nursing as their main work. The idea became so popular that many tertiary orders emerged, and this prompted Gregory at the Council of Lyons (1272) to reduce them to four: the Dominicans, Franciscans, Carmelites, and Augustinians.

The Third Order epitomized the ideals of St. Francis. It represented a revival of the early Christian spirit. Religion was carried into everyday life, and unselfish and useful service was rendered to humanity. Many famous nursing saints were enrolled in this order of St. Francis: Elizabeth of Hungary (1207–1231), Louis of France (1214–1270), Elizabeth of Portugal (1271–1336), Isabelle of France, Anne of Bohemia, and Bridget of Sweden (Tuker and Malleson, 1900).

St. Elizabeth of Hungary was probably the most renowned among the women tertiaries of St. Francis. Her virtues have been set forth in prose, poetry, art, and music. Elizabeth, the daughter of the Hungarian king Andreas II, was married at the age of fourteen to Ludwig of Thuringia. She became the mother of four children. With her husband's support she built hospitals in Thuringia and humbly ministered to the sick with her own hands. Daily she distributed alms to the poor, fed the hungry, nursed the lepers, and bathed newborns and comforted their mothers with special tenderness. Hers was a life of extreme piety, asceticism, and austerity. Elizabeth was the heroine of beautiful tales, which were accepted as either fact or fiction. The story of the miraculous roses is perhaps the most well known. It is said that one winter day while Elizabeth was carrying a basket of food to the poor she met Ludwig. (In some accounts it is her father-in-law whom she met.) Irritated by complaints against Elizabeth by his family, Ludwig demanded to see what she was carrying. When she opened her cloak, Ludwig saw an armful of blooming white and red roses.

Upon Ludwig's death during the Crusades, Elizabeth was driven from her husband's castle, the Wartburg, by her in-laws. She became a member of the Third Order of St. Francis and built the Franciscan hospital at Marburg, where she spent the remaining years of her short life nursing the sick. Elizabeth was considered to be an excellent organizer, administrator, and nurse. Her conception of social service carried a modern ring, since her service to the needy "was tempered with discretion; and instead of encouraging idleness such as were able to work, she employed them in a way suitable to their strength and capacity" (Butler, 1934, vol. 10, p. 43). Always frail, Elizabeth died at the age of twenty-four. Considered the patron saint of nursing, she is honored on November 19. Elizabeth is regarded by some as the forerunner of the visiting and public health nurses of the twentieth century. The Gray Nuns of the thirteenth century, who were also Tertiaries of St. Francis, were often called Sisters of St. Elizabeth, since they had chosen her as their patron saint.

This stamp is one of Hungary's 1932 set of four stamps commemorating the seven hundredth anniversary of the death of St. Elizabeth (1207–1231). During the famine of 1226, Elizabeth organized food distribution and devoted her life and strength to helping the sick and poor. She had hospitals built where she cared for lepers and comforted prisoners. When her husband of six years died, she moved to Marburg and spent the rest of her young life nursing the sick. She died at twenty-four years of age. *(Courtesy of Howard B. Hurley.)*

Interior of St. Elizabeth's Church looking east to the choir and altar, c. 1233–1283. *(Foto Marburg, Art Resource, New York.)*

St. Louis IX was another saint whose endeavors with lepers was well known. His special care of their needs was recognized and respected by his subjects, who mourned his death during one of the Crusades. France flourished under Louis's rule and experienced peace and prosperity. Louis personally tended to the sick and devoted his life to humane treatment for all individuals. He was interested in education, particularly for health care workers, and attempted to assist with its provision. His efforts resulted in the establishment of the Saint-Chapelle in Paris and the Sorbonne College of the University of Paris. Louis belonged to the Franciscan Tertiaries.

The Third Order of St. Dominic was originally formed to recover Church property. The Tertiaries, however, performed other services and assisted the poor and the ill as regular functions of their religious duty. They were patterned after the Third Order of St. Francis. There are at least hints that some competition existed between the two groups. Robinson presents an interesting account of this rivalry:

> Dominic was the imitator, Francis always the originator; and the story of Dominic lacked the emotional fire of the Francis legend. Moreover, the Franciscans had the inestimable advantage that only upon the body of their founder had been miraculously inflicted the Five Wounds which Christ received at his crucifixion: after the death of Francis, Clara saw the wounds in his feet, but could not

extract the nails which had been driven through them. In the contemporary rivalry between the Franciscans and the Dominicans, Catherine came to the rescue of the latter: Christ put a ring on her finger as proof that she was to be his heavenly spouse; and, as she knelt in a church in Pisa, she received the crowning glory of the wounds of the Lord. . . . The Franciscans coldly denied, while the Dominicans fervently accepted, the stigmatization of St. Catherine.

— Robinson, 1946, pp. 46–47

The first members of the Third Order of St. Dominic were known as the Mantellate. They wore the Dominican habit—a white tunic bound by a leather belt, a white veil, and a black cloak (mantella). Margaret of Metola (1287–1320) was the first young woman to join the Mantellate. She was the daughter of wealthy parents who abandoned her because she was blind and deformed. Margaret gave her life to the needs of others. She had a special affinity for prisoners and visited them daily, giving them food, clothing, medicines, and bedding. Other remarkable personalities joined the Dominican Tertiaries.

St. Catherine of Siena (1347–1380), a favorite subject of painters, is often portrayed in the act of expelling demons or in an ecstatic state with a lily, thorn, or book. She is also frequently pictured carrying a lighted lamp, which

Hans Memling, *Altarpiece of St. John the Baptist and St. John the Evangelist*, (The Mystic Marriage of St. Catherine), 1479. Approx. 172.5 × 172.5 cm. *(Memlingmuseum, Brugge.)*

she carried on her nightly visits to La Scala hospital. (Her lamp was as famous as the Nightingale lamp of later years.) Catherine Benincasca was the daughter of a wealthy merchant and the last of twenty-five children. Her twin died at birth. At the age of seven, Catherine devoted herself to Christ. She became a member of the Third Order of St. Dominic at eighteen. The literature identifies Catherine as a hospital and visiting nurse, social welfare worker, reformer of society and of the Church, peacemaker, stateswoman, and great mystic.

When the Black Death (bubonic plague) swept over Siena, Catherine personally cared for the victims. For more than a year she rarely went home but spent her nights and days in the La Scala wards tending to the afflicted. Although there was little that could be done for the victims of the plague, she exhibited her willingness to comfort them. She organized groups of young men as stretcher bearers to transport the stricken from all over the city to wards of the hospital, which she supervised. Catherine's prominence, however, lies in her influence in the political affairs of the day. She never hesitated to speak out to the highest and mightiest in the land and had some part in persuading the Pope to end the Babylonian Captivity and to return to Rome from Avignon. Catherine attempted to start another Crusade to rescue Jerusalem from the Muslims. She was also instrumental in healing breaches between members of prominent families in Genoa.

Secular Nursing Orders

At the same time that the military knights and the first, second, and third orders were developing, groups of workers banded together in semireligious orders. These orders were not bound by vows to monastic life and have been referred to as *secular nursing orders*. They made many contributions to nursing and served the sick, the poor, foundlings, and orphans in their own communities. At times they also did hospital nursing. The development of these orders marks a significant step in the secularization of nursing. Their success was in part a result of their "freedom" in the community.

Another order of men in this period was the Antonines (Hospital Brothers of St. Anthony), founded about 1095 and issued a rule in 1218. Houses were established in France, Spain, and Italy. The members devoted themselves to sufferers of "St. Anthony's Fire," which was probably the condition of ergotism. This disease was caused by a fungus growth on rye, which was a staple grain of the Middle Ages. Hospitals were developed for the victims of this disease, who were lovingly cared for by the brothers. The hallucinatory manifestations of ergotism have been vividly described in the literature. An interesting account of an outbreak of ergotism in 1951 in Pont Saint-Esprit in France is described by Fuller (1968) in his book *The Day of St. Anthony's Fire*. Eventually this order also cared for victims of other diseases. They were also in charge of the papal household until their suppression in the eighteenth century.

The origin of the Beguine movement is uncertain, and the derivation of its name is obscure. It is usually credited to a priest of Liège, Lambert le Begue, who encouraged the settlement of *Mulieres Sanctae* around his church—among them the daughters of barons, knights, and nobles—in what has come to be regarded as the first beguinage. The Mulieres Sanctae were individual women who identified themselves with a monastery by donating a part of their substance (if they were rich) or voluntary service (if they were poor). They took no vows and lived in their own homes. Eventually these women gathered together into a communal life. They took vows of chastity and obedience for the time they were in residence but did not give up rights to property or possessions. They were free to marry and leave at any time. The Beguines of Flanders were one of the most prominent secular nursing orders. Later, many of these communities became Tertiaries of St. Francis or St. Dominic.

The organization was extremely simple. Two to four women lived together in small houses built in an enclosed precinct and grouped around a church or hospital. Such beguinages were picturesque in their simplicity. Those at Bruges (c. 1184) and Ghent (c. 1234) in Belgium are well known. Each community was self-contained and fixed its own rules, which were approved by the bishop of the diocese. Because there was great diversity in the Beguines, it is difficult to render an adequate description of their work. Their original objective seems to have been religious; they strived for perfection and reform of the Church and the saving of souls. Members ranged from the rich to the poor, the noble to the humble, and their work varied. Their dress varied according to location.

The Beguines supported themselves by teaching, spinning cloth, and other handicrafts, and care of the sick in hospitals. They started a visiting nursing service in the neighborhood homes, and fees were charged if the families were able to pay. Hospital work became one of their chief interests and led to the erection of their own hospitals, where they nursed. One of the most famous is the Hôtel Dieu at Beaune, France, which was founded in 1443. These hospitals were also staffed by the Sisters of Matilda, an order established specifically for this purpose by the Beguines. During wars, famines, and epidemics, members of the order converted their cottages into hospitals; they also served as nurses on battlefields.

The Beguines were always popular with the people, but they met with resistance and suffered a certain amount of persecution from ecclesiastical authorities. Clerics could not tolerate their independence and striking innovations in community life. The Beguines were accused of heresy and in 1215 were forbidden by the Pope to found any more such groups. Despite several periods of persecution, they flourished and expanded. By the end of the thirteenth century there were few communities without a beguinage, and the order had spread to neighboring countries. It is estimated that there were 200,000 Beguines by that time. Gradually a decrease in numbers and size of these organizations occurred for various reasons. The Beguines retain a corporate existence in Belgium today. According to one source, they constitute

> as historically interesting a community of women as can anywhere be found. The freedom and independence of their original mode of existence, their self-supporting character, the irreproachable dignity and quiet, simple usefulness of their lives, continue unchanged. They have passed through vicissitudes and perils, but always safely.
>
> — *Nutting and Dock, 1937, p. 271*

Other groups of women appeared somewhat later. The Sisterhood of the Common Life gathered about Gerhard Groot, who was an idealist and leader of thought. The sisters, like the Beguines, took no binding vows but held no private property. They lived together in a conventional manner and were preeminently visiting nurses in the cities along the Rhine. Their habit was a simple gray dress, and they were self-supporting. The order of men, the Brothers of the Common Life, was also founded by Groot. The brothers devoted themselves to the sick poor and taught children who were bedridden. They became known as the schoolmasters of the time. Thomas à Kempis lived and studied with this community.

Another interesting confraternity was the brotherhood of Misericordia, which was started about 1244 in Florence. Founded primarily as a volunteer ambulance society, it was composed of a group of religious laymen. The members functioned in many Italian cities and became known as the "Masked Brotherhood." This name arose from the members' belief that their contributions would gain spiritual reward only if they prevented themselves from being recognized by others.

The order of the Alexian Brothers was formed in 1348 to assist with the care of the victims of the bubonic plague in the Netherlands. This group of laymen also undertook the burial of the dead. St. Alexius, a fifth-century Roman who nursed the sick in a hospital at Edessa, was chosen as their patron saint. This occurred in 1469, when the group organized under Augustinian rule. The sick continue to be cared for by this order. Several large general hospitals for men and boys, a rest home, and a home for elderly men are supported and serviced by its members. The Alexian Brothers also staff Memorial Hospital and Clinic at Boys Town, Nebraska. At one time the Alexian Brothers' Hospital School of Nursing in Chicago was the largest male nursing school in the United States.

Map of the roads to foreign historic hospitals. (*Redrawn from National League of Nursing Education calendar, 1929.*)

Growth of Hospitals

During the late Middle Ages Pope Innocent III encouraged the development of hospitals in European cities. Church executives or influential citizens who visited with him were invited to study the model Santo Spirito Hospital and were encouraged to organize similar institutions in their own communities. This idea of city hospitals was met with support and approval, and in some cases hospitals passed amicably from ecclesiastical to secular control. The number of hospitals rapidly escalated, and the size of the institutions varied greatly. Several factors contributed to the demand for more hospitals: existing hospitals had been organized as orphanages, hospices for travelers and the sick, and almshouses; communicable disease was uncontrolled; urban life had been hastily developed; and crowded living conditions were contributing to the spread of disease.

In general, the hospitals were erected to care for the sick poor. The wards were large; privacy was frequently provided by the use of cubicles. The structures were usually beautiful, having been constructed at a time when every public building was to be a work of art. The larger ones were similar in architectural form to the churches of the period.

> Indeed, the appearance of a main hall or ward would have suggested an ecclesiastical interior to a modern observer. Straw pallets were replaced by wooden beds, and curtains or partitions supplied some privacy. Linen and woolen supplies became more ample, and a large place would have its own farms to provide food and its own wind or water mills to prepare "corn" (wheat) for the patients. Although the buildings were still cold and dark by modern standards, they were a great improvement over the bare and humble dwellings of the "dark ages."
>
> — *Shryock, 1959, pp. 109–110*

Management and hygienic practices varied from hospital to hospital; they were sometimes good and sometimes bad. The hospitals, which were usually well endowed, were built on carefully chosen sites. Medieval hospitals were a place to keep, not cure, the patients. The aspect of cure evolved slowly and did not become widespread until the late nineteenth century. Nursing care, which was largely custodial, was provided twenty-four hours a day, primarily by monks and nuns, although servants were used part of the time. It is difficult, however, to determine where the division of labor actually occurred. As centuries passed, there were not always enough nurses. Other changes began to occur: the sickbed began to hold more than one patient; patients were sometimes not only dirty but ill fed; and the practice of using individuals of low character to augment inadequate nursing staffs became more common. At least a hint of a decline in nursing was present, a decline that would ultimately occur and persist for a long, dreadful time.

A custom of this period was to display paintings in the hospitals as diversional therapy for patients. St. John's Hospital at Bruges in Belgium offers an example of this practice. Established in 1118 by Augustinian monks and nuns as a hospice for travelers, its older buildings are preserved as a museum. Six paintings by the Flemish master Hans Memling are in this hospital.

The first English hospital was doubtless that at York, built by Athelstane about 936. It was also a poorhouse and had a ward for lepers. St. Giles' Hospital was built by Queen Matilda in 1101 for the care of forty lepers. The queen was also instrumental in the building of the Hospital of St. Katherine in London in 1148. Women of noble birth did the nursing in these hospitals, they did district nursing in the homes of the poor. The charter of these hospitals incorporated both types of nursing service.

Following pages, Pontormo, *Hospital of Saint Mathew,* early sixteenth century. *(Accademia, Florence, Italy. SCALA/Art Resource, New York.)*

Pontormo illustrates women nursing the sick—females only—as the focus of the painting. He has given some of the women halos.

Rahere Ward, 1832. From a contemporary drawing by a patient. *(St. Bartholomew's Hospital, London.)*

Facing page, Designed by Reynolds, Francis, and Rohnstock, "St. Thomas London," c. 1938. Stained glass. Panel from *The Nightingale Window,* Washington Cathedral, Washington, D.C. *(Courtesy of Morton Broffman.)*

Florence Nightingale is shown laying the cornerstone of the hospital building.

St. Bartholomew's Hospital probably has the longest continuous record of service of any hospital in the British Empire. It was founded in 1123 by Rahere, who rose to fame as a jester to Henry I and then joined the Augustinian monks. Rahere became a convert after a pilgrimage to Rome, where he became critically ill. He promised to build a church and hospital in honor of St. Bartholomew if he recovered and reached England safely. During the Reformation the hospital was seized by Henry VIII. The pleas of the lord mayor and citizens of London resulted in a new charter for it to become a hospital once again. Originally a poorhouse and orphanage, St. Bartholomew's was exclusively a hospital by the thirteenth century.

St. Thomas's Hospital was founded in 1213 by Richard, Prior of Bermondsey. This institution was made famous in the nineteenth century, when the first school of nursing was established there by Florence Nightingale. Because of its strategic location in a densely populated area of London on the main route to Rome and other cities, St. Thomas's became a hospital for the sick, a refuge for the poor, and a hospice for travelers and pilgrims. Lepers were not admitted but were sent to the nearby Lock Hospital. (St. Thomas's Hospital paid their bill.) There was a "foule" ward for contagious diseases and a men's and a women's ward; children were also admitted. In addition, there was a lying-in ward for unmarried women, which had been donated by the famous Richard Whittington.

Bethlehem Hospital was the first English institution for the mentally ill. It was founded in 1247 by Simon FitzMary, sheriff of London, as a priory. Originally a hospice of St. Mary of Bethlehem, it was designated a hospital about 1330. During the fourteenth century it was mentioned as a lunatic asylum that rapidly became infamous for the brutal treatment of its inmates. It has been said that once patients responded to treatment they were sent out into the streets to beg for a living. They wore metal armbands to identify themselves as mental patients and were called "Tom o'Bedlams." Violent patients were chained in cells, and they became one of the tourist attractions of London in the eighteenth century. Admission fees provided a source of revenue for the hospital. The name of the hospital was gradually contracted into "Bedlam." This word is used today to describe a place where fools chatter.

Ospedale Santa Maria degli Innocenti was built in 1451 as a foundling asylum for abandoned children. Such children either died or became the property of the person who found them. Many times the children were picked up and sold for money, and they were constantly at the mercy of the

ST THOMAS LONDON

slave traders. This Hospital of the Innocents in Florence was built with funds from a guild of silk merchants. The structure designed by Brunelleschi embodied beautiful architecture. It was adorned with the famous medallions of Andrea della Robbia (1435–1525), a nephew of Luca della Robbia. Luca had created a kind of glaze combined with clay that became known as "Robbia Ware." He produced artworks of enameled terra-cotta for which the della Robbias became famous. Andrea designed the infant figures to fit in the arches of the long arcade of the hospital building. A type of foster-parent plan was initiated by the institution, in which the parents promised to treat the orphans as their own children. Either the hospital or the foster parents taught the children a trade.

William Hogarth, "The Rake In Bedlam," c. 1735. From the series entitled *The Rake's Progress*. (Copyright The British Museum, London.)

Filippo Brunelleschi, Ospedale degli Innocenti. Begun 1419, completed mid-fifteenth century. Piazza della SS. Annuziata in Florence. *(Fratelli Alinari, Florence, Italy.)*

Andrea della Robbia's terracotta tondos from the facade of Filippo Brunelleschi's Ospedale degli Innocenti in Florence. *(Fratelli Alinari, Florence, Italy.)*

Medicine in the Late Middle Ages

As hospitals were built in the cities of Europe, the universities with their medical schools were also developing. The revival of a lay medical profession brought physicians into the hospitals during the later medieval period. The most reputable physicians were those who had attended universities and had received the degree of doctor of medicine. The beginning of a connection between physicians and hospitals occurred as physicians were called into the institution to see or follow a patient. The physician might even be paid a retainer fee if summoned on a regular basis.

> Medicine saw its darkest days in the early medieval period. During the later medieval period, two currents may be seen in medical practice. A vain speculation with little or no concern for obvious facts and search for truth is quite apparent; on the other hand, the foundation for scientific medicine was being laid through the rediscovery and translation of the old masters and through more frequent use of dissection of human bodies to study human anatomy and disease processes in human tissues. Prior to this time, the teaching of anatomy was based almost entirely on Galen. Most of Galen's observations were derived from animal dissections.
>
> — *Frank, 1953, pp. 109–110*

There continued to be an enormous amount of faulty knowledge and superstition during this time. Undoubtedly the majority of it had been passed down from the ancient world and from tribal ancestors.

> Apothecaries prescribed such ridiculous remedies as crocodile dung or cheaper substitutes for the common people who could not afford such an exotic cure. Even the great surgeon, Pare, considered powdered mummy and unicorn's horn as a valuable remedy. In early modern times the potato was used as a medication before it was accepted as a staple food, coffee and tea were thought to prevent acidosis. . . .
>
> — *Sellew and Nuesse, 1946, p. 113*

The use of astrology and alchemy were accepted practices; physicians consulted the horoscopes of their patients as well as medical books to determine treatments. Humoral therapy was still trusted. The astrological signs were used to determine when to take medicine or when to be bled, since the humors were supposedly controlled by the planets. Various other techniques were developed and put into practice by physicians in this period. They included the use of extraordinary medicines such as the horn of the unicorn, a narcotic inhalation for anesthesia, the use of spices for drugs and leeches for bloodletting, and the examination of urine.

St. Hildegarde (1098?–1179), the "Sybil of the Rhine," was a leading medical authority during this time. She was born at Bockelheim of noble, wealthy, and religious parents. At the age of eight, she was sent to be educated at the Benedictine cloister at Disibodenberg. Hildegarde entered this monastery and eventually became its abbess at the age of thirty. She established another Benedictine cloister near Bingen on the Rhine.

During her life of eighty-one years, Hildegarde accomplished many things. Considered to be one of the greatest women of the twelfth century, she was a mystic, poet, prophetess, musician and composer, artist, and physician. She ascribed her extraordinary intellectual powers to a kind of revelation granted to her frequently in a trancelike state. In fact, her writings are among the earliest important mystic works of the Middle Ages. Hildegarde foretold such things as the downfall of the German Empire, the approach of the Reformation, and the disasters of the papacy (Nutting and Dock, 1937). She consistently communicated with kings and princes. Pilgrims frequently sought her advice and counsel; invalids came to her to be cured.

Hildegarde's knowledge embraced medical science, nursing, music, herb gardening, natural science, and spiritual and religious philosophy. She was a prolific writer on many subjects, including theology and physiology. Her greatest achievement, however, was her knowledge of medicine. Hildegarde was more conspicuous as a physician than as a nurse, although she combined the arts of both in her work. (No account of nursing work as such or mention of the care of the sick, however, is found in her biographies.) Whether she actually practiced medicine or nursing is unknown, yet her vast knowledge is certain (Eckenstein, 1896). Hildegarde wrote two medical books between 1151 and 1159, when she was nearly sixty years of age. One of these, *Liber Simplicis Medicinae,* which contained nine books, was edited in the sixteenth century under the title *Physica St. Hildegardis.* The other, *Liber Compositae Medicinae,* contained five books that dealt with the causes, symptoms, and cure of disease. Normal and abnormal psychology were also discussed. Hildegarde referred to anxieties, obsessions, idiocy, phobias, and mental illness and stated: "When headache, vapours, and giddiness attack a patient simultaneously they make him foolish and upset his reason. This makes many people think that he is possessed by an evil spirit, but that is not true" (Butler, vol. 9, 1934, p. 234). Another important work by Hildegarde was *Liber Operum Simplicis Hominis,* which was concerned with anatomical and physiological subjects. The range of subjects contained in these works is amazing. Hildegarde foretold autoinfection, recognized the brain as the regulator of all the vital processes, understood the influence of the nervous system, and discussed the vibration and pulsation of blood in the veins. Her mental distinction gave her a natural supremacy over her contemporaries.

Obstetrics. The care of the pregnant woman and the infant has always been a sensitive index of social progress. Contrary to popular opinion, childbearing has become more difficult as civilization has advanced. This has been particularly true among city populations. The simple outdoor life of primitive women and wives of serfs on feudal manors was substituted in the city by monotonous work that taxed one part of the body. In addition, city life was unhygienic in many ways. In those countries where rickets prevailed, a woman's pelvis was often deformed and cesarean operations were thus necessary to save the mother and child. Often the mother died because medieval surgery was crude. Returning Crusaders spread syphilis, which became an important cause of infant, and sometimes maternal, fatality. Intermarriage occurred and often resulted in the union of a man and woman of different body structures. Thus a woman might give birth to a child too large for the size of her pelvis.

During the Middle Ages the *midwife,* not the physician, delivered infants. Only in difficult cases was a barber-surgeon asked to help with the delivery. The unborn child was sometimes killed and the body removed with crude instruments introduced through the vagina. Reputable physicians attended pregnant women only in rare instances, usually if the woman was of noble birth or was the king's mistress. In fact, the services of a physician in this area were not valued and strong prohibitions existed against their use. A Doctor Wertt of Hamburg was burned at the stake in 1522 for attending a delivery dressed as a woman.

Numerous paintings depict the practice of obstetrics by midwives. The delivery is portrayed in a variety of ways, and different themes are depicted: guarding of the lying-in chamber from medical interference; presence of the midwife and the child's nurse; different positions used for delivery, such as sitting or squatting; and types of appliances (obstetrical chair, V-shaped stool, and beds) used.

Shortly after 1500 several events occurred that affected obstetrical care. The first book on obstetrics, *The Garden of Roses for Pregnant Women,* was written by Eucharius Roslin in 1513 at the request of the Duchess of

Judy Chicago, "Hildegarde of Bingen," plate from *The Dinner Party,* 1979. China-painted porcelain, 35.6 cm diameter. *(Copyright Judy Chicago, 1979. Photo copyright Donald Woodman. Through the Flower, Albuquerque, New Mexico.)*

Hildegarde of Bingen was one of the greatest and most original thinkers of her time. Her knowledge embraced the arts, nursing, medicine, and science, as well as spiritual and religious philosophy. A prolific writer and composer, she corresponded with leading medieval thinkers. She was considered by many to be a mystic and a visionary, which led to her involvement in the political and religious issues of the time. The development of a theory of the universe that emphasized the relationship between the human and the divine became her focus in later years.

Colombia's 1967 eighty-cent air mail stamp was issued in observance of the Sixth Congress of Colombia Surgeons held in Bogota. The color reproductions of Grau's painting, *The First Caesarean Section* (1844), show a nurse as a member of the surgical team. *(Courtesy of Howard B. Hurley.)*

Brunswick. The best-known practices of obstetrical care were reinforced; full of superstitions, this book sanctioned the crudest practices of midwives (Haggard, 1929). The *podalic version* was introduced in France by Ambroise Paré. This technique was used when a child was not in the proper position for a normal delivery; the surgeon's hand was inserted into the uterus and the child was grasped by the feet and turned. A school of midwifery was opened at the Hôtel Dieu in Paris in the sixteenth century. The Chamberlen brothers invented the obstetrical forceps in 1588. This instrument was kept a secret and passed on to the son of one of the brothers.

Epidemics and Plagues

In the fourteenth century a catastrophic disease, Black Death, swept over the European continent and England four times. The worst occurrence was in 1348. Black Death is generally believed to have been a plague of the bubonic type, which results from the bite of an infected parasite. Primarily a disease of rodents, particularly rats, it is transmitted to humans by parasites, such as fleas, that have fed on the diseased rodents. Direct contact with an infected person can also transmit the disease. Rats on vessels that were being used to transport supplies spread the disease over the greater part of Europe. The name *Black Death* derived from the dark hemorrhagic spots that appeared under the skin of its victims. These were generally accompanied by inflammation of the lungs, unquenchable thirst, burning sensations, and inflammation in a variety of body parts. The outbreak of bubonic plague in the fourteenth century is considered one of the most devastating crises that ever occurred in human history. The sudden and unusual character of the disease brought terror to the people.

> The Black Death, which caused the unprecedented mortality of one-fourth of the population of the earth (over sixty millions of human beings), appeared in Europe about 1348, after devastating Asia and Africa. . . . Sweeping everything before it, this terrible plague brought panic and confusion in its train and broke down all restrictions of morality, decency and humanity. Parents, children and lifelong friends forsook one another, everyone striving to save only himself and to come off with a whole skin. Some took to vessels in the open sea only to find that the pestilence was hot upon them; some prayed and fasted in sanctuaries, others gave themselves up to unbridled indulgence, or . . . fled the country to idle away their time in some safe retreat; others lapsed into sullen indifference and despair. The dead were hurled pell-mell into huge pits, hastily dug for the purpose, and putrefying bodies lay about everywhere in the houses and streets.
>
> — *Garrison, 1913, pp. 127–128*

The sweating sickness began in England and spread over the continent about the same time. This virulent disease is thought to have been influenza. Large numbers of people died within a day or a few hours after the first symptoms appeared. The onset was accompanied by chills, fever, headaches, stupor, cardiac pain, vomiting, fatigue, and profuse sweat. Some of the care that was rendered probably hastened the patient's end. It was believed that the patient must sweat continuously for twenty-four hours. Therefore windows and doors were closed, stoves were lighted, and furs were piled on the ill. Attendants stayed with the patients, attempting to keep them awake so that they might retain their senses. Various techniques were used to accomplish this, such as whipping the body with branches or dropping vinegar into the eyes. It was remarked that the patient was "stewed to death" (Jamieson and Sewall, 1950).

Tremendous changes took place in the last centuries of the Middle Ages. The feudal system deteriorated. Cities and a middle class society developed. Luxury and misery, learning and ignorance existed side by side. The changing needs of society prompted the beginning of reforms.

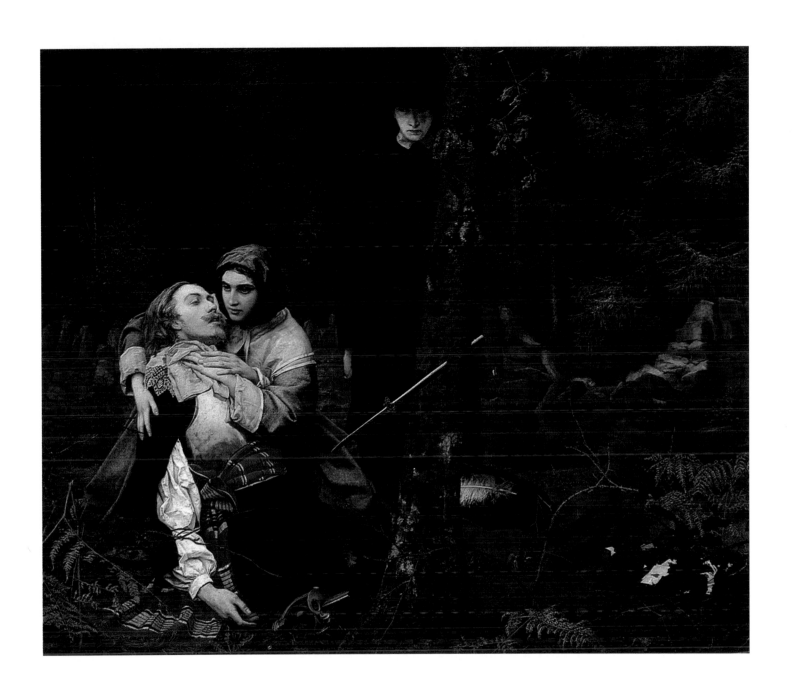

William Shakespeare Burton, *The Wounded Cavalier*, c. 1856. *(The Bridgeman Art Library, Guildhall Art Gallery, City of London.)*

U N I T 5

Nursing in Transition

The Dark Period and the Dawn of Modern Times

The transition from medieval times becomes quite evident toward
the close of the fifteenth century. Among the momentous forces
that again changed the existing social order were movements
whose seeds were planted in preceding centuries and which came
to fruition in this era. Those forces were the Renaissance, the
Protestant Revolt or Reformation, nationalism, the discovery
of a new world, oceanic commercial enterprise, and diffusion
of knowledge through the printed word. All of these forces
influenced the healing arts in one way or another.

— SISTER CHARLES MARIE FRANK

John Morton-Sale, *The Red Cross of Comfort*, 1939. Photogravure of the original painting.
(Copyright Roysia Romanelli.)

John Morton-Sale was commissioned to do the painting in 1939 by the Queen Mother.
He and other artists were asked to create works that would be auctioned to raise money for
the Red Cross. Neither the artist nor his family has knowledge as to the whereabouts of
the original work since all records were apparently lost during the "Blitz." Whether the
painting survived the war and is owned by someone outside of London is unknown.

Nursing in Transition

	1400	1470	1540	1610
DAILY LIFE		**1454** Guttenberg Bible printed **1500** Suppression of monasteries occurs **1517** Reformation begins **1517** Martin Luther pins his ninety-five theses to castle church door at Wittenburg	**1545** Council of Trent meets in Trentino, Italy	**1600** Wigs and dress trains become fashionable **1618–1648** Thirty Years' War
SCIENCE AND TECHNOLOGY		**1473–1543** Nicholas Copernicus' discoveries precipitate Intellectual Revolution	**1561–1630** Henry Briggs promotes use of logarithms **1564–1642** Galileo	**1600** Dutch opticians invent the telescope
THE VISUAL ARTS	**1400** Renaissance begins in Italy **1450** Renaissance spreads throughout Europe **1452–1519** Leonardo da Vinci, Italian artist who drew illustrations of human body **1475–1564** Michelangelo Buonarroti, Italian sculptor **1483–1520** Raphael, Italian painter		**1577–1640** Peter Paul Rubens, Flemish painter **1580–1666** Frans Hals, Dutch painter	**1599–1641** Antony Van Dyck, Dutch painter **1603** Carlo Maderna builds facade at St. Peter's in Rome **1606–1669** Rembrandt van Rijn, Dutch painter
MEDICINE AND HEALTH CARE		**1514–1564** Andreas Vesalius, founder of modern anatomy		**1619** William Harvey describes circulation of blood
NURSING		**1538** Jean Ciudad (John of God) founded Brothers of St. John of God in Spain **1550–1614** St. Camillus De Lellis founded Nursing Order of Ministers of the Sick **1550–1850** "Dark Period of Nursing" **1576–1660** St. Vincent de Paul founded Dames de Charité		**1633** Sisters of Charity founded

1680	1750	1820	1890

1665 Great plague in London

1700 Factory system of production gains popularity

1738 First cuckoo clocks in Black Forest district of Germany

1750 Industrial Revolution begins in England

1789–1795 French Revolution

1797–1815 Napoleonic wars

1800–1825 Latin American Revolution

1817 Elizabeth Fry establishes association to improve Newgate Prison conditions

1846 Irish potato famine

1848–1849 Extensive immigration to America from Europe

1854–1856 Crimean War

1864 Treaty of Geneva signed by twelve governments, establishing International Red Cross

1865 First carpet sweeper comes into use

1642–1727 Isaac Newton discovers laws of gravity

1742 Celsius invents centigrade thermometer

1752 Benjamin Franklin invents lightning conductor

1793 Eli Whitney invents cotton gin

1865 Gregor Mendel enunciates Law of Heredity

1656 Academy of Painting established in Rome

1697–1764 William Hogarth, British painter and engraver

1806 Claude Clodion begins Arc de Triomphe, Paris

1846 First painted Christmas card designed by John C. Horseley

---

1632–1723 Anton van Leeuwenhoek discovers protozoa, bacteria, and human spermatozoa

1641 Arsenic prescribed for medicinal purposes

1668–1751 Thomas Coram labors to establish the Hospital for Foundlings in London

1775 F.A. Mesmer uses hypnosis for health purposes

1798 Edward Jenner discovers a vaccine against smallpox

1802–1887 Dorothea Dix focuses on care of criminals and mentally ill in the United States

1805 Sartürner isolates morphine

1818 René Laënnec develops the stethoscope

1822–1895 Louis Pasteur lays foundation for science of bacteriology

1843–1910 Robert Koch discovers causes of cholera and tuberculosis

---

1634 St. Louise de Marillac becomes first Sister of Charity of St. Vincent de Paul

1809 Mother Elizabeth Seton establishes Sisters of Charity in America

1815 Mother Mary Aikenhead establishes order of Sisters of Charity in Ireland

1820–1910 Florence Nightingale, pioneer and founder of modern nursing

1836 Deaconess Institute, Kaiserswerth, established

1840 Elizabeth Fry establishes Society of Protestant Sisters of Charity as visiting nurses

1844 Dickens' *Martin Chuzzlewit* depicts nursing conditions through characters of Sairey Gamp and Betsy Prig

1854–1856 Death rate of British Army reduced from forty-two percent to two percent with nursing care

1857 Longfellow immortalizes Nightingale in poem *Lady with a Lamp*

1859 *Notes on Nursing* published

1860 Nightingale training school for nurses opens at St. Thomas Hospital, London

The centuries that immediately followed the Crusades were marked by great social changes. These changes began as early as 1250, tended to accelerate about 1450, and by 1750 had become dominant as the modern characteristics in Western Europe. Between the fall of Constantinople (1453) and the Battle of Waterloo (1815), a variety of revolutions served to expand people's idea of the universe and the meaning of human life. Yet these forces also threatened to destroy the social recovery that had been accomplished thus far. The economic, industrial, intellectual, political, and religious revolutions inevitably had far-reaching effects on every aspect of life, including the treatment of the sick and the sick poor, the management of hospitals, and the status of nursing. These movements demonstrated the currents of popular feeling that increased tensions in most of Europe: the dominant Church with its large temporal power had become oppressive; the intellectuals were criticizing the doctrines of extreme ecclesiasticism; the laboring classes were bitter toward serfdom and oppression; and the religious were yearning for a return to a simpler faith with greater observance of ceremonials. The time was ripe for change.

Samuel Luke Fildes, *Application for Admission to a Casual Ward,* 1874. Canvas. *(Royal Holloway College, London, England.)*

RENAISSANCE AND REFORMATION

To the sixteenth century belong two great movements, the Renaissance and the Reformation. Each was a result of the spirit of revolutionary change and the human quest for new knowledge and beauty. Probably the same social forces that produced the intellectual movement known as the Renaissance brought a split within the Church that eventually divided Christianity into warring sects. Together, these movements ushered in the "modern era" in which society was aware of the new world of Columbus, the old world of the Near and Far East, the new laws of Newton, and the old learning of the Graeco-Roman ages. The scientific method of inquiry was initiated, and secularism became the modern spirit. All established institutions were affected during this transition period, which produced new institutions and also modified the old ones. Those having to do with the care of the sick were, perhaps, affected the most. Reforms promoted by the changing needs of the society began to occur, although in some instances they were slow in coming.

The Renaissance

The chaos of the Middle Ages subsided with the unparalleled phenomenon known as the Renaissance. Its exact time frame varies slightly depending on particular source materials; dates span a period from 1400 to 1700. Changes, although fairly rapid, came about at different times in different countries. The

Joost van Geel, *Mother With Nurse and Child*. Panel. 35.5 × 29.5 cm. (*Museum Boymans-van Beuningen, Rotterdam, Netherlands.*)

155

Renaissance is generally viewed, however, as the primary period of transition from medieval to modern times. This period in history was called a *rinascita,* or rebirth, by Giorgio Vasari (1511–1574), a Florentine artist and architect who believed that the major motivation for its evolution was a return to the cultures of ancient Rome and Greece. It was a period characterized by shifts in standards that were evident in literary and intellectual circles. Of primary importance was the decline in the power of the Church in temporal matters accompanied by a rise in intense secular interest in worldly affairs. The dominant spirit of the Renaissance was an interest in the things of the earth without reference to God.

> In the sixteenth century men rejected the Church but held on to their belief in Christ. In the seventeenth century the intellectuals rejected the divinity of Christ but retained their belief in the Deity. . . . In the eighteenth century, the Age of Enlightenment, the "philosophers" openly rejected God Himself and substituted Reason. In the nineteenth century religious indifferentism, materialism, general unbelief and atheism spread among the masses.
>
> — *Devane, 1948, p. 55*

With this lost sense of relationship to God, the movement became characterized by both gullibility and skepticism, which led to a renewal of pagan superstitious practices and witchcraft. Yet outstanding Christian humanists emerged during this time, and renowned saints lived exemplary lives.

The Renaissance, indeed, has been viewed as both a blessing and a curse. It brought about a tremendous renewal of interest in learning in the areas of classical literature, humanism, and expressions of beauty. It was therefore also known as the period of humanism or the revival of learning. This renewal of interest in the arts and the sciences had a positive influence on the medical advancement in the Renaissance period. The learning, however, engendered materialistic, secularistic, and individualistic tendencies in the people. The society divided into two classes, the intelligentsia, who lived luxurious lives, and the working classes, who were oppressed because of their lack of knowledge and worldly possessions. Intellectual superiority and moral laxity emerged and drastically affected the political and religious character of the European people.

The Renaissance began in Italy about 1400 and permeated western Europe during the ensuing century. The new state of mind reflected itself in literature, painting, sculpture, and architecture. In addition, increasing wealth made it possible for art to penetrate the middle class. Painting, which had been limited to religious subjects and idealized themes from the Christian tradition, expanded to include the depiction of contemporary life. It was a realistic type of painting that sought to represent natural objects as they actually appeared. Artists even began to devote themselves to scientific studies. In Italian Renaissance painting, however, religious subjects still predominated. Renaissance painting, noted for its human quality, was "realistic" and attempted to reproduce natural objects as they actually appeared. During this era prominent and innovative artists portrayed real people with increasing skill in perspective and color. Students from the school of Florentine art who left an indelible mark in this field included Leonardo da Vinci (1452–1519), Michelangelo (1475–1564), who painted frescoes in the Sistine Chapel, and Raphael (1483–1520). Titian (1477–1576) led a second group of students from the Venetian school. The Florentine school was noted for form and grace of line; the Venetian school, for its mastery of color.

Leonardo da Vinci was perhaps the most versatile of the artists of the Renaissance. His masterpiece, *The Last Supper,* was painted on a wall of the refectory in a monastery at Milan. Although not a physician, he belonged to a guild comprising artists, apothecaries, physicians, and surgeons. Da Vinci was the first artist to consider anatomy for reasons other than its practicality.

Facing page, Leonardo da Vinci, *Embryo in the Womb,* c. 1510. Pen and ink, 30.1 × 21.4 cm. *(The Royal Collection. Copyright Her Majesty Queen Elizabeth II.)*

Da Vinci was the first to draw the single-chambered uterus at a time when it was generally believed that it was made up of several compartments, which was thought to explain the mystery of twin births. He was also the first to correctly describe the fetus in utero tethered by an umbilical cord. His ideas, however, that the cord was equal in length to the body at each stage of the child's development and that the child did not breathe since it was in water proved to be wrong. The majority of da Vinci's anatomical drawings were produced between 1506 and 1513.

Leonardo himself made anatomical preparations from which he produced drawings, of which more than 750 are extant, representing the skeletal, muscular, nervous, and vascular systems. The illustrations were often supplemented with annotations of a physiological nature. Leonardo's scientific accuracy was greater than that of Vesalius, and his artistic beauty remains unchallenged. His correct assessment of the curvature of the spine went otherwise undiscovered for more than a hundred years. He depicted the true position of the *fetus in utero* and first noted certain anatomical structures. The sketches were seen by only a few contemporaries and were not published until the end of the last century.

— Petrucelli, 1978, p. 410

Da Vinci painted marvelous variations in expressions on the faces of his subjects. Reactions of fear, frustration, pain, joy, and happiness appeared natural and lifelike. His anatomical drawings and sketches were advanced for his time, perhaps because of the one hundred human dissections he performed.

The northern schools of painting, notably the Dutch and the Flemish, gave rise to artists such as Peter Paul Rubens (1577–1640), Anthony Van Dyck (1599–1641), and Rembrandt van Rijn (1606–1669). The Dutch and Flemish masters tended to abandon religious themes and devote themselves to merchants, princes, or scenes from everyday life. In addition, the Dutch masters were interested in human dissection and left excellent examples of this, as in Rembrandt's classic *Lesson in Anatomy*. Dissection was practiced in their medical schools.

The Reformation

The Reformation (Protestant Revolt), which began in 1517, started as a reform and ended as a revolt. It was a religious movement that resulted in a division in Christianity. The Reformation was precipitated by two major factors: (1) the widespread abuses that had become a part of Church life and practice, such as the selling of indulgences and pardons, the veneration of relics, and the ignorance and depravity of the clergy, and (2) doctrinal difficulties. Essentially, a showdown occurred between the philosophy of St. Augustine, which dominated the early Church, and that of St. Thomas Aquinas, which gained preeminence in the thirteenth century. The more liberal doctrine of Aquinas permitted humans free will to choose between good and evil and to achieve grace through both good works and faith. Reform had been advocated for many centuries by influential individuals from within and without the Church. Erasmus scoffed at the ridiculous abuses, and Thomas More prayed for internal revision. The Church, however, did not take action and thereby paved the way for drastic intervention. By the time Martin Luther (1483–1546) pinned his Ninety-Five Theses to the castle church door at Wittenburg in 1517, many people were ready to oppose the established regime.

The rebellion against the Pope and the patriarchal rule of the Church was led by Martin Luther. Luther, once a German mendicant monk, became the leader of a group of dissatisfied people who broke away from the Catholic Church. These separatists were called *Protestants* ("those who protested"), a group that was to comprise many religious denominations. The followers of Luther were called Lutherans, and the Lutheran Church of today still adheres to his doctrine. The Lutherans rapidly declared both the independence of their congregations from the Pope and the right of each state to choose between the new Church and the old. Where there had been only one Europe, there were henceforth two. The Western world was divided into Catholics, who adhered to the teachings of Christ as dictated by the Church, and Protestants, who rejected the authority of this Church.

Within a few years northern Germany, Norway, Sweden, and Denmark were Lutheran. In addition, the success of Lutheranism encouraged other revolts against Catholic authority. During the next century many sects arose, such as Anabaptists, Mennonites, Quakers, Calvinists, Presbyterians, Puritans, and Anglicans. Each interpreted the doctrine in a slightly different way; each was certain of the absolute truth necessary for salvation. Although this division weakened Protestantism, it enhanced society by insisting upon each individual's right to think for himself or herself. Some of these groups ultimately established churches that were as intolerant of opposition as was Catholicism.

Correction of abuses within the Church finally came with the Council of Trent, a general council of church authorities called at Trentino in northern Italy, in 1545. To identify means of removing causes of criticism and clarify the Church's position, this council continued its sessions for eighteen years, until 1563. Serious abuses were altered, a popular and simple prayer book was adopted, and an even more rigorous discipline pervaded nursing orders and other groups.

> The Council defined attacked points of Christian theology, established disciplinary measures for clergy, religious and laity, and prepared a catechism of Christian doctrine for parish use. The means taken to bring about the real reform are sometimes referred to as the Counter-Reformation.
>
> — *Frank, 1953, p. 130*

However, efforts to reconcile Catholicism and Protestantism failed, and Europe drifted into a tragic struggle between the two groups. The result was an era of hatred, civil conflict, the development of multiple factions to foster individuality, and an international conflict known as the Thirty Years' War (1618–1648). People had also begun to depart for the New World, where they might ensure for themselves a true freedom in religion.

After Thomas Rowlandson, *Interior at Middlesex Hospital, London*, c. 1808. Etching and aquatint. *(National Library of Medicine, Bethesda, Maryland.)*

The Doorkeeper at Toicuses Hospital. (From Picture Book of Graphics Arts 1500–1800, *volume 6. Compiled by Georg Hirth, published in Munich by Knorr & Hirr, 1882. By permission of The British Library, London, England.)*

The Reformation had no direct effect on hospitals in Catholic countries, and some hospitals did, indeed, survive in Protestant countries. Yet the majority of hospitals operated by the Catholic religious orders were closed or controlled by the Protestants. Monks and nuns were driven out of the institutions in the Protestant countries, which caused a tremendous shortage of people to care for the sick and the poor. The plight of the unfortunates became unbearable as they were reduced to a state of disgraceful pauperism. (Under Catholicism the poor had been esteemed.) Hospitals became places of horror, since there was no qualified group to take the place of the nursing religious orders. The most serious consequences occurred in England, where Henry VIII suppressed all the religious orders and confiscated the property of some six hundred charitable endowments. Women were recruited from all sources to fill the nursing ranks. Many of these women were assigned nursing duties in lieu of serving jail sentences. This "Dark Period of Nursing," between 1550 and 1850, saw nursing conditions at their very worst.

The seeming ambivalence of Protestant countries toward their sick and poor was the result of two conflicting influences: the desire to make money, to be rich and powerful, and the desire to be the chosen of God by doing works that would provide a state of "grace." Laws and customs discouraged the humane care of the downtrodden and the weak, yet tremendous efforts were made to raise money to open hospitals and provide the necessities of life. This dichotomy had the most serious effect on nursing.

The Reformation had a profound effect on nursing. Nursing suffered a great setback as monastic institutions were closed and nursing orders were eliminated. Even in some Catholic countries kings seized monasteries to accumulate more wealth and possessions. The most extreme impact on nursing in both Protestant and Catholic countries, however, was the almost entire removal of men from nursing. Thereafter, the majority of Catholic nursing orders were for women; nursing in Protestant countries became a woman's occupation.

The Nurse, c. 1840. Cartoon illustrating the popular idea of the nurse of the day. (The Mansell Collection Limited, London, England.)

Albrecht Dürer, *Four Apostles ("Die vier Apostel")*, 1526. Panel, approx. 214.6 × 76.2 cm (each). *(Alte Pinakothek, München.)*

The four apostles symbolize the four temperaments. *From left to right,* St. John represents the sanguine temperament; St. Peter, the phlegmatic; St. Mark, the choleric; and St. Paul, the melancholic.

THE AGE OF REVOLUTIONS

The intellectual, political, industrial, and economic revolutions were strong motivators for changing human ideas and activities, as was the religious revolt. These movements—complex, varied, and interrelated—all were influences that brought about the Renaissance. It was a time of flux, and these factors were crucial to the development of new necessities and new circumstances in the life that had evolved. The modern world was being born, but it would experience severe labor pains and harsh growing pains.

The Political Revolution

The political life that was characterized by feudal institutions in medieval times gave way to the establishment of national states during the Renaissance. These national states developed in the part of Europe that had previously been unified under the Holy Roman Empire. Unity was achieved through monarchs who gradually overthrew feudal lords. Authority was centralized in the monarchy; a system of private ownership and private enterprise took shape. Individuals and nations sought power through the accumulation of wealth and the grasping of opportunity.

Other changes occurred as nationalism progressed. The language and customs of the capital were spread throughout the entire kingdom. The trend toward a national language had begun and fostered a growing pride in the land. Individuals in the literary field began to work in their own tongue instead of using Latin. This patriotism was also stirred by wars against other peoples, which were initiated by the ambition of kings. National competition developed and resulted in armed interventions. One great struggle followed another until the Seven Years' War (French and Indian War) in 1754, which earned first place for England. However, poverty and discontent followed the wars, and a series of revolutions erupted in an endeavor to create more democratic forms of government. The American Revolution (1775–1783), the French Revolution (1789–1795), and the Latin American Revolution (1800–1825) reflected a reaction against human inequality and placed an emphasis on individual rights. Finally, the Napoleonic Wars began in 1797 and ended in 1815 with the Battle of Waterloo. This particular conflict suppressed dictatorship for a time.

The Economic Revolution

The physical world was explored by England, France, Spain, Portugal, and Holland over the space of three centuries (1450–1750). New lands were discovered. North and South America, New Zealand, and the ocean islands were seized from less civilized peoples and colonized. India, China, and Africa were rediscovered and forced into trade with Europe. The world of humans was doubled in size, and their dream of wealth expanded proportionately. Vast riches from trade with the Old and New Worlds poured into Europe. Particularly significant was the bullion carried from the Americas by Spain, which put more gold and silver into circulation in western Europe than ever before. It is estimated that the circulating gold and silver in 1500 was worth two million dollars; by 1600 its worth had increased to two billion. (Bullion could also have included precious stones.) A revolution in economic thought and practice was thus created. A capitalistic economic system, sometimes referred to as *merchant capitalism,* began to take form.

Mercantilism developed in response to economic activity for national ends. It began to emerge as early as the fourteenth century and was dominant during the seventeenth and early eighteenth centuries. This system held that a nation's wealth was determined by the amount of precious metals in its treasury. Government regulated industry, agriculture, and labor. Furthermore, government controls would ensure the maintenance of a stable economy and an increase in the stockpile, particularly through a favorable balance of trade. The state would create laws to force an excess of exports over imports and reap the profit in bullion. Businessmen became the dominant class in their community and were led by merchant princes. (Shakespeare's title character in *Merchant of Venice* [1596] impressed men of England as the dynamic business leader.) Private enterprise, competition for markets, and expectations of gains were vital components of this system.

The Industrial Revolution

The industrial revolution began in England at approximately 1750 and drastically upset traditional life-styles. With the rise of the capitalist economic system, medieval craftsmen became dependent upon capitalists for wages. At first, craftsmen labored in their own homes, but by 1700 the factory system of production had gained popularity.

> The factory system is marked by the wage relationship between the employer and employees, by mass production, and by the tendency to enlarge steadily the size of the productive units. This system requires centralized direction and elaborate financial outlays.
>
> — *Sellew and Nuesse, 1946, p. 143*

A belief prevails that the industrial system was suddenly introduced during this time because of inventions in the textile industry. The real revolution, however, was under way before the occurrence of such inventions, which served to accelerate the process. Machinery did, however, standardize quality, and master craftsmen were forced to give up their crafts and lands and become laborers (factory hands) for rich individuals. All types of industries were affected, and efficiency became the key to success. In addition, as the era of invention unfolded, the number of manufacturing cities grew. Along with these cities came various social problems including poverty, overcrowding, and disease.

The Intellectual Revolution

The intellectual or scientific revolution was precipitated by the discoveries of Copernicus (1473–1543), Galileo (1564–1642), and Newton (1642–1727). Their work demonstrated that the earth was not the center of the universe but revolved in accordance with universal laws over which humans had no control. Experimentation, measurement, and instruments to improve sight or hearing became important aids to observation and the development of the new science, "experimental philosophy." The inductive method of thought was introduced as scholars began to observe facts and phenomena and determine solutions to the mysteries of life through a process of reasoning.

Numerous discoveries occurred in the physical sciences that seemed to revolutionize human thought. Nicholas Copernicus demonstrated that the earth turns on its axis and moves in an orbit around the sun. Johannes Kepler (1571–1630) further developed this theory. Isaac Newton discovered the law of gravitation. Simon Stevin (1548–1620) developed the use of decimals. John Napier (1550–1617) and Henry Briggs (1561–1630) promoted the use of logarithms. René Descartes (1596–1650) invented analytical geometry. A number of other individuals were also instrumental in advancing the physical sciences. These sixteenth-century discoveries led to the invention of the telescope, microscope, thermometer, barometer, and pendulum clock.

The field of the biological sciences was also advancing and would become basic to the progress of medical science. The work of Andreas Vesalius (1514–1564), the founder of modern anatomy, was thought to be revolutionary. His findings were based on investigation rather than speculation. William

Harvey (1578–1657) described the circulation of the blood, proof of which was published in 1628 in his *Exercitatio Anatomica de Motu Cordis et Sanguinis in Animalibus* (*On the Movement of the Heart and Blood in Animals*). Robert Hooke (1635–1703) described the cellular structure of plants. Anton van Leeuwenhoek (1632–1723), using the recently invented microscope, discovered protozoa and bacteria and described human spermatozoa.

Advances in technology interfaced with progress in the sciences. This was particularly evident with the greatest of the Renaissance inventions, the printing press. Letters could be stamped on paper by movable type, and after the year 1500 manuscripts were rapidly superseded by printed volumes. The first complete book printed in this manner was the famous Gutenberg *Bible* (1454). Books became cheaper and more available to all educated persons. Scientists were thus able to read one another's books, exchange ideas promptly, build on published works, and communicate findings.

William Hogarth, *An Operation Scene in a Hospital,* mid-eighteenth century. Pencil and grey wash over chalk. *(The Pierpont Morgan Library, New York.)*

NEW DIRECTIONS IN MEDICINE

The birth of the scientific method of inquiry profoundly influenced the development of medicine in the Renaissance period. Medical scientists, like other scientists, benefited from the development of experimentation. Indeed, the majority of scientists *were* physicians. Yet the line between science and magic remained blurred. Quacks and charlatans continued to appear and appeal to the poor and the ignorant, who depended on this type of "medicine man" and self-medication. This was necessary because physicians were the elite group during this period and they took care of only the upper classes.

The Nurse Old Style, c. 1879. Cartoon illustrating the drunken nurse dozing at the bedside of an alarmed patient. *(The Mansell Collection Limited, London, England.)*

After Thomas Rowlandson, *While Confined to Your Bed by a Sickness: The Humours of a Hired Nurse,* c. 1807. Hand colored etching. *(From Rowlandson's* Miseries of Human Life. *National Library of Medicine, Bethesda, Maryland.)*

The New Anatomy

The first movement in the advance of medical science was the growth of anatomical knowledge and its application to surgery. The Flemish anatomist and surgeon Andreas Vesalius was undoubtedly the leader in this area. His work, which was based on human dissection, replaced crude medieval concepts and corrected more than two hundred mistakes in the works of Galen (Shryock, 1959). Vesalius's *De Humani Corporis Fabrica* (*The Fabric of the Human Body*) of 1543 illustrated both in words and pictures the dissected parts of the human body—the skeleton, muscles, vascular system, abdomen, and so forth. The findings of Vesalius were revolutionary and were not well received by his colleagues, who derided him and ignored his work. He eventually decided to leave academic life after suffering bitter disappointment and disillusionment. After Vesalius's death his students continued his work. They included Gabriele Fallopio (1523–1562), the discoverer of the fallopian tubes.

Ambroise Paré (1510–1590), a Parisian surgeon, transformed the practice of surgery by applying anatomical knowledge with the scientific method. He began his career as a barber's apprentice, became an assistant at the Hôtel Dieu, and finally was a surgeon in the army. Based on his military experience, he reinstituted the use of ligatures for bleeding vessels caused by gunshot wounds. (His colleagues treated such wounds with boiling oil.) Paré brought together the surgeons of the universities and the barber surgeons who were relied upon by the people. He believed that anatomy was a necessary prerequisite to a surgeon's skill. His practical genius included improvements in artificial limbs, trusses, hernia operations, and the glass eye. A man of many talents, he was also involved in dentistry; he restored missing teeth, reimplanted teeth, and invented a palatal obturator. His collected writings, *Oeuvres,* were first published in 1575. Paré always credited his success with patients to God, which was clearly evident in his motto: "Je le pansay. Dieu le guérit," that is, "I treated him. God cured him."

Aureolus Theophrastus Bombastus von Hohenheim (1493–1541), better known as Paracelsus, was one of the most unusual individuals in medical history. Paracelsus viewed the body as a sort of glorified chemical retort and initiated the chemical approach to physiology. This often led others to view him as an ignorant, itinerant quack. He stressed that alchemists should stop attempting to make gold and start making medicines. Paracelsus particularly advocated the use of mercury, arsenic, lead, iron, sulfur, and antimony. He thus earned the title of Father of Pharmacology, even though he combined the use of chemicals with astrology. Paracelsus, an eccentric Swiss physician who had trained in Italy, consistently rebelled against authority. It is said that he publicly burned the books of Galen and other classical works. Paracelsus was one of the few surgeons of his time who renounced the accepted theory that pus was normal in the healing process. His was a daring approach to the field of medicine (Haggard, 1933).

The value of the new methods and the transition from anatomy to physiology was clearly illustrated by work done in the area of the heart and blood vessels.

> Galen had declared that the vascular system centered in the liver, and that blood ebbed and flowed through the body via a septum between one side of the heart and the other. But anatomists now found that no such septum existed and this cast doubt on the whole theory.
>
> — *Shryock, 1959, p. 140*

William Harvey (1578–1657) solved the problem by demonstrating with animals the actual circulation of the blood with the heart acting as a central pump. These findings were published in his *Exercitatio Anatomica de Motu Cordis et Sanguinis in Animalibus* (*On the Movement of the Heart and Blood in Animals*), one of the most important works in medicine and biology. He demonstrated that the heart was both a muscle and a pump, that blood flowed continuously in one direction along the arteries, and that the blood returned to the heart through veins, thereby completing a circle or cycle. Harvey was ridiculed and became known to some as the "circulator." To others, he was known as the Father of Modern Medicine, since his most valuable contribution was the establishment of physiological experimentation.

The value of anatomical studies was demonstrated during the Renaissance. Wide-reaching effects of these studies occurred in medicine, particularly in the areas of surgery and physiology. In addition, they logically led to the acceleration of the field of pathology.

Three Centuries of Progress

The seventeenth century saw the beginnings of attempts to explain the mechanics of the human body. Jerome Fabricus (1537–1619) was the first embryologist. Athanasius Kircher (1602–1680), a Jesuit monk, used a microscope and connected microorganisms with contagion. Anton van Leeuwenhoek perfected the microscope and described bacteria and protozoa. The development of the clinical method was the contribution of Thomas Sydenham (1624–1689), who advocated the subjection of old theories to new scientific observation. His efforts to observe cases and to experiment with treatments led him to propose new methods of handling the sick. His thought was that specific diagnosis might lead to specific therapy. Sydenham provided detailed descriptions of prevalent diseases such as dysentery and measles and influenced the trend of medicine by emphasizing fresh air to replace the stuffiness of the sick room. The autopsy was also found to be useful during this period.

The real importance of these discoveries was the provision of frameworks for thought about normal and deviant functioning of the human body. These innovations served to illustrate a specific trend in medical thought, the readiness of enlightened persons to discard old ideas for new ones. Increasingly, medical and scientific names of renown began to emerge:

> Marcello Malpighi, the greatest of the microscopists and founder of the science of histology; Willis, de Graaf, Peyer, Brunner, Stensen, Glisson, Van Deventer, the father of modern midwifery; Priestley who isolated oxygen; Lavoisier who discovered the interchange of gases in the process of respiration; Port, John Hunter, the surgical pathologist; Pringle, founder of modern military medicine . . .
>
> — *Frank, 1953, p. 132*

In addition, this century witnessed the changing of alchemy to chemistry by Robert Boyle (1627–1691). His knowledge of the nature of a pure substance overturned the ancient, long-revered theory that the four elements are earth, air, fire, and water. With this change the old humoral theory of health and illness was no longer relevant and a new theory was needed. One of the first new models was offered by René Descartes (1596–1650), whose *De Homine* was the original modern attempt at a physiology text. Descartes was perhaps the most influential intellectual of his generation.

It took the first fifty years of the eighteenth century for all of this new knowledge to be organized and digested. Advances continued to be made during this new century, but they were not as bold or as conspicuous as those of the previous one. They were, nevertheless, important in improving the standards of medical practice. Albrecht von Haller (1708–1777) systematized the new discoveries and made them available to practitioners. Giovanni Morgagni (1682–1741) correlated diseases of the organs with symptoms arising from impaired organic functioning. John Hunter (1728–1793) used his studies in comparative anatomy in new operative procedures and developed a simple, safe operation for aneurysm.

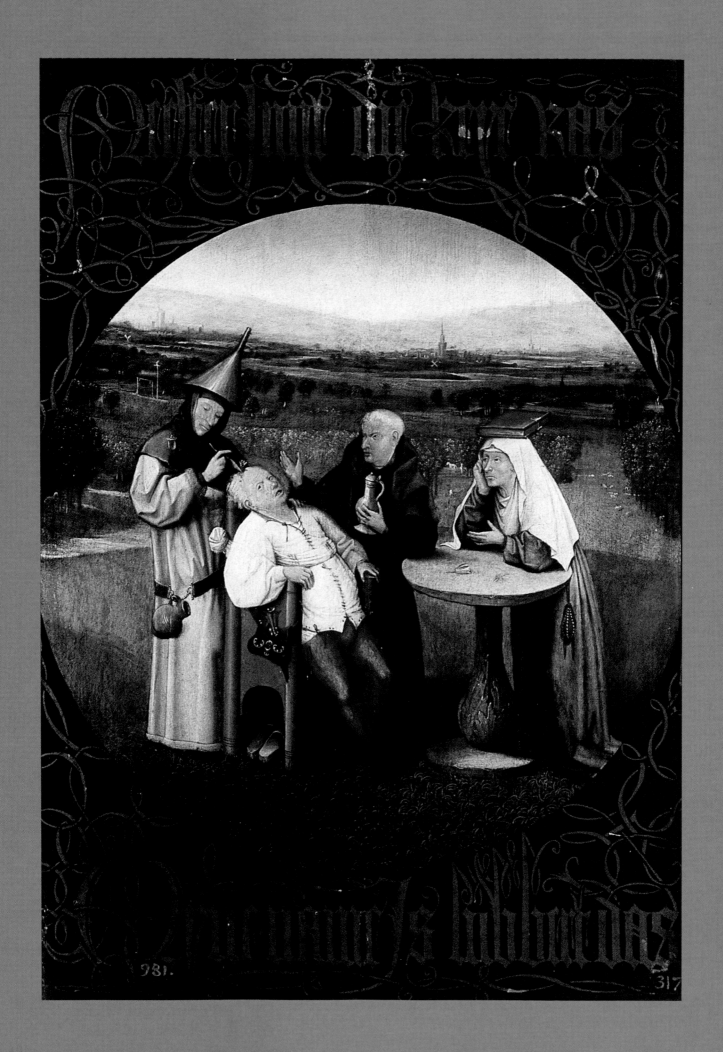

In the eighteenth century smallpox was prevalent and took many lives. Edward Jenner (1749–1823), an Englishman, discovered a satisfactory method of vaccination against smallpox in 1798. This procedure, with certain modifications, is still used today. Despite its proven efficiency and effectiveness, however, vaccination has been avoided by some people.

Psychiatry developed as a separate branch of medicine in the latter part of the eighteenth century. The mentally ill had received cruel, inhumane treatment in the sixteenth and seventeenth centuries. Vicious practices were associated with the idea that the mentally ill were "possessed" of a demon or even the Devil himself. Hogarth, the English artist, vividly portrayed these conditions through such works as *The Rake in Bedlam*. Attempts were made to rectify conditions by certain physicians who protested that mental disease was a medical problem and that the mentally ill should be treated in a humane fashion. Vincenzo Chiarrigi (1759–1820) established sound treatment of the mentally ill in the hospital that he directed. A Quaker, William Tuke, introduced more understanding methods in a retreat (York Retreat, managed by the Society of Friends) that he had established. Philippe Pinel (1745–1826), a physician and director of two hospitals in Paris, was probably the most famous leader in this area. He abandoned the use of restraining chains and advocated acceptance of the mentally ill as human beings in need of medical assistance, nursing care, and social services. His treatises on insanity were an effort to promote both scientific and humane treatment of the mentally ill.

During this same period instruments were invented for measurement and inspection of the body. A pulse watch was made by Sir John Floyer (1647–1734) in 1707. This watch ran for exactly one minute and then stopped, allowing the physician to obtain an accurate pulse count. Leopold Auenbrugger (1722–1809) initiated the use of percussion. This technique had

Facing page, Hieronymus Bosch, *Extraction of the Stone of Madness (The Cure of Folly). (Copyright Museo del Prado, Madrid, Spain.)*

The quack operation for removal of stones in the head is illustrated in this painting. A barber-surgeon who is wearing the "funnel of wisdom" operates on a fat old man who is deranged. The slang expression "rocks in the head" arises from this concept that insanity or lunacy is caused by objects in the head.

Philippe Pinel Ordering the Chains Removed From the Mentally Ill, c. 1793. *(World Health Organization, Geneva, Switzerland.)*

been unique to innkeepers, who tapped wine kegs to determine the remaining volume. René Théophile Laënnec (1781–1826) devised the stethoscope after listening to heart sounds through a tube of rolled-up paper tied with a string. This was followed by a cylinder made of light wood, about twelve inches long, that could be taken apart by unscrewing it into two pieces. (Dr. Cammann of New York developed the binaural stethoscope.)

Advances in medicine continued into the nineteenth century. One of the greatest contributions was the result of the work of Louis Pasteur (1822–1895). His discoveries laid the foundation for the science of bacteriology. The principles relating to attenuation of viruses, preventive vaccination against disease-producing organisms, treatment of rabies, and the discovery of the process of "pasteurization" were all significant works that enhanced the practice of medicine and the prevention of disease. Robert Koch (1843–1910), one of Pasteur's contemporaries, discovered the causes of cholera and tuberculosis. Joseph Lister (1827–1912) became one of the greatest men in the history of surgery. He introduced the use of antiseptics in operating rooms as a preventive measure against infection. During Lister's time "hospitalism" was accepted as an unavoidable evil in surgery. This name was applied to the infectious epidemics that stalked the hospital wards and took many lives. Anyone who was fortunate enough to recover from surgery often regained only partial health. Such morbidity and mortality were not acceptable to Lister, who scientifically studied their causes and perfected his techniques. Other very important discoveries were facilitated by the work of Pasteur.

> In 1879, Neisser discovered the gonococcus; in 1880, Eberth described the typhoid bacillus; in 1882, Koch reported the discovery of the tubercle bacillus; in 1883, Klebs and Loeffier discovered the *Bacillus Diphtheriae* and Salvioli described the pneumonococcus that he found in thoracic exudates and tissues; in 1892, Welch and Nuttal first described Welch's bacillus (gas infection); and in 1897, Shiga discovered the dysentery bacillus.
>
> In 1895, Röentgen discovered x-rays; in 1896, Marie and Pierre Curie isolated radium, and Widal introduced his agglutination test for diagnosing typhoid fever.
>
> — *Frank, 1953, p. 213*

By the middle of the nineteenth century other instruments of diagnosis came into being. The stethoscope, the mercury thermometer, and x-rays had become important adjuncts to the practice of medicine. The introduction of ether and chloroform as general anesthetics greatly aided the practice of surgery. The science of bacteriology had become the basis for modern medicine and surgery. Indeed, medicine had made revolutionary progress. Many individuals, only a few of whom have been mentioned here, had made significant contributions. A rapid series of discoveries had occurred over the three centuries, and these would forever change the direction of medicine.

Obstetrics and Infant Welfare

The serious problem of infant and maternal death rates in the eighteenth century was tackled in Europe and the British Isles. Since exact statistics were not available, however, it is difficult to assess the change with any accuracy. The maternal death rate had many causes, including poor or no prenatal care, poor nutrition from ignorance and poverty, infectious disease in early pregnancy, and the dreaded hospital infection—puerperal fever. In some instances it was also precipitated by delivery at the hands of ignorant, unwashed midwives.

In the eighteenth century all but the wealthy used midwives for delivery in normal cases; surgeons were called in for difficult cases. The destruction of the child and removal of its body, however, were less frequently done by the surgeons because of Paré's introduction of the podalic version and the inven-

A MIDWIFE GOING TO A LABOUR

Thomas Rowlandson, *A Midwife Going to a Labour,* 1811. *(Copyright The British Museum, London.)*

tion of the obstetrical forceps by Peter Chamberlen. Yet surgeons tended to interfere with the deliveries, either with instruments or manually, so that their efforts to relieve mothers often brought death to both the mother and the infant. In the latter part of the eighteenth century, particularly in England, physicians assumed the care of pregnant women. They replaced surgeons in difficult cases and even attended some normal deliveries. The "consultant in midwifery," the predecessor of the obstetrician, became a specialist who was separate from both physicians and surgeons. Two other events occurred that assisted with the improved status of the mother: the addition of the study of obstetrics to the medical curriculum and the advent of lying-in hospitals. In the lying-in hospitals, however, improved maternal death rate was dependent on the conditions that existed. In some, where conditions were the worst, the rate fluctuated between ten and twenty percent of the mothers who delivered.

As an answer to the problem of puerperal fever, William Hunter (1718–1783) proposed noninterference during delivery. During his time the number of cases of puerperal fever had increased to tragic proportions. Since the cause of the infection was unknown and the danger of contracting it was high, Hunter's solution seemed plausible. However, some of his followers

171

became so adamant about noninterference that some patients were allowed to die who might have otherwise been saved.

Ignaz Philipp Semmelweis (1818–1865) also became concerned about the problem of puerperal fever. Born in Budapest, he received his doctor's degree and the degree of master of midwifery from the University of Vienna. Semmelweis was granted a position as assistant director of the obstetrical clinic at the Lying-in Hospital in Vienna, where he was appalled by the high maternal mortality rate resulting from puerperal sepsis (childbed fever). He began to observe and analyze patient care and noticed a curious fact. He noted a difference between the maternal mortality rates of two clinics. The incidence of the fever and death was lower in the clinic where midwives practiced, but it was higher in the one where medical students practiced. Semmelweis determined that the spread of infection occurred because of the careless habits of the medical students, who went directly from the dissecting (autopsy) table to deliveries or to examinations of prenatal or postpartum patients. Therefore he demanded that the students wash their hands with soap and water, then wash them with chlorinated lime. As a result of this practice, there was a remarkable decrease in death rate, from ten percent to a little over one percent. *The Cause, Concept, and Prophylaxis of Childbed Fever*, published in 1861, provided an account of this valuable research. The work of Semmelweis was ridiculed and was not accepted by his colleagues. The criticism he suffered apparently led to his eventual mental illness. In 1865 he died of blood poisoning, a condition that he had fought to eliminate.

Oliver Wendell Holmes (1809–1894), a graduate of Harvard, also fought to eliminate childbed fever. Holmes, who abandoned the study of law for medicine, in 1829 wrote the essay, "The Contagiousness of Puerperal Fever," now considered a medical classic. This work was published five years before the research of Semmelweis became known and was bitterly attacked by the medical community. Like Semmelweis's theory, Holmes's idea regarding the cause of puerperal fever was correct. He republished the essay in 1855 with an introduction that criticized what he thought were unjust remarks. Gradually the cause of the disease as identified by both Holmes and Semmelweis was accepted.

The plight of the child in this time was vividly depicted by the extremely talented British painter and engraver William Hogarth (1697–1764). Hogarth criticized the social problems of his day, which were present in a world craving the pleasures of life. His pictures were stories of the frailties of human nature, usually displayed in a scene of horrible devastation. In the *Works of Charles Lamb*, a section entitled "On the Genius and Character of Hogarth" explains the extraordinary gift of this artist with the observation that most "pictures are looked at—his prints we read" (Lamb, vol. 1, 1818, p. 70).

The abandoned child had become a serious problem in the eighteenth century. There was public callousness and indifference to the practice of extensive infanticide. This attitude needed to be changed before strides could be made to reduce infant mortality. Evidence was also available that demonstrated infant death from neglect, cruelty, and illness.

> The exact statistics are not available, but in the early part of the century, the infant mortality rate for children under five years of age was 50 per cent. In London between 1730 and 1750, 75 per cent of all the babies christened were dead before the age of five. Of 10,272 infants admitted to the Dublin Foundling Hospital during 21 years (1775–1796) only 45 survived, a mortality of 99.6 per cent. Many famous foundling hospitals of the period had similar records. Even Queen Anne, who presumably received the best of care, lost 18 children in early infancy.
>
> — *Dolan, Fitzpatrick, and Hermann, 1983, pp. 111–112*

The infant death rate was also caused by factors other than neglect and cruelty. These included *headmouldshot*, the overriding of the sutures of the cranium; *horseshoehead*, the separation of the sutures usually associated with con-

Facing page, William Hogarth, *Gin Lane,* c. 1750. Engraving. *(Copyright The British Museum, London.)*

Hogarth's paintings vividly depicted the frailties of human nature. His criticism focused on society's emphasis on a world in which people craved the "pleasures of life." Numerous activities are taking place in this illustration, which is a masterpiece of excesses. One mother reaches for a pinch of snuff while another, at right, pours gin into her baby's mouth to pacify him; all around her are rowdy drinkers. The pawnbroker is extremely busy with those in need of money to buy liquor. In the background, a barber has hanged himself because no one in Gin Lane cares about personal grooming. At this period in history, gin and other hard liquors were cheap and could be sold without a license. Distillers functioned with government approval because they bought surplus grain, thereby swelling farm income.

GIN LANE.

Gin cursed Fiend, with Fury fraught.
    Makes human Race a Prey;
It enters by a deadly Draught.
    And steals our Life away.

Virtue and Truth driv'n to Despair,
    It's Rage compells to fly,
But cherishes with hellish Care,
    Theft, Murder, Perjury.

Damn'd Cup! that on the Vitals preys,
    That liquid Fire contains,
Which Madness to the Heart conveys,
    And rolls it thro' the Veins.

Alfred Roll, *The Wet Nurse.* (*Musée des Beaux-Arts, Lille/Bridgeman Art Library, London. Giraudon/Bridgeman Art Library.*)

The rearing of children was often entrusted to a wet nurse just as their birth was often attended by a midwife. Since wet nurses and midwives were rarely adequately trained or supervised, their services at times were fatal for infants and, in the case of midwives, for the mothers as well. Nevertheless, midwifery and wet nursing were among the principal female occupations in the eighteenth century.

genital cranial defects; and *overlying,* the practice of nurses sleeping with infants. In addition, wet nurses were frequently hired, and they sometimes transferred disease to the child. Just as there were nurses who infected their sucklings, there were also infants who infected their nurses (Robinson, 1946). Bottle-feeding, too, was a potential contributor to infant death through the contraction of disease from contaminated milk and water. Some sources indicated the death rate of bottle-fed infants to be three times that of breast-fed infants. Another cause of infant death was the common occurrence of "dropping," the practice of abandoning the infant on doorsteps of wealthy homes or simply leaving them to freeze or starve in the street. Infanticide continued into the nineteenth century.

As in most complex social movements, it is difficult to establish all the reasons for improvement in the infant death rate. However, this improvement was in no small part a result of the efforts of several individuals who wished to alleviate the high infant mortality. Among these were Thomas Coram (1668–1751) of England, who labored to establish the Hospital for Foundlings in London (1738); Jonas Hanway (1712–1786), who was involved with the parish workhouse movement in England and persuaded Parliament to enact

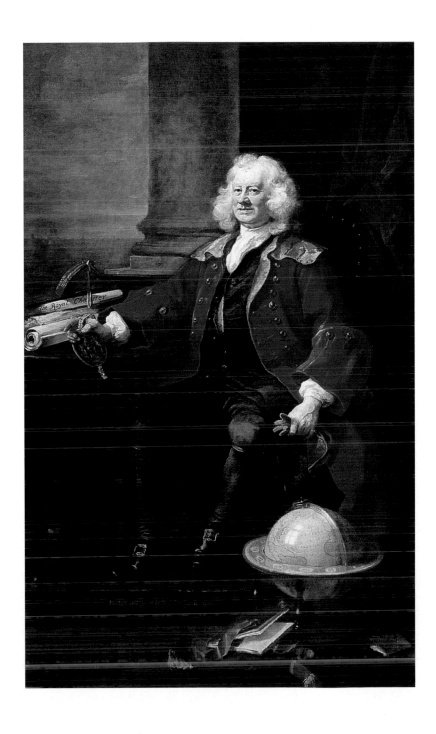

William Hogarth, *Captain Coram,* 1740 Canvas. *(Thomas Coram Foundation for Children, London, England.)*

Designed by Thomas Stothard, R.A., *The Work of Charity Schools, Children Rescued From Want and Misery, To Be Clad and Educated*, c. 1790. Engraving. *(Copyright British Museum, London, England.)*

laws for relief of infants of the poor; and George Armstrong (died 1781), one of the first English pediatricians, who was a staunch advocate of infant welfare and the prime leader in the dispensary movement that culminated in the establishment of the Dispensary for the Infant Poor on April 24, 1769. Perhaps the most significant development was a work titled "An Essay Upon Nursing and Management of Children," which appeared in London in 1750. It was written by William Cadogan (1711–1797), who became a physician to the Foundling Hospital after receiving master of arts, bachelor of medicine, and doctor of medicine degrees at Oxford. Cadogan was the first to write a simple, understandable book of instructions addressed to mothers about the care and feeding of infants and young children. Some might consider him the Doctor Spock of the era! A now–familiar passage dealt with Cadogan's plea for maternal feeding:

> There would be no fear of offending the husband's ears with the noise of the squalling brat. The child was it nurs'd in this way would be always quiet, in good humour, ever playing laughing or sleeping. In my opinion a man of sense cannot have a prettier rattle (for rattles he must have of one kind or another) than such a young child. I am quite at a loss to account for the general practice of sending infants out of doors to be suckled or drynursed by another woman, who had not so much understanding, nor can have so much affection for it as the parents: and how it comes to pass that people of good sense and easy circumstances will not give themselves the pains to watch over the health and welfare of their children: but are so careless as to give them up to the common methods, without considering how near it is to an equal chance that they are destroyed by them. The ancient custom of exposing them to wild beasts or drowning them would certainly be a much quicker and more humane way of despatching them.
>
> — *Quoted in Robinson, 1946, p. 83*

Cadogan was an apostle of maternal breast-feeding; no other woman's milk was good enough for the child. He also stressed daily baths for infants and frequent changes of clothing. But of particular importance was his influence in removing all swaddling clothes from babies and emphasizing the use of loose clothing.

Disease Epidemics

Epidemics continued to ravage Europe from the sixteenth through the nineteenth centuries. Devastating outbreaks of typhus and bubonic plague occurred and reduced the masses of the population to a pitiful state. These plagues were particularly ravaging because of the social decay that had resulted from urban industrialism. The epidemics of this early modern period forced physicians to accept a realistic view of medicine. Advances in medical knowledge and sanitation were frequently offset by the health hazards that existed in the large cities.

It is clear that health conditions were probably no better or worse than those that had existed in previous centuries. Yet urban living conditions facilitated the precipitation of diseases: sanitation was poor, sanitary facilities were lacking, sewage disposal was inadequate, cities were filthy, public health laws were lacking, water supplies were impure, and dirt and congestion inevitably brought pests such as rats, lice, and bedbugs, which carried infection. Congestion had increased, but its implications for health had been ignored. Epidemics of typhus were evidently spread to the European nations through foreign trade. Dark rooms served to increase the rate of tuberculosis. Since the value of fresh air was not understood, doors and windows were closed when someone was ill. Windows in hospitals and homes were frequently blocked up or bricked over for economical reasons.

Approximately one third of the population of London died in the plagues that swept England in 1603 and 1625. Other diseases were equally destructive: typhus caused a large proportion of deaths in the eighteenth century; smallpox was responsible for the death or disfigurement of one of every ten people in Europe. Conditions resulting from smallpox were even worse in new settlements, where immigrants carried the infection to natives. At one point Cotton Mather wrote that nine of ten, "nay 99 out of 100," of the American Indians perished of smallpox. Cholera epidemics occurred frequently, with the greatest severity in the slum areas. During the nineteenth century major outbreaks of this disease occurred in 1832, 1849, and 1866.

The home of the person who contracted plague was boarded up, and the well members of the family became prisoners of the house and the disease. The imprisonment usually lasted at least a month after all trace of the disease had disappeared. The plague physician wore an elaborate dress—a long red or black leather gown, leather gauntlets, a mask with glass-covered openings for the eyes, and a long beak filled with fumigants and antiseptics. He carried a container of sweet-smelling spices, a meager attempt to thwart the stench in the air. Fires were burned continuously in the streets to help purify the air. The dead were buried at night, usually with great precautions.

The spread of syphilis became so far-reaching that it could truly be called one of the great plagues. Although it was differentiated from epidemic diseases by the close of the fifteenth century, it was thought to be spread in the same manner, through proximity to an infected person. At first the sexual nature of this disease was unknown and no social stigma existed. Social attitudes changed very rapidly, however, as people became aware that syphilis was transferred through sexual relations. Secrecy was common among those who had contracted the disease and led to the foregoing of treatment and the spread of the disease through marriage. At this time barber-surgeons treated syphilitic sores with salves that contained mercury; this treatment was extremely painful.

Urban life, trade, and industrialism contributed to the overwhelming health hazards that existed during these centuries. The situation was confounded by the lack of an adequate means of social control. Reforms were desperately needed. Eventually the organization of physicians, hospitals, and public health activities arose from the alterations brought about by the industrial revolution.

Jean-Honoré Fragonard, *The Visit to the Nursery,* before 1784. Oil on canvas, 73.7 × 92.1 cm. *(Copyright 1995 Board of Trustees, National Gallery of Art, Washington, D.C., Samuel H. Kress Collection.)*

The affectionate attitude toward young children that appeared to be developing in the eighteenth century among Europe's upper-class parents is portrayed in this painting. Previously, these parents tended to shield themselves against the potential loss of several children. It is possible that decreasing mortality rates may have influenced emotional changes and prompted greater intimacy in family life. Here, the father and mother demonstrate genuine love for their child.

HOSPITALS AND REFORMERS

The Reformation brought about the widespread movement toward suppression of monasteries that was led by Martin Luther and Henry VIII. The immediate result of monastic dissolution was that established hospitals and inns were taken away from the public, who had been dependent on them for many years. This was followed by a period of rapid deterioration in the care of the sick and the poor. A decline in the quality of public service, particularly for the sick, thus occurred and created a long period of stagnation and decay. As wars were waged for religious opinion, the sick and the poor were being neglected. The unselfish devotion of the religious orders was no longer available in Protestant countries, where these orders had been oppressed. In this age of callousness and brutality, neither officials nor physicians took any particular interest in elevating nursing or in improving the conditions of hospitals.

Hospital Decay

After the Protestant Revolt, charitable activities were usually divided along religious lines or delegated to secular authorities. The religious struggles had no direct effect on hospitals in Catholic lands such as Spain and Italy. Many small institutions, however, were closed in Protestant countries when the nursing orders were suppressed, and this led to either the necessity for modifications in the large city establishments or the development of city hospitals. Severe utility replaced the beauty that previously had been associated with institutions for the sick.

W.A. Delamotte, *Rahere Ward,* 1844. Drawing. *(St. Bartholomew's Hospital, London, England.)*

This picture has unfortunately been labeled as depicting a "Gamp" type nurse simply because she wears the usual dress of her class at that period. The Dickens character Sairey Gamp was a monthly nurse who attended the sick in their homes, and although hospitals—by no means excluding this one—undoubtedly had many nurses who were uncaring gin-swillers, it is recorded that the Sister of Rahere Ward at the time of this picture was: "stout, ruddy, positive and very watchful . . . she could report correctly the progress of a case; and from her wages she saved all she could and left it in a legacy to the hospital."

Bleeding Knife With Three Blades and Lancing Pin With Ivory Handle and Cover, c. 1790. *(Private Collection/Bridgeman Art Library, London.)*

The hospitals of cities were like prisons, with bare, undecorated walls and little dark rooms, small windows where no sun could enter, and dismal wards where fifty or one hundred patients were crowded together, deprived of all comforts and even of necessaries. In the municipal and state institutions of this period the beautiful gardens, roomy halls, and springs of water of the old cloister hospital of the Middle Ages were not heard of, still less the comforts of their friendly interiors.

— *Nutting and Dock, 1937, p. 500*

Unsanitary conditions that prevailed in these hospitals led to outbreaks of epidemics. Diseases were seldom segregated. "It was not uncommon for the sick to be thrown into beds already occupied by several bedfellows—the dead or the delirious, side by side, perhaps, with those who still lived and retained their reason" (Jamieson and Sewall, 1950, pp. 268–269). Beds were so close together that cleaning was almost impossible. Consequently, all types of rubbish remained under them. Bed baths were not attempted; bleeding and purging were the usual treatments for all conditions. The following description of a late eighteenth century hospital was rendered by Max Nordau:

> In one bed of moderate width lay 4, 5, or 6 sick persons beside each other, the feet of one to the head of another. . . . In the same bed lay individuals inflicted with infectious diseases beside others only slightly unwell; on the same couch, body against body, a woman groaned in the pains of labor, a nursing infant writhed in convulsions, a typhus patient burned in the delirium of fever, a consumptive coughed his hollow cough, and a victim of some diseases of the skin tore with furious nails.

— *Quoted in R. Dalton, 1900, pp. 17–27.*

Mismanagement, inadequate staffing, and exploitation were common occurrences within these facilities. Men who were civil appointees assumed leadership and withheld authority from the women (matrons), who were placed in charge of the secular help doing the "nursing" of the day. Control of nursing was thereby lost by women. This was truly a period of the most complete and general masculine supremacy in the history of nursing. Women were without a voice in both hospital management and nursing organization. In addition, the typical nurses were usually the dregs of society, those individuals who were immoral, drunken, and illiterate. The actual squalor of the times is evident in a portion of the regulations (1789) of the Royal Hospital at Haslar, which were hung in the wards:

III. That no dirt, bones, or rags, be thrown out of any window, or down the bogs, but carried to the places appointed for that purpose; nor are any clothes of the patients, or others, to be hung out of any of the windows of the house.

IV. That no foul linen, whether sheets or shirts, be kept in the cabins, or wards, but sent immediately to the matron, in order to its being carried to the wash-house; and the nurses are to obey the orders of the matron in punctually shifting the bed and body linen of the patients, *viz,* their sheets once a fortnight, their shirts once in four days, their nightcaps, drawers, and stockings once a week, or oftener if found necessary.

V. That no nurse or other person do wash in the water closets. . . .

VIII. That no nurse do admit any patients, on any pretense whatsoever, into her cabin, nor suffer any person to remain in it at night, not even her husband or child.

IX. That any person concealing the escape of any patient from her ward, or that has not made due report, at the agent's office, of her having missed such patient, be discharged the hospital, upon proof thereof.

X. That all nurses who disobey the matron's orders, get drunk, neglect their patients, quarrel or fight with any other nurses, or quarrel with the men, or do not prudently or cautiously reveal, to the superior officers of the house, all irregularities committed by the patients in their wards (such as drinking, smoking tobacco in the wards, quarrelling, destroying the medicines, or stores, reigning complaints and neglecting their cure) be immediately discharged the service of the house, and a note made against their names, on the books of the hospital, that they may never more be employed.

— Howard, 1791, pp. 180–182

In some hospitals nurses were dismissed for abusing the patients. In other hospitals they were reprimanded or dismissed for abuses of various types such as entertaining men at night in wards, scolding patients, or in general patient neglect. Some attempts were thus made to develop qualifications for nurses or sisters who would function in the hospitals. Thomas Fuller (1654–1734), an English physician, developed the first set believing that the nurse should be:

1. Of middle age, fit and able to go through with the necessary Fatigue of her Undertaking.
2. Healthy, especially free from Vapours, and Cough.
3. A good Watcher, that can hold fitting up the whole Course of the Sickness.
4. Quick in Hearing, and always ready at the first Call.
5. Quiet and Still, so as to talk low, and but little, and tread softly.
6. Of good Sight, to observe the Pocks, their Colour, Manner and Growth, and all Alterations that may happen.
7. Handy to do every Thing the best way, without Blundering and Noise.
8. Nimble and Quick a going, coming, and doing every Thing.
9. Cleanly, to make all she dresseth acceptable.
10. Well-tempered, to humour, and please the Sick as much as she can.
11. Cheerful and Pleasant; to make the best of Every Thing, without being at any time Cross, Melancholy, or Timorous.
12. Constantly careful, and diligent by Night and by Day.
13. Sober and Temperate; not given to Gluttony, Drinking, or Smoaking.
14. Observant to follow the Physician's Orders duly; and not be so conceited of her own Skill, as to give her own medicines privately.
15. To have no Children, or other to come much after her.

The English Scene

The most serious consequences in health care occurred in England. It must be remembered, however, that an inward and religious revolution had taken place in England, especially in London, long before Henry VIII legalized its outward and visible form. Many people were ready for the break with Rome, the divorce between Henry and Catherine, and the suppression of the monasteries. This sovereign used the Protestant Revolt to free himself from papal authority with the excuse of the Church's refusal to sanction his divorce. An ulterior motive was based in the fact that monastic properties represented one fifth of his kingdom. Henry VIII suppressed all orders and confiscated the property of more than six hundred charitable endowments. Many of these had been devoted to beggars, orphans, the elderly, and the poor, as well as to those who were acutely ill. Eventually the civil government was forced to take over the general public relief, and this culminated in a "Poor Law" system developed during the reign of Elizabeth.

All the London hospitals were closed in two waves, the smaller ones in 1538 and the larger ones (income over two hundred pounds per annum) in 1540. The fate of the larger English hospitals was particularly important, since they essentially limited their work to the care of the sick. Decisions about their outcome ultimately affected the future of both medicine and nursing. The effect was immediate because "England alone among European countries possessed no hospital system" (Evans and Howard, 1930, p. 69). It was not long before the citizens begged that hospitals be given to the city to be financed and run by civil authorities. In 1547 the city of London petitioned Henry VIII's son, Edward VI, who reigned from 1547 to 1553, for permission to take over the largest hospitals—St. Bartholomew's, St. Thomas's, Bridewell, Bethlehem, and Christ's.

The city arranged to govern these hospitals through a "court" of governors, undertook to add to their endowments, maintained them through private subscription and "rates" (taxes), and assigned to each a specific responsibility for the solution of one social problem. St. Bartholomew's and St. Thomas's hospitals were to care for the sick poor; Bridewell, the unemployed; Bethlehem, the insane; and Christ's, the orphans. With the passage of time the individual functions changed. St. Bartholomew's and St. Thomas's hospitals progressed toward the cure aspect of the general hospital as opposed to the medieval custody function. Bridewell became a workhouse and a house of correction. Knowledge regarding treatment of the insane was lacking, and the conditions in Bethlehem Hospital were dreadful. Over time, the term "Bedlem"—a contraction of "Bethlehem"—came to indicate a state of confusion. Christ's Hospital became one of the leading schools of England. Such was the beginning of the civilian control of hospitals and the advent of lay nursing in England. Care of the sick in these institutions gradually deteriorated for about three hundred years, since England possessed no nursing class. Other Protestant countries followed trends similar to those in England with reorganization of city hospitals.

Religious Nursing Orders

The sixteenth century also saw renewed activity in nursing within the Church itself. Various religious orders devoted to this cause originated in this period. More than a hundred female orders were founded specifically to do nursing. In fact, orders multiplied so rapidly and some had so little permanence that information about them is unavailable. Most prominent among these was an order of men, the Brothers of St. John of God, or the Brothers of Mercy. The name was derived from the inscription on their almsboxes: "Brothers, do good" (*"Fate bene, fratelli"*). This order was founded in Spain in 1538 by a Portuguese, Jean Ciudad (1495–1550), known as John of God (Juan di Dios). After spending eighteen years as a soldier, he vowed to devote his life to God if he recovered from a wound received in battle. In 1540 John opened a hospital in Granada and invited a group of friends to assist with the nursing care. At first these brothers were laymen, not monks, and they worked without a rule until 1570. They were mendicants who devoted themselves to nursing, hospital work, the distribution of medicines, the tender care of the mentally ill and abandoned children, and the visitation of the sick at home. Those in need were cared for in a very loving and special way. Homeless vagrants, the crippled, and even derelicts received devoted nursing service. It is said that St. John himself carried on his back the deformed who were unable to walk or crawl to the hospital. The Brothers of St. John eventually opened hospitals at Madrid, Cordova, Toledo, Naples, and Paris. This order spread over a large part of the civilized world within fifty years of its founding. Its members were probably the best-known nursing brothers *(baumherzigen Brüder)* in Catholic Germany by the eighteenth century. Paintings of Juan di Dios frequently show wards of a hospital in the background.

Another notable nursing order of men, the Nursing Order of Ministers of the Sick, was founded by St. Camillus De Lellis (1550–1614). St. Camillus was totally committed to alleviating the sufferings of human beings, a service that was dependent on love. He achieved success in the care of the dying and eventually opened a hospital for alcoholics in Germany. His Nursing Order of Ministers of the Sick, an Italian order, did hospital work and specially cared for those stricken with the plague in Rome in 1590. Conflicting information exists regarding the early life of St. Camillus. What is important, however, is that a series of illnesses that necessitated his hospitalization stirred him to devote himself to the care of the sick. The members of his order, popularly known as the Camillian Fathers and Brothers, took the three regular vows plus a fourth, a pledge to the work of nursing. They wore a red cross on their cassocks.

Perhaps the most interesting of these later organizations and one that has maintained importance until the present day is the Sisters of Charity founded by St. Vincent de Paul (1576–1660). This order developed at a time when destitution and disease from continual wars were overcoming France. Political unrest was also great. St. Vincent offered solutions to these problems that were both revolutionary and visionary. He was a quiet, unassuming French Catholic priest (Franciscan) whose experiences in his earlier life prepared him to assist with the sufferings of humanity. Of particular note were his capture by Barbary pirates and his sale as a slave to the Turks. St. Vincent described this experience in a personal letter:

> This is how they set about disposing of us. After having stripped us naked, they bestowed on each of us a pair of breeches, a linen doublet and a cap, and marched us through the streets of Tunis, whither they had come in order to sell us. After having perambulated the town five or six times with chains round our necks, we

Jacob Jordaens, *The Sisters of Charity of Antwerp*, c. 1635. 226 × 269 cm. *(Koninklijk Museum voor Schone Kunsten, Antwerpen [België].)*

In seventeenth century Catholic Flanders, the artistic use of the nurse was a means of illustrating social tensions in a society that was both intensely religious and intensely secular. The image of the nurse was used to clarify religious and social relationships and in a sense explained more about the society than about the nurses. Jacob Jordaens painted this group of nursing sisters at work for the Hospice of St. Elizabeth in Antwerp. Hospitals and the arts were supported by the wealth of Flanders, which permitted the perpetuation of the tradition of the nursing sister in paintings and sculpture in the seventeenth and eighteenth centuries. The Catholic obligation to perform good or charitable works was validated through paintings.

Jean Restout II, *St. Vincent de Paul Appointed as Almoner to the Sisters of the Visitation,* c. 1729. *(Church of Saint Marguerite, Paris, France. Photographie Bulloz.)*

St. Vincent was instrumental in reforms for the poor and hospital reforms. Groups of men and women who formed under his counsel constituted the first societies for organized charity.

St. Vincent de Paul, nineteenth century. Engraving. *(The Bettmann Archive, New York.)*

were taken back to the boat for the dealers to come and see who could eat and who could not, by way of proving that our wounds were not mortal. When this was over they led us into the marketplace, where the dealers came and inspected us precisely as one does when one is buying a horse or an ox, opening our mouths to examine our teeth, feeling our sides, probing our wounds, making us walk, trot and run, carrying burdens the while, then setting us to wrestle in order to judge of our respective strength, and indulging in hundreds of other brutal proceedings.

— *Quoted in Robinson, 1946, p. 63*

Eventually, St. Vincent was able to return to Paris, where he was appalled at the conditions of the poor and the sick poor in such a large town. He began to assist the Brothers of St. John of God with the care of patients in the Charité Hospital in Paris. His interests soon reached out into provincial communities, and in 1617 he moved to the country parish of Châtillon-en-Bresse. Here St. Vincent was asked to appeal on behalf of a destitute family, and he became distressed at the indiscriminate relief that was called forth. The family was inundated by well-meaning individuals. This event vividly demonstrated charity's waste from lack of control. It proved to be the motivating force for St. Vincent's institution of a society of ladies called the Confrérie de la Charité (Dames de Charité), whose members visited the sick in their homes to render both nursing care and spiritual consolation. This was the first society for organized aid in which a service was offered to as many people as possible, with a minimum of duplication. The membership of eleven women took no vows and did not make any kind of promises. From this simple beginning, associations arose in numerous towns and villages. At first, all the branches were composed of women, but later a branch for men was founded at Folleville. With the extension of services into homes in the centuries that followed, St. Vincent became a regular feature of the work of certain communities. Sympathy for the poor was combined with a genius for organized reform and led to a system of social service, a method to help people help themselves.

Mlle Le Gras (1591–1660) became the first supervisor of these community nurses. St. Louise de Marillac, as she was later known, was a woman of noble birth and a widow when she became associated with the work of St. Vincent. In 1629 and 1631 she was sent on tours of the provincial associations to investigate their work and assist them with improvements in their care. A secular nursing order called Les Filles de Charité, or the Sisters of Charity, was founded in 1633, and St. Louise became its superior. The Filles were initially under no written rule but merely followed a few regulations that had been drawn up by Mlle Le Gras. Young single girls were recruited; they were required to be intelligent, refined, and sincerely interested in the sick poor. An educational program was established to include experience in the hospital, home visits, and care of the sick. Such was the modest and humble beginning of the now famous Sisters of Charity. (They, perhaps, should be called Daughters of Charity, since St. Vincent always referred to them as "Filles.")

On March 25, 1634, approximately one year after this community was formed, St. Louise formally took a vow to devote herself to this life. She thus became the first Sister of Charity of St. Vincent de Paul. In the year 1642 the first four sisters took vows that were, and still are, only annual. This order was a tremendous innovation because it was active yet uncloistered. (The Church insisted that consecrated virgins be cloistered.) St. Vincent was adamant in this regard and expressed his ideal quite eloquently:

> Their convent must be the houses of the sick; their cell the chamber of suffering; their chapel the parish church; their cloister the streets of the city or the wards of hospitals; in place of the rule which binds nuns to the one enclosure, there must be the general vow of obedience; the grating through which they speak to others must be the fear of God; the veil which shuts out the world must be holy modesty.

> — *Nutting and Dock, 1937, p. 436*

The sisters' spiritual training was in the hands of St. Vincent, who provided a weekly lecture conference. These talks were written down by St. Louise, and about one hundred and sixty have been preserved. "They are a model of simplicity and clearness and remain the earliest as well as one of the best series of addresses on nursing ethics" (Seymer, 1932, p. 54). The organizational pattern of this order was composed of the following:

- A selected group, with set regulations restricting acceptance
- A common home with experienced supervision
- A system of instruction
- A probation of two months followed by a training period of five years
- Protection by the use of uniform dress of a type which would distinguish them from the people about them, and at the same time be secular
- Annual renewal of vows, or freedom to leave for marriage or change of occupation

> — *Jamieson and Sewall, 1950, p. 323*

The dress of the Sisters of Charity did indeed become distinctive—a gray-blue gown and apron of rough woolen cloth, a stiff white collar, and a white, spreading headdress called a cornette. In 1809 the sisters were introduced into America by Mother Elizabeth Seton (1774–1821), the first American-born person to be canonized. A community was established at Emmitsburg, Maryland, after the rule of the Motherhouse in France had been obtained. It was not until 1815 that Mother Mary Aikenhead organized a community in Dublin.

The work of the society was ever expanding into new fields. One important role was the development of special skills in caring for abandoned children. With the encouragement of St. Vincent the women went into action to save these doomed children. They wandered the dark streets and gathered the babies who had been thrown away. Unwanted infants were frequently brought

Nicaragua's 1963 issue of a three-stamp set, to which this stamp belongs, marked the three hundredth anniversary (in 1960) of the deaths of St. Vincent de Paul and St. Luisa de Marillac. Known as "the nurse of the poor," St. Luisa de Marillac was founder of the Sisters of Charity of St. Vincent de Paul. She was canonized in 1934. *(Courtesy of Howard B. Hurley.)*

A semi-postal emission from Austria in 1937 consisted of four denominations, each with a surcharge for charitable purposes. Included were stamps depicting nurse and infant, nursing of the aged, and the illustrated value showing a Sister of Mercy with patient. *(Courtesy of Howard B. Hurley.)*

This 1958 Irish stamp honors Mother Mary Aikenhead (1787–1858), the first Sister of Charity of the Irish order of St. Vincent de Paul. Among the earliest visiting nurses, she organized a community in Dublin; a lay school for nurses was established in 1892. *(Stamp courtesy of Medical Economics Publishing, New Jersey.)*

Robert Vickrey, *Sister of Charity*, 1965.
Tempera. 45.8 × 60.9 cm. *(Copyright Robert Vickrey/VAGA, New York.)*

The Sisters of Charity were organized by St. Vincent de Paul and were perhaps the most widespread and best loved of all nursing orders. They took charge of hospitals, the poor, asylums, and parish work. They became widely known as visiting nurses, since they also cared for the poor and the sick in their homes.

St. Vincent de Paul Being Shown Three Small Children, eighteenth century. From a painting in the old Paris Foundling Asylum. *(Musée de l'Assistance Publique-Hopitaux de Paris, France.)*

to the Hospice des Enfants Trouvés et Orphelins, established by Vincent's disciples, where the Sisters of Charity served as nurses. This organized relief for the foundlings of Paris led to the portrayal of St. Vincent with orphans in his arms, wrapped in his cloak. The sisters also took charge of hospitals, foundling asylums, and homes for the insane, and they engaged in general parish work. They taught in schools, gave heroic service during many wars, and offered care to lepers. The modern principles of visiting nursing and social service were sown during this time.

Humanitarian Efforts

The existence of actual deterioration in hospitals during this time is beyond dispute. A period of stagnation had set in, and little or no progress in the art of nursing was made, particularly in Protestant countries. There is evidence of the squalor of the hospitals and the inferiority of the attendants within them. The era of reform, however, was on the horizon. A number of humane individuals were stirred by the painful social conditions of the eighteenth century and began to labor for change. Of those reformers who lived before the nineteenth century, one of the best known was John Howard (1727–1789). Howard, an English philanthropist, spent his life and fortune examining and reporting on the conditions of prisons, dungeons, pesthouses, hospitals, and asylums. His series of investigations were probably the most powerful factor in the improvement of public institutions in this era. Howard's writings depicted the story of the degradation of often forgotten human beings. Although prisons and lazarettos were his chief concern, he left graphic notes of what he observed in hospitals. His reports on hospitals were the most authentic of the time and emphasized the necessity for fresh air and cleanliness. Howard's only praise was extended to the Sisters of Charity and the Beguines. His accounts were varied, sometimes limited to a few sentences and other times consisting of long commentaries, as in the case of the Knights of St. John's Hospital at Malta:

One ward is for patients dangerously sick or dying; another for patients of the middle rank of life; and the third for the lower and poorer sort of patients. In this last ward (which is the largest) there are four rows of beds; in the others, only two. They were all so dirty and offensive as to create the necessity of perfuming them; and yet I observed that the physician, in going his rounds, was obliged to keep his handkerchief to his face. . . .

From the kitchen (which is darker and more offensive than even the lower hall, to which it adjoins) the broth, rice soup and vermicelli are brought in dirty kettles first to the upper hall, and there poured into three silver bowls, out of which the patients are served. . . .

The number of patients in the hospital during the time I was in Malta (March 28th to April 19, 1786) was from five hundred and ten to five hundred and thirty-two. These were served by the most dirty, ragged, unfeeling and unhuman persons I ever saw. I once found eight or nine of them highly entertained with a delirious *dying* patient. The governor told me that they had only twenty-two servants, and that many of them were debtors or criminals, who had fled thither for refuge.

— *Howard, 1791, pp. 58–60*

The writings of John Howard were serious and had their effect. However, they penetrated society slowly, and for another generation or two shameful conditions continued in both hospitals and nursing. Through Howard's efforts vast prison reforms ultimately occurred and conditions were vastly improved.

Interest in reform grew steadily, and the movement brought about many changes that influenced health care and nursing. Humanitarian leaders emerged and dwelt on a sense of social responsibility for the welfare of others. One of these was the notable social reformer, Elizabeth Gurney Fry (1780–1845), who was closely identified with practical reforms and the revival of nursing. Elizabeth Gurney was a deeply religious Quaker who married Joseph Fry and settled in London. She was beautiful, a gifted speaker, and the

This satirical aquatint was published to portray Elizabeth Fry's "unwomanly" public role, which sometimes evoked censure and hostile gossip, c. 1825. *(Religious Society of Friends, London, England.)*

"AN HOUR IN NEWGATE" *Exhibiting* Mrs. FRY *and her friends; as published by the* QUAKERS.

mother of eleven children. She, too, gave conspicuous service in prison reform based on principles similar to those of John Howard. She visited Newgate Prison in 1813 and was appalled by the conditions and treatment of the incarcerated prisoners. Murderers, sex offenders, thieves, and the mentally ill and retarded were all housed together in dark, damp, and poorly ventilated living quarters. Even children were inmates of this prison; they accompanied their parents if there were no relatives who could or would care for them. Such children were thus raised in an environment where there was a scant supply of food and little adequate clothing. Although the exterior of Newgate was beautiful, conditions within the walls were deplorable, as a description of the women's quarters illustrates:

> They occupied two long rooms, where they slept in three tiers, some on the floor and two tiers of hammocks over one another. . . . When I first entered, the foulness of the air was almost insupportable; and everything that is base and depraved was so strongly depicted on the faces of the women who stood crowded before me with looks of effrontery, boldness and wantonness of expression that for a while my soul was greatly dismayed.
>
> — *Whitney, 1936, p. 193*

> The infirmary was not much better: On going up, I was astonished beyond description at the mass of woe and misery I beheld. I found many very sick, lying on the bare floor or on some old straw, having very scanty covering over them, though it was quite cold; and there were several children born in the prison among them, almost naked.
>
> — *Whitney, 1936, p. 184*

In *David Copperfield* Charles Dickens vividly portrayed Newgate using humorous, pointed descriptions of the existing evils. Few who read his story realized that it was one of personal experience. Dickens's father had been locked up in debtors' prison, where the entire family had resided until a fortunate legacy set them free. This novel brought the conditions of the English gaols to the attention of groups that may have ignored the reports of Elizabeth Fry.

In 1817 Elizabeth Fry established an association for improving the lot of women prisoners in Newgate Prison. She began a program of instruction for

Elizabeth Fry Reading to the Prisoners in Newgate Prison, 1823, nineteenth century. From an engraving after Jerry Barrett. *(Religious Society of Friends, London, England.)*

the children, arranged for sewing rooms for the women, found books for those who wanted to read, and was instrumental in developing a prison shop where materials produced in the prison could be sold outside. (Income from the sales would go to the workers.) In 1818 she visited other prisons in the British Isles and became known for her investigations of prison conditions and her attempts to arouse public opinion.

Elizabeth Fry, who became widely known as a philanthropist, eventually founded a society for visiting nursing that had its origin in her prison work. This group of ardent workers was called the Society of Protestant Sisters of Charity (1840). They were not, however, affiliated with any church and later were known as the Institute of Nursing Sisters. The members were prepared for private nursing only, to nurse the sick of all classes in their homes. These women received no classroom or theoretical instruction; for several hours a day for a few months' period, they visited Guy's Hospital in London, where they obtained a minimum of practical experience. A similar organization was founded among the Quakers in Philadelphia at a later date.

Elizabeth Fry kept in close contact with other leaders of humane thought. Among these was Amalie Sieveking (1794–1859) of Hamburg, Germany, a well-known author who was prominent in the "women's movement." Sieveking wished to develop a Protestant counterpart of the Sisters of Charity but was not successful. She therefore formed a group of volunteers, the Friends of the Poor, who visited the poor and the sick and gave nursing care in homes. Both men and women were originally included in this organization, and the women were called "nurses" rather than "deaconesses." Amalie Sieveking was also interested in the establishment of better housing for low-income groups, distribution of food, finding employment for the disabled, and other types of social service for the poor. She enlisted the aid of women who were interested in a larger sphere of women's work outside the home. From this time, social work and nursing thus became closely connected to feminist movements.

More than a century later, the efforts of Dorothea Lynde Dix (1802–1887) on behalf of the insane in the United States were comparable to the work of Howard and Fry. She focused on two distinct problems: the care of the criminal and the care of the mentally ill. Dorothea Dix found that many of the prisoners were actually mentally ill and their treatment was negligible. Her efforts, begun at the age of thirty-nine, eventually earned her the title of "The John Howard of America." Her constructive work in surveying the needs of the mental patients and prisoners in Massachusetts led to the establishment of more than thirty psychiatric hospitals in the United States. One of these, Butler Hospital, was founded in Rhode Island with the backing of a wealthy and influential gentleman named Cyrus Butler.

The accomplishments of Dorothea Dix were many, including the construction of the first state psychiatric hospital in Trenton, New Jersey; the elevation of standards of care for the mentally ill in the United States and Canada; and the systematic and careful recording of observations to be presented to the legislature to elicit support for humane treatment of the mentally ill. Dix had personally observed the incredible practices associated with these patients: some were confined in cages, closets, and cellars; other patients were chained and naked; and some were beaten into submission with rods or other implements. Her crusades continued for approximately twenty years and resulted in a system of mental hospitals under government control. Legal commitment based on medical diagnosis, abolition of restraints, and expertness of supervision provided the backbone of these institutions.

Dorothea Dix was the pioneer crusader for the mentally ill in the United States. Before her endeavors, few people realized that the mentally ill needed humane treatment or that they were classified by law as comparable to criminals. Frequently the mentally ill were used as entertainment for the public, who paid a fee to witness their antics. In some locations they were kept in almshouses or jails. The most unfortunate aspect of this situation was that mental illness was thought to be incurable. Consequently, incentives for reform were lacking, and efforts toward change were not understood. It thus took a persistent individual such as Dorothea Dix to initiate a movement to correct an unpardonable situation.

Francisco y Lucientes Goya. *The Madhouse,* c. 1812–1819. Canvas. *(Real Academia de Bellas Artes de San Fernando, Madrid/Bridgeman Art Library, London/SuperStock.)*

SOCIAL REFORMS AND NURSING

The great revival of learning left the care of the sick untouched and unimproved. This was probably because of the prevailing thought that nursing was a religious rather than an intellectual occupation. Therefore scientific improvement was not considered necessary. Yet the religious motive was lacking in the lay persons who were employed to care for the sick after the Reformation had occurred. Intelligent persons could not be persuaded to undertake nursing in the offensive municipal hospitals. Nursing slipped back into its ancient position of menial work, and the disagreeable features of nursing assumed prominence.

The latter half of the period between 1500 and 1860 saw nursing conditions at their worst. The "Dark Period of Nursing" had indeed arrived. In general, the lay attendants or nurses were illiterate, rough, and inconsiderate, oftentimes immoral or alcoholic. When a woman could no longer earn a living from gambling or vice, she might become a nurse. Nurses were drawn from among discharged patients, prisoners, and the lowest strata of society. They scrubbed, washed, cleaned, worked long hours (sometimes twenty-four to forty-eight hours at a stretch) and essentially led a life of drudgery. Roaches, other insects, and vermin plagued the nurses in the hospitals of this period. Pay for nurses was poor and was frequently supplemented in any way pos-

"Sairey Gamp," a Nurse of Sixty Years Ago, c. 1907. *(Illustration from the Wellcome Trustees' Professional Nurse Diary. Wellcome Institute Library, London, England.)*

191

The Monthly Nurse, c. 1840. *(The Mansell Collection Limited, London, England.)*

This illustration appeared around 1840 in *Tristram Shandy*. The following passage descibes the household staff's feelings of relief as the "monthly nurse," or midwife, arrives to deliver the mistress's baby: "From the very moment the mistress of the house is brought to bed every female in it, from my lady's gentlewoman down to the cinderwench, becomes an inch taller for it."

Facing page, Frederick Barnard, *Mrs. Gamp.* From Charles Dickens' *Martin Chuzzlewit,* first published in 1844. *(The Bettmann Archive, New York.)*

Sairey Gamp was the best-known literary image of a nurse until contemporary times. She clearly reflects Dickens' attitude toward nurses, those women who "care for the sick" by neglecting them, stealing from them, and at times physically abusing them. According to Dickens, Mrs. Gamp not only cared for the sick but also delivered babies and prepared bodies for burial. These functions were exclusively the function of women before the evolution of male obstetricians and funeral directors.

sible. The nurses expected and took bribes whenever they could be obtained. This deplorable status of nurses and nursing continued throughout this period. There was little organization associated with nursing and certainly no social standing. No one would enter nursing who could possibly earn a living in some other way. As nurses, even the sisters of the religious orders came to a complete standstill professionally because of a persistent sequence of restrictions from the middle of the sixteenth century (Nutting and Dock, 1937).

The search into the social evils of the eighteenth century included an examination of nursing. Hogarth's cartoons and Charles Dickens's later descriptions of nurses were effective caricatures. In *Martin Chuzzlewit* (1844) Dickens depicted nursing conditions through the immortal characters of Sairey Gamp and Betsy Prig. Mrs. Gamp represented the hired attendant for the sick, the private duty nurse; Mrs. Prig portrayed the hospital nurse. Sairey Gamp was, in reality, not a fictitious character but an actual nurse Dickens's friend had hired for a member of his family. Both of these women cheated their employers, tricked their patients, and stole their rations and possessions. They demanded that the patients pay for extra little services, and they were deliberately cruel to the sick who were at their mercy. In a later preface to the novel (November 1849), Dickens remarked:

> Mrs. Sarah Gamp is a representation of the hired attendant on the poor in sickness. The Hospitals of London are, in many respects, noble institutions; in others, very defective. I think it not the least among the instances of their mismanagement, that Mrs. Betsy Prig is a fair specimen of Hospital Nurse; and that the Hospitals, with their means and funds, should have left it to private humanity and enterprise, in the year Eighteen Hundred and Forty-nine, to enter on an attempt to improve that class of persons.
>
> — *Dickens, 1910, p. xxviii*

Mrs. Gamp's first appearance in the novel occurred when she was summoned by Mr. Pecksniff to prepare the body of Anthony Chuzzlewit for burial:

> She was a fat old woman, this Mrs. Gamp, with a husky voice, and a moist eye, which she had a remarkable power of turning up and showing the white of it. Having very little neck, it cost her some trouble to look over herself if one may say so, to those to whom she talked. She wore a very rusty black gown, rather the worse for snuff, and a shawl and bonnet to correspond. In these dilapidated articles of dress she had, on principle, arrayed herself, time out of mind, on such occasions as the present; for this at once expressed a decent amount of veneration for the deceased, and invited the next of kin to present her with a fresher suit of weeds: an appeal so frequently successful, that the very fetch and ghost of Mrs. Gamp, bonnet and all, might be seen hanging up, any hour in the day, in at least a dozen of the second-hand clothes shops about Holborn. The face of Mrs. Gamp—the nose in particular—was somewhat red and swollen, and it was difficult to enjoy her society without becoming conscious of a smell of spirits. Like most persons who have attained to great eminence in their profession, she took to hers very kindly; insomuch, that setting aside her natural predilections as a woman, she went to a lying-in or a laying-out with equal zest and relish.
>
> — *Dickens, 1910, pp. 312–313*

Leigh Hunt, a contemporary of Dickens, also gave his version of the midwife specialist, which Sairey also professed to be. (Mrs. Gamp considered herself a monthly nurse, or, as her signboard boldly stated, "midwife.")

> Her greatest pleasure in life is, when lady and baby are both gone to sleep, the fire bright, the kettle boiling, and her corns quiescent. She then first takes a pinch of snuff, by way of pungent anticipation of bliss, or as a sort of concentrated essence of satisfaction; then a glass of spirits—then puts the water in the teapot—

takes another glass of spirits (the last having been a small one, and the coming tea affording a "counteraction")—then smoothes down her apron, adjusts herself in her arm-chair, pours out the first cup of tea, and sits for a minute or two staring at the fire, with the solid complacence of an owl—perhaps not without something of his snore, between sneeze and snuffbox.

— *Hunt, 1889*

Help was needed for the prevailing nursing situation, and public interest in its improvement began to be demonstrated among various groups. Doctors, clergy, and philanthropic citizens advocated the establishment of nursing systems of a different character. Some favored a system under religious auspices, others a secular plan involving paid nurses. This public concern resulted in the beginning of significant changes that directed steady reform in nursing.

The Birth of Modern Nursing

One of the most important factors in the regeneration of nursing was the Deaconess Institute at Kaiserswerth, Germany, established in 1836 by Pastor Theodor Fliedner (1800–1864). The deaconess orders, which had existed at the time of Christ, were revived by the Protestant churches during the nineteenth century. This movement was sparked by the recognition of the need for the services of women. In a number of instances women were prompted by religious motives to perform social services, and the care of the sick became their chief duty. Kaiserswerth became the most significant organization of Protestant deaconesses for nursing service; it is credited with creating the first modern order of deaconesses.

This institute was started on a modest scale, yet made an indelible impression on the whole of nursing that was to follow. It indirectly influenced individuals such as Florence Nightingale, who stayed there for a brief time. Pastor Fliedner, who had been appointed to the parish of Kaiserswerth in 1822, began his social work by founding a German Prison Association (Rheinisch-Westfälischer Gefängnisverein) in 1826. The first of its kind in Germany, it

Mrs. Gamp Proposes a Toast. From Charles Dickens' Martin Chuzzlewit. (The Bettmann Archive, New York.)

The Deaconess Institute at Kaiserswerth, c. 1848. Engraving. (The Bettmann Archive, New York.)

was inspired by the work already done in prison reforms in England and Holland. Fliedner had traveled abroad to raise money for his struggling parish and observed these changes firsthand. He met Elizabeth Fry and was impressed with her work at Newgate Prison. He inspected hospitals, almshouses, and prisons in Holland, where he observed the work of deaconesses. He married Friederike Münster (1800–1842) in 1828, and their joint activities in prison reform led to the start of a small refuge for discharged prisoners in 1833. This asylum, as it was called, was the first of many units that formed the institute.

The Fliedners next turned their attention to the care of the sick and opened a small hospital with a training school for deaconesses. This hospital was started in a house, and the first deaconess, Gertrude Reichardt, the daughter of a physician, was admitted in 1836. By the end of the first year, six other women joined her for training. These deaconesses took no vows but simply promised to work for Christ. Although they received no salary, they were taken care of for life, an arrangement known as the *motherhouse system*. It was an offspring of the monastic system and offered security, since the deaconesses were provided with a permanent home and protection. They were sent out to district, hospital, and private duty assignments or to distant mission fields. Their dress was a plain blue cotton gown with a white apron and a large turned-down collar. A white muslin cap with a frill around the face was tied under the chin with a large white bow. Long black cloaks and black bonnets over their caps were worn outdoors.

The movement of the institute expanded rapidly, and "by 1840 the work at the Kaiserswerth hospital had grown so much that two other adjoining houses were bought; by 1842 the total bed capacity was over two hundred, and the institute itself, now too small to house all the Deaconesses, had to be rebuilt" (Seymer, 1932, p. 63). The training of the deaconesses was designed to prepare them for both teaching and nursing. The program in nursing included a rotation in hospital clinical services (experience on wards for men, women, and children, as well as on wards for communicable disease, convalescents, and sick deaconesses), instruction in visiting nursing, theoretical

The Children's Hall in the Deaconess Institute at Kaiserswerth, c. 1850. Engraving. (The Bettmann Archive, New York.)

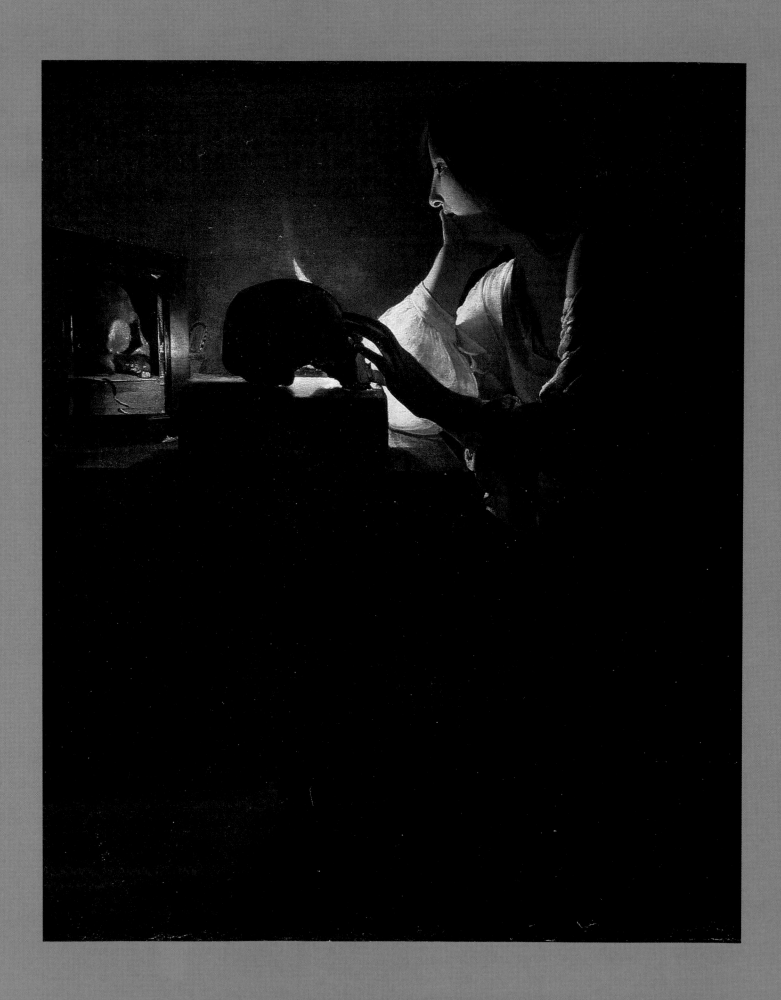

and bedside instruction in the care of the sick, instruction in religious doctrine and ethics, and enough pharmacy to pass the state examinations for pharmacists. This program of study took three years. An interesting principle was enforced in that the nurses were required to follow the physician's orders exactly and that the physician alone was responsible for the outcome.

> It is interesting to see how much of their system and detail our modern training schools have inherited from the Motherhouse—the probationary system, and the school for preparatory training; the letters from clergyman and physician as to character and health; the allowance of pocket-money; the grading of work, from easy to difficult; the chain of responsibility; the grading of pupils from probationer to head nurse, with the superintendent at the head; the class-work and lectures; and every principle of discipline, etiquette, and ethics. The combination of a semi-military form of professional discipline with social equality, found in the Motherhouse, gave the pattern to the early American schools even more than did the English schools, whose system of class distinctions was never established in America.
>
> — *Nutting and Dock, vol. 2, 1907, p. 40*

A framework of organization evolved at Kaiserswerth that incorporated many facets of service. These were divided into four areas: nursing, relief of the poor, the care of children, and work among the unfortunate women who were prisoners and "Magdalens." The institute became so well known that many individuals came to study its methods. Friederike Fliedner, the ambitious, energetic cofounder of Kaiserswerth, died in 1842. After her death, Pastor Fliedner married Caroline Bertheau (1811–1892), who had acted for three years as superintendent of the female surgical department of the Hamburg Hospital. Her nursing experience proved to be extremely valuable to the continuation of the work at the institute. The Kaiserswerth influence spread far beyond the German boundaries. In 1849 Fliedner escorted four deaconesses to Pittsburgh, Pennsylvania, where they were to assume responsibility for the Pittsburgh Infirmary (currently Passavant Hospital); other branches were founded in Jerusalem, Smyrna, Constantinople, Beirut, and Alexandria. Graduates of the program went to all corners of the globe to assist with the care of the sick and the needy. These beginnings set the stage for the founding of a new system of nursing by Florence Nightingale, whose reforms drastically changed the care of the sick throughout the world.

The Nightingale Revolution

> Miss Nightingale introduced sanitary science through female nursing in military hospitals by reducing the death rate of the British Army from 42 to 2 per cent (1854–55); protested against the corridor system of hospitals and fought for pavilions (1856); printed her extensive octavo on the health of the army (1858); issued the anonymous blue book on military sanitation in which she demonstrated the frightful but preventable mortality of the recent war (1859); showed the relationship of sanitary science to medical institutions (*Notes on Hospitals,* 1859); wrote the authoritative text of modern nursing (*Notes on Nursing,* 1859); established the Army Medical School at Fort Pitt, Chatham, and chose its faculty (1860); and founded the first training school for nurses (St. Thomas's Hospital, 1860). Florence Nightingale epitomized her lifework when she wrote in a private note: 'I stand at the altar of the murdered men, and, while I live, I fight their cause.' Florence Nightingale was the greatest war nurse in history.
>
> — *Robinson, 1946, p. 129*

It is doubtful whether any woman's story has been repeated more often than that of Florence Nightingale. Yet existing accounts fall short in efforts to document totally her place in the sphere of social progress. Unquestionably, she was a significant individual in nursing's history and has been identified as the pioneer and founder of modern nursing as well as a reformer of hospitals.

Facing page, Georges de La Tour, *The Repentant Magdalene,* c. 1640. Oil on canvas, 113.3 × 92.7 cm. *(Copyright 1995 Board of Trustees, National Gallery of Art, Washington, D.C., Ailsa Mellon Bruce Fund.)*

Unfortunate women were often referred to as "magdalens." They were usually women who were prisoners and/or were reformed prostitutes. The term *magdalen* also evolved to indicate a house of refuge or reformatory for prostitutes.

influence on her life, since it was through him that she later went to the Crimea and with him that she formed "the little war office." On this particular journey she also became familiar with the nursing of Roman Catholic sisterhoods. Her travels took her to Egypt, Greece, and eventually Germany, where she spent a fortnight at Kaiserswerth. Later in 1847 she enrolled in the program for nursing at Kaiserswerth and finished the three-month program. She spoke of this institute as her "spiritual home," although she would not admit that she had "trained" there. In her opinion the hospital work of the deaconesses was not on a level with the rest (Cook, 1913). In 1853 Nightingale studied in Paris under the Sisters of Charity at the Maison de la Providence. Returning to London, she assumed an administrative position as superintendent of the Establishment for Gentlewomen During Illness, a charity hospital for governesses that was run by titled ladies. She remained for a year and succeeded in creating a model institution by the standards of the day. However, she was disappointed that she was unable to initiate a formal training school for nurses. As she began to plan and prepare for the superintendent's position at King's College Hospital, British and French troops invaded the Crimea in support of Turkey's dispute with Russia. This event precipitated an unexpected opportunity for achievement.

The hour and the woman. In his biography of Florence Nightingale, Cook (1913) used the chapter heading "The Hour and the Woman" to express the period of Nightingale's life during the time of the Crimean War. No other phrase could better describe the union that occurred between the national need and the woman who was most fit to meet it. Soon after the outbreak of the Crimean War, England rang with the stories of the base at Scutari. With the British army was the first war correspondent, William Howard Russell of The *Times* (London), who quickly dispatched vivid reports of conditions of soldiers and the utter inadequacy of their care in October 1854.

Designed by Reynolds, Francis, & Rohnstock. "The Crimea," c. 1938. Stained glass. Panel from *The Nightingale Window.* *(Washington National Cathedral, Washington D.C. Courtesy of Morton Broffman.)*

The great work for which Nightingale is best remembered is symbolized by the well known subject, "The Lady of the Lamp," immortalized by Henry Wadsworth Longfellow in his 1857 poem.

It is with feelings of surprise and anger that the public will learn that no sufficient preparations have been made for the proper care of the wounded. Not only are there not sufficient surgeons . . . not only are there no dressers and nurses . . . there is not even linen to make bandages . . . it is found that the commonest appliances of a workhouse sick-ward are wanting, and that the men must die through the medical staff of the British army having forgotten that old rags are necessary for the dressing of wounds. . . . The manner in which the sick and wounded are treated is worthy only of the savages of Dahomey. . . . Here the French are greatly our superiors. Their medical arrangements are extremely good, their surgeons more numerous, and they have also the help of the Sisters of Charity, who have accompanied the expedition in incredible numbers. These devoted women are excellent nurses.

— Woodham-Smith, 1951, p. 85

An appalling picture of the army's inefficiency was thus presented to the public; it illustrated the high death rate from wounds, infections, cholera, and lack of adequate care. The country was seething with rage, and a letter in The *Times* demanded angrily, "Why have we no Sisters of Charity?"

Sir Sidney Herbert, by then the secretary of war, decided to defy precedent and for the first time in English history send a contingent of female nurses to military hospitals. He knew of one woman capable of bringing order out of the chaos and immediately wrote his remarkable letter (October 15, 1854) to Florence Nightingale, requesting her services. It contained a plea to supervise the military hospitals in Turkey:

There is but one person in England that I know of who would be capable of organising and superintending such a scheme. . . .

The selection of the rank and file of nurses will be very difficult: no one knows it better than yourself. The difficulty of finding women equal to a task, after all, full of horrors, and requiring, besides knowledge and goodwill, great energy and great courage, will be great. . . . My question simply is, Would you listen to the request to go and superintend the whole thing? You would of course have plenary authority over all the nurses, and I think I could secure you the fullest assistance and co-operation from the medical staff, and you would also have an unlimited power of drawing on the Government for whatever you thought requisite for the success of your mission. . . . but I must not conceal from you that I think upon your decision will depend the ultimate success or failure of the plan. Your own personal qualities, your knowledge and your power of administration, and among greater things your rank and position in Society give you advantages in such a work which no other person possesses.

— Woodham-Smith, 1951, pp. 87–89

Florence Nightingale was appointed "Superintendent of the Female Nursing Establishment of the English General Hospitals in Turkey." She left for the base hospital at Scutari on October 21, 1854, accompanied by thirty-eight nurses. (She realized that several were unfit, but time was of the essence.) They included ten Roman Catholic sisters from Bermondsey, eight Anglican sisters from the Sellonite order, six nurses from St. John's House, and fourteen from various hospitals. The vast Barrack Hospital, which resembled a hollow square with a tower at each corner, was crowded with four miles of beds. It was designed to accommodate seventeen hundred patients, but between three thousand and four thousand were packed into it. Candles sticking in empty beer bottles lit up endless scenes of human agony. An open sewer that attracted rats and vermin was immediately under the building. There was no water, no soap; there were no towels, few utensils of any sort, no knives or forks, and putrid food. It took four hours to serve a meal that for all practical purposes was not edible. Men lay practically naked or in ragged uniforms clotted with blood. When available, canvas sheets were used; these were so coarse that the wounded men begged to be left in their blankets. Essential surgical and medical supplies were lacking, and there was no dietary or laundry equipment of any kind. The death rate was 42.7 percent.

Designed by Reynolds, Francis, & Rohnstock. *The Nightingale Window*, c. 1938. Stained glass. *(Courtesy Washington National Cathedral, Washington D.C.)*

The window was dedicated in 1938 and portrays the theme of "The Glorification of Nursing." The six medallions are wrought in richly glowing colors and depict six phases of Florence Nightingale's life: childhood, education, hospitals, the Crimea, St. Thomas London, and Notes on Nursing.

Nightingale demonstrated her skill as an administrator. She was, however, hampered by military authorities who resisted every change that she suggested. They resented that her authority was independent of the armed services, that she was a civilian, and that she was a woman. In addition, she had to reckon with the unreliability of many on her nursing staff. Yet none of her difficulties with doctors was as wearing as those with her nurses. In the midst of appalling horror, this type of situation occurred:

> I came out, Ma'am, prepared to submit to everything, to be put on in every way. But there are some things, Ma'am, one can't submit to. There is the Caps, Ma'am, that suits one face and some that suits another. And if I'd known, Ma'am, about the caps, great as was my desire to come out to nurse at Scutari, I wouldn't have come, Ma'am.
>
> — *Woodham-Smith, 1951, p. 119*

Overcoming these obstacles and obtaining the obvious necessities, Nightingale transformed a place of horror into a haven where patients could truly convalesce. She set up five diet kitchens, a laundry, coffee houses that provided music and recreation (canteens), reading rooms, and organized classes. In the evening, after the other nurses had retired, she made solitary rounds. She stopped to observe the condition of the sickest patients. These rounds were made with her famous lamp or lantern, which had a wind shield that prevented the candle within it (placed in a candlestick) from being extinguished. Henry Wadsworth Longfellow immortalized this "Lady with a Lamp" in his poem of 1857, "Santa Filomena":

Whene'er a noble deed is wrought,
Whene'er is spoken a noble thought,
Our hearts, in glad surprise,
To higher levels rise.

The tidal wave of deeper souls
Into our inmost being rolls,
And lifts us unawares
Out of all meaner cares.

Honour to those whose words or deeds
Thus help us in our daily needs,
And by their overflow
Raise us from what is low!

Thus thought I, as by night I read
Of the great army of the dead,
The trenches cold and damp,
The starved and frozen camp—

The wounded from the battle plain,
In dreary hospitals of pain—
The cheerless corridors,
The cold and stony floors.

Lo! in that house of misery,
A lady with a lamp I see
Pass through the glimmering gloom,
And flit from room to room.

And slow, as in a dream of bliss,
The speechless sufferer turns to kiss
Her shadow, as it falls
Upon the darkening walls.

A.G. Walker, R.A., *The Lady With the Lamp.* Stone. *(Crimean Memorial, London, England. By permission of the Royal College of Nursing of the United Kingdom.)*

The Florence Nightingale Lamp. Appeared on the cover of the *AARN Newsletter,* Vol. 48, No. 6, June, 1992. *(Courtesy of the Alberta Association of Registered Nurses, Museum and Archives, Edmonton, Canada.)*

This rare Turkish candle lamp or "Kelly lamp" was donated to the AARN Museum and Archives by Dr. Winston Backus and Mrs. Backus of Sylvan Lake, Alberta. This lamp was carried by Mary Stanley, a nurse who, during the Crimean War, rather annoyed Florence Nightingale. The lamp was originally given by a patient (the granddaughter of Mary Stanley) to the late Mrs. Valmai Backus when she was a student at the London Hospital in London, England. Three lamps of this specific design are known in the world: an identical lamp to this one located in the Florence Nightingale Museum Trust in London; another situated in a different museum in London and reported as "not being of the same quality." The lamp "has a circular shaped brass base linked by a linen concertina supported by wire to a circular shaped brass cover with a heat shield and hook. The cover contains some lattice design. The lamp is thus used as a lantern when extended or a candle holder when collapsed."

Miss Nightingale used the folding candle lanterns, not the "Aladdin type" or "Greek lamp of knowledge" with which she is so often depicted.

As if a door in heaven should be,
Opened, and then closed suddenly,
The vision came and went—
The light shone and was spent.

On England's annals, through the long
Hereafter of her speech and song,
That light its rays shall cast
From portals of the past.

A lady with a lamp shall stand
In the great history of the land,
A noble type of good,
Heroic womanhood.

Nor even shall be wanting here
The palm, the lily, and the spear,
The symbols that of yore
Saint Filomena bore.

The greatest measure of Nightingale's success was the overall drop in the mortality rate—to 2.2 percent—that occurred within six months' time. When the conditions at the Barrack Hospital were reasonably satisfactory, Nightingale went across the Black Sea to the Crimea, where two British hospitals were located near the seaport of Balaclava. On horseback or in a carriage the army had given her, she covered the distances between them. She visited the front and the hospitals but contracted "Crimean Fever" and nearly died. The English soldiers wept at the news of her illness, and all of England waited patiently for her recovery. The strain from the illness and the nursing care she had provided undermined her health to the point that she was never able again to work with her former vigor. For the rest of her life she remained a semi-invalid. Nightingale returned to England in July 1856, four months after the end of the war. By that time she had supervised 125 nurses. A testimonial was presented to her by the English public in the form of fifty thousand pounds. This sum was obtained by compulsory subscription from the soldiers of the Crimea and donations from the public. It was deposited into the Nightingale Fund, which later was used for a training school for nurses.

Two figures emerged from the Crimea as heroic, the soldier and the nurse. In each case a transformation in public estimation took place, and in each case the transformation was due to Miss Nightingale. Never again was the British soldier to be ranked as a drunken brute, the scum of the earth. He was now a symbol of courage, loyalty, and endurance, not a disgrace but a source of pride. . . . Never again would the picture of a nurse be a tipsy, promiscuous harridan. Miss Nightingale had stamped the profession of nurse with her own image . . . in the midst of the muddle and the filth, the agony and the defeats, she had brought about a revolution.

— *Woodham-Smith, 1951, p. 179*

Before departing from the Crimean theater, Florence Nightingale made a pledge to the dead soldiers to fight for their cause. She insisted on a formal investigation of military health care, which led to the establishment of a Royal Commission on the Health of the Army in 1857. Nightingale published her own views in an 800-page book titled *Notes on Matters Affecting the Health, Efficiency and Hospital Administration of the British Army,* which included a section of statistics accompanied by diagrams. She called the diagrams "coxcombs" because of their vivid colors; these polar-area charts depicted the statistic being represented in proportion to the area of a wedge in a circular diagram. These statistics were Nightingale's most compelling argument for the improvement of medical care in military and civilian hospitals. After five years of hard fighting for reforms, her efforts were realized. Army hospitals and barracks were reconstructed on a sanitary basis, a sanitary code for the army was developed, a military medical college was established, recreational clubs were founded, and the army's procedures for gathering medical statistics were reorganized.

Florence Nightingale exercised a somewhat similar influence over British administration in India. Vast irrigation projects and economic reforms were enacted by the government on the strength of two of her reports, *Observations on the Sanitary State of the Army in India* (1863) and *Life or Death in India?* (1873). This revolution in the military hospitals was carried over into civilian hospitals. The work was aided by *Notes on Hospitals* (1859), an exhaustive study on hospital planning and administration. Nightingale also drew up a standard nomenclature on diseases and devised a Model Hospital Statistical Form that was approved at the International Congress of Statistics, held in London in the summer of 1860. As a recognized authority, she was frequently consulted about the plans for new hospitals in England, Australia, the United States, and Canada. Plans for the Johns Hopkins Hospital in Baltimore were taken to England for her criticism.

The Nightingale School. Florence Nightingale developed the first organized program of training for nurses. The Nightingale Training School for Nurses opened in 1860 as an entirely independent educational institution financed by the Nightingale Fund. A council of distinguished persons had been appointed to administer the fund and negotiate the establishment of the school. The members investigated the existing London hospitals and chose St. Thomas's Hospital, where the resident medical officer, R.G. Whitfield, was sympathetic and the matron, Mrs. Wardroper, had made her mark by exhibit-

Miss Nightingale's Carriage at the Seat of War. Illustration from the *Illustrated London News,* August 30, 1856. *(The Illustrated London News Picture Library, London, England.)*

ing an upright character, an unremitting devotion to her task, and success in reforming hospital abuses. An overwhelming majority of London physicians opposed the project. Of one hundred physicians queried, only four favored the school. Strong opposition came from within St. Thomas's itself through John Flint South, a senior consulting surgeon. South vehemently opposed the school and published a pamphlet, *Facts Relating to Hospital Nurses* (1857), in which he asserted: "As regards the nurses or ward-maids, these are in much the same position as housemaids, and require little teaching beyond that of poultice-making." Nightingale's ill health prevented her from taking charge of the program, but she acted as a chief adviser for many years.

The aims of the Nightingale school were to train hospital nurses, to instruct nurses in the training of others, and to train district nurses for the sick poor. Consequently, students went into homes as well as into hospitals to care for and teach patients and families about the preservation and maintenance of health. The length of the program was one year, after which the nurses were drafted on the staff of a hospital for two years' further experience. A distinction was made between ordinary probationers and "lady nurses," which reflected the British class consciousness. The former were drawn from relatively uneducated levels, and their expenses were paid by the Nightingale Fund; the latter were gentlewomen who paid their own way (tuition fees) and were expected to become future matrons. The graduates of this program were destined to become nursing leaders on an international scale. As soon as they were available, they were in demand at other hospitals.

The Nightingale school was extremely important to nursing. It served as a model for other schools, sent graduates to foreign lands, and raised nursing from degradation and disgrace to the rank of a respectable occupation for women. The opening of the school was the opening of a new way of life for women. Gone forever, at least in England, was the reign of Sairey Gamp and Betsy Prig.

A small book of seventy-seven pages written by Florence Nightingale, *Notes on Nursing* (1859), held special interest for nurses. It was used as a text

Facing page, Home! Return From the Crimea, nineteenth century. Engraving. (Copyright The Board of Trustees of the Victoria & Albert Museum, London, England.)

Designed by Reynolds, Francis, & Rohnstock. "Notes on Nursing," c. 1938. Stained glass. Panel from *The Nightingale Window. (Washington National Cathedral, Washington, D.C. Courtesy of Morton Broffman.)*

Miss Nightingale is shown writing *Notes on Nursing*, the work that provided an enormous motivation for the study of nursing. It was not, however, her only book dealing with aspects of health care. *Notes on Hospitals* was an exhaustive study on hospital planning and administration.

Designed by Reynolds, Francis, & Rohn-stock. "Hospitals," c. 1938. Stained glass. Panel from *The Nightingale Window. (Washington National Cathedral, Washington D.C. Courtesy of Morton Broffman.)*

Florence Nightingale visited hospitals at home and abroad. Here she takes notes at the bedside of a patient in the hospital of St. Vincent de Paul in Paris.

in the Nightingale school and in many schools founded by the nurses who studied there. In 1860 the book was rewritten, enlarged, and translated into Italian, German, and French. Concern over the meager number of available copies prompted a reprinting in 1946. The fundamental principles that were set forth in this book remain as true today as when they were written. Their scope is described in the preface:

> The following notes are by no means intended as a rule of thought by which nurses can teach themselves to nurse, still less as a manual to teach nurses to nurse. They are meant simply to give hints for thought to women who have personal charge of the health of others.
>
> — *Nightingale, 1859, p. iii*

After the founding of the school, fifty years remained, for Nightingale survived until the age of ninety. This half-century was spent in constant, fruitful activity. She died in August 1910 and was buried in the family plot at East Wellow, near Romney, in Hampshire. A small cross with her initials and dates marks the site of the grave. The family refused burial in Westminster Abbey in respect of Nightingale's wishes. There are numerous monuments to her in various places in the world: in London, Derby, Milbank, Florence, and Calcutta and in St. Paul's Cathedral, St. Thomas's Hospital, the Royal Infirmary, and the Episcopal Cathedral in Washington, D.C. In this last structure is the famous and beautiful stained glass "Nightingale Window," composed of six panels that depict the events in the life of Florence Nightingale.

One need not review all the "causes" to which Florence Nightingale gave of herself to appreciate her role as a creative social force. She was a living memorial to a new type of thought that would forever influence the direction of nursing.

The definite dividing-line between the old nursing and the new, is the demarcation between pre-Nightingale nursing and Nightingale nursing. In the sense that

G. Scharf, *Florence Nightingale at Embley,* 1857. Pencil drawing. *(By courtesy of the National Portrait Gallery, London, England.)*

Hippocrates (460–370 BC) was the father of medicine, Florence Nightingale (1820–1910) was the founder of nursing: systematized medicine is thus an ancient art, while organized nursing is a recent art. Miss Nightingale hewed a new profession out of centuries of ignorance and superstition. The greatness and the goodness of Florence Nightingale combined to emancipate woman from the curse of not finding her work: Florence Nightingale gave to woman the blessed work of the trained nurse of the human race.

— *Robinson, 1946, p. 129*

Judy Waid, *Nursing: A Tradition of Caring,* 1990. *(Copyright Judy Waid and District Three, Ohio Nurses Association, Youngstown, Ohio.)*

The Birth of the Red Cross

A further stimulus for nursing reform culminated in the development of the International Red Cross organization. Its founder was J. Henri Dunant, an investment banker from Geneva, Switzerland. A humanitarian, Dunant had journeyed to Italy to secure a meeting with Napoleon III of France but found himself at Solferino, where he was a witness to the horrors of the bloodiest battle of the war between France and Austria. He was depressed by the lack of medical services; only two physicians were attending to nearly six thousand wounded men. Dunant enlisted local people to give whatever aid and nursing care was possible. He subsequently appealed to various European governments to set up an international organization that would provide volunteer nursing aid on battlefields.

Dunant repeatedly referred to Florence Nightingale and her work in the Crimea as the inspiration behind his crucial trip to Italy. Her work had also

This first edition of the "Nursing: A Tradition of Caring" medallion is dedicated to the contributions that nurses have made to health and humanity, both past and present. The medallions were envisioned by the 1700 members of District Three as their contribution to the profession toward the goal of improving the image of nursing. The medallion depicts Florence Nightingale.

Battle of Solferina, June 24, 1859, which gave cause to the foundation of the Red Cross by Jean Henri Dunant. *(The Bettmann Archive, New York.)*

Jerry Barrett, *Florence Nightingale Receiving the Wounded at Scutari,* c. 1856. Canvas, 141 × 212.7 cm. *(By courtesy of the National Portrait Gallery, London, England.)*

fortified his belief in the feasibility of such an organization. In 1862 he published the famous *Recollections of Solferino* (*Un Souvenir de Solferino*), which contained the idea for the birth of the Red Cross. He first presented his plan to the Society of Public Utility in Geneva (1863). After five years of hard work, Henri Dunant observed the gathering of a national congress at Geneva to consider the ways and means of accruing volunteers to serve in the event of another war. On August 22, 1864, twelve governments signed what is now known as the Treaty of Geneva. It contained principles to govern and protect those wounded in war, the supplies needed for their care, and the personnel attending the wounded through the use of a single determined emblem. The design chosen for the common flag of the organization was that of the flag of Switzerland with its colors reversed—a red cross on a white background. (The

Red Cross societies of Muslim nations use a red crescent on a white background for their flag. Iran has a red lion and sun, which for many years has been the Persian national symbol.) Each government agreed to honor Red Cross nurses as noncombatants and to respect their hospitals and other facilities. In addition, societies in neutral countries would be permitted to render humanitarian services to either side.

National Red Cross societies were built up in many countries, and some older groups that had carried on relief work in the earlier wars of the nineteenth century became affiliated with it. The Geneva treaty was signed by England in 1870. The United States refrained from confirming it until 1882; it was confirmed only after Clara Barton, with rugged determination, paved the way for Congress to ratify it.

UNIT 6

The Development of Nursing in America

In the early nineteenth century, the status of nursing in the United States was not unlike that in England prior to the influence of Florence Nightingale. Large city hospitals were in existence and nurses were haphazardly trained in the hospital. There were few trained nurses and no formal training programs. The Civil War, much like the Crimean War in the case of England, brought the need for skilled nurses to the attention of government agencies, and brought about the first major reforms in nursing in this country. In the latter half of the century, the growing sense of social responsibility for health, the improved status of women in society, and the influence of the Nightingale concept, all contributed to the development of nursing education and improved nursing practice. The United States produced many women who greatly influenced nursing during the same period that Florence Nightingale made her reforms, and later.

— GLORIA M. GRIPPANDO

Joan Maynard, *Harriet Tubman*, 1977. (*U.S. Army Center of Military History, Washington, D.C.*)

Harriet Tubman was called the "Moses of her people." After her own escape to the North, she became active with the Underground Railroad and assisted more than three hundred slaves in their quest for freedom. During the Civil War, she held the position of "nurse" or "matron" at the Colored Hospital in Fort Monroe, Virginia, where she cared for those who needed her ministrations.

213

	1500	1575	1650
DAILY LIFE	**1492** Columbus lands in America **1519** Hernando Cortez conquers Mexico **1535** Jacques Cartier sails into the St. Lawrence River	**1605** First permanent French settlement at Port Royal in Nova Scotia **1607** First permanent English settlement in America at Jamestown **1620** Pilgrims land in Plymouth **1626** Dutch East India Company establishes "New Netherlands"	
SCIENCE AND TECHNOLOGY	**1492** Leonardo da Vinci draws a flying machine **1525** Dürer compiles first German manual on geometry **1540** G.L. de Cardenas discovers the Grand Canyon **1547** First predictions of astrologer Nostradamus **1595** Mercator's Atlas published **1596** Galileo invents thermometer	**1631** William Oughtred proposes symbol "X" for multiplication **1656** Thomas Wharton describes anatomy of glands	
THE VISUAL ARTS		**1644** Last age of fine Chinese porcelain **1647** Dresden Academy of Arts founded **1656** Rembrandt declares bankruptcy **1662** André Le Nôtre designs park and gardens of Versailles	
MEDICINE AND HEALTH CARE	**1524** Cortez establishes first hospital on American continent, built in the Tenochtitlan capital **1528** Hospital of Santa Fe built	**1578** First medical school established at the University of Mexico **c. 1600** Medical School at University of Lima established	**1639** Hôtel Dieu at Quebec opens **1642** Hôtel Dieu at Montreal founded **1658** Bellevue Hospital precursor founded by the Dutch West India Company
NURSING		**1606–1673** Jeanne Mance, one of the most romantic figures in Canadian nursing **1617** Maria Hubow, first woman to nurse in North America **1639** Three Augustinian Sisters staff Hôtel Dieu at Quebec **1657** Three hospital nuns of Society of St. Joseph de la Flèche staff Hôtel Dieu in Montreal	

1725	1800	1875

1775–1781 American Revolution

1861–1865 American Civil War

1865 United States abolishes slavery

1888 Yellow Fever epidemic in Florida

1889 Johnstown flood

1893 World's Fair in Chicago

1898–1899 Spanish-American War

1714 D.G. Fahrenheit constructs mercury thermometer with temperature scale

1775 Priestley discovers hydrochloric and sulfuric acids

1816 Laënnec invents the stethoscope

1699–1779 Jean Chardin, French painter

1715 Early beginnings of Rococo

1738–1815 John Singleton Copley, American painter

1738–1820 Benjamin West, American painter

1793 The Louvre, Paris, becomes national art gallery

1834 Statue of Liberty by F.A. Bartholdi, French sculptor

1836–1910 Winslow Homer, American painter

1844–1915 Thomas Eakins, American artist, illustrates scientific basis of patient care

1875 *Gross Clinic* painted

1889 *Agnew Clinic* painted

1731 Philadelphia Almshouse erected

1737 Charity Hospital of New Orleans founded

1745–1813 Benjamin Rush, most renowned physician of colonial times

1751 Pennsylvania Hospital designed solely for care of the sick

1765 Medical school established at College of Philadelphia

1783 Medical school at Harvard established

1786 Quakers establish Philadelphia Dispensary for home care of the sick

1791 New York Dispensary opens

1810 Medical school established at Yale

1847 American Medical Association (AMA)

1861 United States Sanitary Commission established

1869 Bellevue Hospital establishes ambulance service

1876–1901 Clara Maass, nurse who gave her life to conquer yellow fever

1893 Medical school established at Johns Hopkins

1910 *Flexner Report* published

1727 Ursuline Sisters arrive from France to nurse at L'Hôpital des Pauvres de la Charité in New Orleans

1739 Order of Grey Nuns becomes Canada's first district nurses

1774–1813 Mother Elizabeth Seton, first native-born American canonized for charitable work

1797–1881 Sojourner Truth, early feminist and volunteer Civil War nurse

1817–1901 Mother Bickerdyke, volunteer Civil War nurse

1820–1913 Harriet Tubman, abolitionist and volunteer Civil War nurse

1821–1912 Clara Barton, volunteer Civil War nurse and founder of American Red Cross

1839 Nurses Society of Philadelphia organized for home maternity services

1862 Louisa May Alcott serves as a volunteer Civil War nurse

1862 Walt Whitman serves as a volunteer Civil War nurse in Washington, D.C.

1873 Linda Richards becomes the first trained nurse in the U.S.

1873 Bellevue, Connecticut, and Boston Training Schools established

1874 St. Catharine's, Ontario, begins nurse training school

1879 Mary Eliza Mahoney becomes America's first Black professional nurse

1886 Spelman Seminary in Atlanta establishes training for Black nurses

1889 Johns Hopkins Hospital Training School opens

1899 Teachers College program for nurses established

*T*he social movements that had characterized several centuries in Europe had their American counterparts. The time of the Reformation, which had split European nations into Catholic and Protestant, was also a period of great discoveries and early emigration to America. Groups from the Old World migrated to various regions of the New World, bringing their customs with them. These customs included those related to the care of the sick. The earliest evidence of nursing, however, in the Western Hemisphere was among the preliterate peoples who inhabited North, Central, and South America. Even before the Jesuit fathers of France had pioneered in medicine and the Catholic sisters had established mission hospitals, the American Indians had practiced crude methods of medical and surgical treatment. They had their own folk and magic medicine and could care for their sick without knowledge of medical science. The newcomers were often impressed by the native "medicine men," who served in the role of doctors, and herbwomen. (The latter assumed the functions of nurses.) According to Nutting and Dock (vol. 2, 1907), the Aztecs and the Incas had built their hospitals and taken care of their sick in the very dawn of history. In *Native Races of the Pacific States of North America,* Bancroft states that in all of the larger cities of ancient Mexico there were endowed hospitals attended by physicians, surgeons, and nurses and that the Mexicans had studied and practiced medicine from ancient times; women physicians were common and obstetricians were women. Shryock, however, makes the statement that "even the civilized Indians of Mexico and of Peru had developed nothing in the way of such institutions . . . of hospitals and nurses there was no evidence" (Shryock, 1959, p. 170).

Although discoveries had been made in the New World before the time of Columbus, no lasting colonies had been established. A northwest passage to India was being sought by navigators and sailors. Thus Columbus named the natives he encountered in the Western world *Indians,* since he thought they were on a land that was part of India. As new lands were discovered, they were generally bestowed on the sovereigns who had financed the expeditions. It was hoped by specific governments that the expeditions would lead to the attainment of wealth and trade from the new lands. Ultimately, kingdoms would be extended and empires created. Columbus, Vespucci, Balboa, Hudson, Cartier, Drake, and others were supported in their endeavors by their homelands. Other factors compelled individuals to journey far from their native lands: freedom from religious persecution and a desire by missionaries to convert the so-called heathens to Christianity.

SETTLEMENTS OF THE NEW WORLD

The settlements of the New World were closely tied to the mother countries of Spain, France, and England. The new territories or colonies were thought to exist for the advantage of the homeland, and trade with them was organized from that perspective. Adventurers who were fascinated by tales of the strange new lands and the fabulous wealth that supposedly existed there left their homelands to explore and conquer. Many of the colonists also included members of religious orders who became the teachers, nurses, and physicians.

> Need for additional provision for care of the sick was created when the first boatload of adventurers started out from Europe. Crude conditions of travel led to deadly outbreaks of scurvy, as well as of disease contracted before leaving the homeland. On his second trip, Columbus was careful to bring a physician. Explorers, conquerors, and conquered—all were exposed to infections for which they had no immunity. Unfortunately, it was almost simultaneous with this need that the period of depression in European nursing was being induced by the Renaissance and the Protestant Revolt—a depression to be prolonged by revolutions to establish religious freedom and the civil rights of man. A great era of

discovery opened up and facilitated the spread of disease, at a time when opportunities for its control were becoming fewer and less adequate than ever.

— *Jamieson and Sewall, 1950, p. 279*

Paul Gauguin, *Sister of Charity,* 1902. Oil on canvas, 64.8 × 76.2 cm. *(Courtesy of the McNay Art Museum, San Antonio, Texas; Bequest of Marion Koogler McNay.)*

The problems of medical care and nursing were met in different ways by the different colonists and were usually dependent upon the customs of the homelands. Spain was best prepared because Protestantism had not weakened her Church. Religious orders of the Catholic Church accompanied the Spaniards to America. In addition to protecting the public health, they explored and converted pagans to Christianity. Nursing was clearly a function of the religious, which included devoted service and the salvation of souls. As hospitals were erected, they were also controlled by the religious, who supported the institutions through gifts they had received. France also used the Dominicans, Franciscans, and Jesuits and, later, the nursing orders, but England had no comparable support. Organization was lacking, and individuals were given the responsibility for medicine and nursing. Eventually, in those colonies settled by Protestant countries nursing was done by persons hired at low wages or supplied by inmates of houses of correction.

Spanish America

Spain rapidly established colonies from Mexico to Peru during the 1500s. These colonies became a large, energetic realm nearly one hundred years before the first permanent settlements of other Europeans were established. In some areas native peoples were able to mingle their culture with that of the conquerors. In others, particularly in the chief centers such as Lima and Mexico City, Spanish civilization followed the pattern of the homeland. The University of Mexico and the University of Lima were founded in 1551, and the various departments of theology, arts, rhetoric, grammar, Scripture, canon law, civil law, and medicine were present. Here the medical science of the Renaissance was cultivated and the first medical schools appeared: the first at the University of Mexico in 1578, the second affiliated with the University of Lima before 1600.

In 1519 Hernando Cortés conquered what we now call Mexico. His conquest brought into Spanish possession the great wealth of the Aztecs, Toltecs, Mayas, and Incas. The well-meaning reigning chief of the Aztecs, Montezuma, had received Cortés into his palace. Montezuma had been taught to believe in a white god, whom he thought had appeared in the form of Cortés. Montezuma was met, however, with cruelty. He was imprisoned and his capital of Tenochtitlán was seized. The Aztecs had risen to a high degree of culture; their temples and pyramids are thought to predate those of Egypt. They had acquired large amounts of gold, silver, and precious stones, which were seized and shipped back to Spain. The American Indians were cruelly treated and in some cases nearly decimated. Where they proved to be unfit for work in the mines, black slaves were introduced. Missionaries protested the inhumane treatment of the natives and slaves and tried to improve their situation.

The medicine of the Aztecs was highly developed. The Aztecs had hospices for the care of the sick, used minerals as drugs (they had knowledge of three thousand plants) and soporifics to deaden pain, and had midwives for prenatal and postpartum instruction and for assistance at deliveries (Frank, 1953). The god of medicine was Tzapotlatean. So skilled were the Aztec surgeons and physicians that Cortés asked the Spanish government to refrain from sending medical practitioners from Spain; he preferred the American Indians because he believed they were superior. The Incas were not as advanced. They used purging, bloodletting, trephining, amputation, and potions made from a single herb. The Incas believed that the cure for a particular disease would be found in the area in which the disease was prominent; therefore quinine from the cinchona tree was found in the malaria-infested jungles.

The devoted missionaries followed the conquerors and established a church in every American Indian and Spanish town. Missions were founded along the outposts of Spanish claims. These extended from California to Texas, and to Paraguay and Chile. They were also founded in Spanish Florida. Junipero Serra, a Franciscan friar, was responsible for this extensive project, which eventually reached as far north as the Mission San Francisco. These missions were government supported and operated schools and manual training centers.

Beautiful churches, buildings, bridges, roads, and aqueducts were built under Spanish rule. Gratitude to God for success found expression in the development of charitable institutions, frequently in the form of hospitals. Approximately thirty hospitals were erected between 1524 and 1802, and the majority of them were staffed by religious men and women. The first hospital on the American continent was built in the Tenochtitlán capital (later renamed Mexico City) by Cortés in 1524. According to legend, this hospital was built on the site where Cortés first met Montezuma. It was originally named the Hospital of the Immaculate Conception (*Hospital de Nuestra Senora o Limpia Concepcion*); it is now called the Hospital of Jesus of Nazareth (*Hospital de Jesus Nazareno*). This building is a reflection of the beauty and spaciousness of Spanish hospital architecture under Muslim influence. Cortés donated funds for the completion of the hospital and also built a convent and a seminary. In his will he left an endowment for the hospital to thank God for his successes and to expiate his sins. This institution was to care for rich and poor alike. In 1528 the hospital of Santa Fe (Holy Faith) was built in what is now New Mexico. In Lima several institutions were built, including almshouses, hospitals, and lazarettos for those afflicted with contagious diseases. Hospital care, however, was reserved for the sick poor, and most of the nursing was done by the Sisters of Charity of St. Vincent de Paul.

The French in America

The first permanent settlement of the French was established in 1605 at Port Royal in Nova Scotia. The Canadian area of North America had been visited earlier: Norwegians had landed there about 1000. John Cabot, a Venetian under King Henry VII, sighted land near the Gulf of the St. Lawrence; Frenchmen arrived in the area early in the sixteenth century. In 1534 Jacques Cartier, under Francis I, sailed for the North American continent. He returned to France after finding neither gold nor a northwest passage to the Orient. When Cartier returned a year later, he sailed into the St. Lawrence River, where he found established American Indian villages. According to Frank (1953), Cartier questioned the natives about the name of the country. Thinking that he was referring to the village, they answered "Kanata," which meant "the place where we live." Therefore Cartier called the land *Canada,* its present-day name. This land has also been referred to as *New France.*

Cartier was followed to Canada by explorers, Franciscan friars, Jesuits, Dominicans, and other settlers. The French priests soon summoned help from the motherland for religious women to teach the children and care for the sick. The first woman to nurse in this new land, however, was Maria Hébart Hubou (the name of her second husband). She was the wife of the surgeon-apothecary Louis Hébart, whom Samuel de Champlain, the famous explorer, brought with him in 1617 (Gibbon and Mathewson, 1947). The Jesuits published reports of the need for aid in the *Jesuit Relations.* They sought to establish schools for American Indian children, build hospitals for the sick, and

Map of the early Canadian settlements.

make general improvements in all social conditions. The Europeans had transmitted measles, smallpox, and tuberculosis to the natives, who blamed the white people for the destruction of their race. The priests found it almost impossible to combat the diseases with the prevailing conditions of the land. They were thwarted in their attempts by dirt, cold, crowded living conditions, lice, and the savagery of the natives.

Great interest arose in the men and women of France through Jesuit publications and reports. Duchess d'Aiguillon, a niece of Cardinal Richelieu, was moved to action. She signed a contract in 1637 with the Augustinian Hospitallers of Dieppe for their services as hospital sisters and sent workers to lay the foundations for the first hospital in New France. The Hôtel Dieu at Quebec opened in 1639 and was staffed by three sisters of the Order of St. Augustine (Augustinian Sisters) upon their arrival on August 1, 1639. These Augustinian nuns belonged to a cloistered order and had been prepared to care for the sick. They wore white woolen dresses with black leather belts and black veils. All three were from good French families: Marie Guenet de St. Ignace; Anne Lecointre de St. Bernard; and Marie Forestier de St. Bonaventure de Jésus. They encountered many hardships, and within eight months one of the sisters had died.

> The Hospital Nuns arrived at Kebec on the first day of August of last year (1639). Scarcely had they disembarked before they found themselves overwhelmed with patients. The hall of the Hospital being too small, it was necessary to erect some cabins, fashioned like those of the savages, in their garden. Not having furniture for so many people, they had to cut in two or three pieces part of the blankets and sheets they had brought for these poor sick people. In a word, instead of taking a little rest and refreshing themselves after the great discomforts they had suffered upon the sea, they found themselves so burdened and occupied that we had fear of losing them and their hospital at its very birth. The sick came from all directions. . . . [t]heir stench was so insupportable, the heat so great, the fresh food so scarce and so poor. . . . In brief, from the first of August until the month of May, more than one hundred patients entered the hospital, and more than two hundred poor savages found relief there.
>
> — Kenton, 1925, pp. 169–170

J. McIsaac, *Hôtel Dieu Sisters Nursing Indians In Montréal*, 1747. *(Archives des Religieuses Hopitalières de Saint-Joseph, Montréal, Canada.)*

Repeated attacks by the Iroquois Indians occurred in the colonies. The Sisters cared for both the colonists and the Indians, and at frequent intervals the hospital was a place where the Indians were fed and lodged and treated kindly.

The hospital in Quebec had a facility similar to an outpatient department that was used for the treatment of American Indians who were not sick enough to be hospitalized. Native American women were trained by the sisters to assist with the care of the sick, but their duties were chiefly domestic, such as cooking, cleaning, and preparing supplies. From 1640 to 1644 the Augustinians went to Sillery, the Jesuit mission not far from Quebec, to care for the natives, but they returned when the Iroquois became hostile.

The Ursuline Sisters accompanied the Augustinians on the voyage from France. They were an order of teaching nuns enlisted by Madame de la Peltrie, who had undertaken the establishment of a mission school for the American Indians. However, they were soon schooled in the care of the sick in order that they might assist during the epidemics. Smallpox broke out in the school, and the Ursuline dwelling was rapidly turned into housing for the infected. In this emergency hospital many American Indians died until the disease finally ran itself out. This short-term instruction in the care of the sick could be regarded as the earliest training and supervision of nurses in America. As soon as it was feasible, the Ursuline Sisters returned to the work for which they had initially been prepared.

A second settlement was founded about two hundred miles farther up the St. Lawrence. Included in the original plans for "Montreal" were a school and a hospital, with the latter deemed to be an immediate necessity. The establishment of this hospital is the story of Jeanne Mance (1606–1673), a roman-

Philip Hebert, *Jeanne Mance.* (*Archives des Religieuses Hopitalières de Saint-Joseph, Montréal, Canada.*)

tic figure in Canadian nursing and considered to be the founder of the Hôtel Dieu of Montreal as well as the co-founder of Montreal itself (Gibbon and Mathewson, 1947). She was the daughter of wealthy French parents and had been educated at an Ursuline convent. From her earliest childhood, Jeanne Mance had demonstrated a religious inclination. She received instruction in nursing care while assisting the Ladies of Charity in 1638 during a severe epidemic. Upon her arrival in Canada, she was also permitted to enter the Augustinian cloister at Quebec, where she waited for completion of the construction of the fort at Ville Marie, the future Montreal. Here Jeanne Mance was provided an excellent opportunity to learn more about nursing and the administration of a hospital. She arrived in Montreal on May 17, 1642, under the financial sponsorship of a wealthy philanthropist, Madame de Bullion, who wanted her to erect a hospital there.

The inhabitants of the settlement lived in peace for about a year. The floods and then the warring Iroquois followed. More than half of the settlers met death at the hands of the Iroquois. In a tiny cottage hospital inside the fort, Jeanne Mance tended to men wounded by arrows. She compounded her own medicines, treated chilblains and frostbite, practiced bloodletting, and cared for the Iroquois Indians as well as the colonists. By October 1644 a larger hospital had been established in a building sixty by twenty-four feet; it was divided into two wards, servants' quarters, a kitchen, and a room for Mance.

Claire Fauteux, *Jeanne Mance. (Collection of the Religieuses Hopitalières de Saint-Joseph, Montréal, Canada.)*

Mlle. Mance earned the reputation of being the "first lay nurse of Canada." She never took vows; she believed that she could contribute more to the community by being a layperson.

Jeanne Mance Window. Stained glass. *(The Notre-Dame Basilica, Montréal, Canada.)*

Jeanne Mance was one of the most romantic figures in the history of Canadian nursing. In the central panel she is depicted surrounded by patients. In the left panel, the first three sisters, Hospitallers of St. Joseph, leave France in 1659. The right panel depicts two sisters praying for and offering sustenance to a sick patient in Montréal.

The hospital was surrounded by a palisade and protected by a moat because of the ever-threatening Iroquois. For almost fifteen years Jeanne Mance did all the nursing here with the help of a few assistants. She earned the reputation of being the "first lay nurse of Canada" and of North America as well.

Jeanne Mance returned to France in 1657 to seek financial support and recruit personnel. Three hospital nuns from the Society of St. Joseph de la Flèche (Hospitallers of St. Joseph) returned to Montreal to staff the Hôtel Dieu with Jeanne Mance as the administrator, a position she held until her death in 1673. The sisters suffered from a variety of misfortunes during the first century of the hospital's existence—American Indian attacks, severe poverty, fire, earthquake, and famine. They persevered and eventually experienced considerable prosperity and recognition for their good work. The next century saw all French developments at Montreal and Quebec pass into English control as a result of the Seven Years' War.

A number of other hospitals and orders were organized in Canada. One of particular note was the order of Grey Nuns established by Madame Marguerite Marie d'Youville in 1739. The members were not cloistered and were thus able to carry their work into the homes of the needy. The Grey Nuns were Canada's first district nurses. However, they were misunderstood because people were not comfortable with nuns walking freely on the streets.

Early nursing in Canada did not particularly affect the development of nursing in the country that later would become the United States. The French settlements of New Orleans and those farther up the Mississippi River, however, had an influence on American nursing. This territory was called Louisiana in honor of France's king. It, too, was ravaged by epidemic diseases, particularly yellow fever and smallpox. All the scourges of a seaport area were encountered. New Orleans needed teachers and nurses. An almshouse had been built there and housed criminals, indigents, the mentally ill, and the sick poor. This inspired Jean Louis, a French sailor, to leave twelve thousand livres upon his death to "Serve in perpetuity to the founding of a hospital for the care of the sick of the City of New Orleans . . .and to secure the necessary things to succor the sick" (Henrietta, 1939, p. 249). Ursuline Sisters arrived

Theophile Hamel, *Grey Nuns, Sisters of Providence and Hôtel Dieu Sisters Caring for the Irish Immigrants. (Chapelle Notre-Dame-de-Bonsecours, Montréal, Canada.)*

This painting is in honor of the nuns and priests who died caring for the Irish immigrants arriving in Montréal suffering from a fatal epidemic in 1847.

from France in 1727 to nurse in the new hospital, the first in the United States established through a private gift. The hospital, which was legally named L'Hôpital des Pauvres de la Charité, developed slowly and went through several name changes. It eventually became the great and famous Charity Hospital of New Orleans. The Ursuline Sisters were very active throughout Louisiana. They opened numerous hospitals and performed many heroic deeds that reached a peak with the nursing done during the Battle of New Orleans. In later years they restricted themselves to teaching, and their work was carried on by the Daughters of Charity.

The English Colonies

Europeans emigrated to the English colonies for a variety of reasons, including freedom from religious oppression, a spirit of adventure, and the chance to start again. It is said that approximately a quarter of a million came as indentured servants. They committed themselves to work for a number of years to pay for their passage. Many of them came from the gaols and debtors' prisons, seeking an opportunity to begin a new and rewarding life.

England laid claim to that portion of the Atlantic coast that was between the claims of Spain and France. Colonization was a private affair in that the English government granted permission to an individual or a chartered company to establish a colony. Royalties were paid to the Crown; profits and losses were assumed by the proprietors. The first permanent English settlement in America was made in Jamestown in 1607 by the London Company. The area was named *Virginia,* after the virgin queen, Elizabeth. The colony faced many hardships and suffered American Indian massacres, illness, starvation, and a heavy mortality. Medical care was lacking, and little of what could be called nursing was available. The first three years in the new colony were a period of human devastation. All but sixty of the original five hundred settlers died of malnutrition or dietary insufficiency. A shipload of women arrived in Jamestown in 1619 to be auctioned off as wives. During that same year the first slaves were brought from Africa.

A succession of colonies followed Jamestown. A group of Separatists, who were later known as Pilgrims, sailed on the *Mayflower* and landed at New Plymouth in 1620. This group was augmented by the Puritans, who were being persecuted in England. (The Plymouth Company was later incorporated as the Massachusetts Bay Company, which became identical with the Massachusetts colony.) In 1626 the Dutch East India Company established a colony called *New Netherlands,* which was located in what is now Staten Island, Manhattan, and Delaware. The principal town, called *New Amsterdam,* was located on Manhattan. Maryland was founded as a refuge for English Catholics in 1633 by Lord Baltimore, Cecil Calvert, a group of Jesuits, and three hundred carefully selected colonists. Connecticut and Rhode Island were founded as a result of grievances among members of the Massachusetts colony. Pennsylvania was given to William Penn by Charles II in payment of a debt to Penn's father. This Quaker colony was noted for tolerance and religious freedom. English colonization became a reality as other equally important settlements developed. There was, however, little similarity and unity among them. Each colony was self-governed, and there was no central power to coordinate them. They remained isolated and even antagonistic toward one another for almost a century and a half. Their differences were particularly caused by religious beliefs, although varying temperaments and the prevalence of bigotry played a role.

The Pilgrim Fathers brought a stern philosophy with them to the New World, and it was not conducive to the development of institutions for the care of the sick. They took it for granted that welfare work was a function of private charity or the state. It was assumed that families would look after their

Charles C. Hofmann, *Berks County Almshouse*, 1878. Metal, 82.55 × 99.69 cm. *(Gift of Edgar William and Bernice Chrysler Garbisch, copyright 1995 Board of Trustees, National Gallery of Art, Washington, D.C.)*

The growth of hospitals in colonial America was slow. The earliest were not hospitals in the truest sense of the word but almshouses, with the care of the sick incidental. The indigent, the insane, the infirm, prisoners, and orphans were often given lodging in these "poor houses." Infirmaries were usually set up where the sick poor were attended by inmates.

TUE, LIBERTY & INDE PEN DENCE!

Western View of the new Hospital.

Tenant House No. III.

Kitchen supplying Spring & Reservoir.

F THE BUILDINGS & SURROUNDINGS
RKS COUNTY ALMS HOUSE. 1878.

Grain Barn.

Winslow Homer, *New York Charities—St. Barnabus House, 304 Mulberry Street.* Engraving, approx. 22.9 × 33.7 cm. (Harper's Weekly, *April 18, 1874.*)

own unfortunates and therefore that public refuge was unnecessary. Early treatments of diseases consisted largely of prayer intermingled with much superstitious medical practice. Samuel Fuller, a deacon, acted as a physician in New England for thirteen years after his arrival on the *Mayflower.* Physicians did not need a degree; the educated individuals among the colonists (clergy, governors, or schoolteachers) were thought to be well equipped enough to handle the role of a physician. Ignorant quacks were in abundance. American Indian folklore soon became incorporated into the overall scheme.

> Obviously this clerical and lay medicine would have to be very primitive. It was a peculiar mixture of religious medicine, folk-medicine, and scientific principle. One invoked the word of God, let blood, or prescribed drugs, to the best of one's understanding. We must not forget that at this period European medicine, even when practiced by physicians, was effective only in exceptional cases.
>
> — *Sigerist, 1934, p. 37*

The English settlers lacked the organized service of the convent or the mission, the experience of nuns and priests. Consequently, hospitals developed slowly in the original thirteen colonies. Social welfare was considered the responsibility of the individual, the family, or the neighborhood. Relatives or friends supplied nursing care when needed. Otherwise, nursing fell to those persons who were inclined to do it. When the settlements reached a certain size, however, some sort of public refuge had to be provided. The colonists followed the pattern of the homeland and ultimately organized institutions for the sick and the poor. This was not done out of Christian charity as much as for social convenience. The poorhouse and the hospital were placed under one roof, and the conditions were similar to those found by Elizabeth Fry in Britain.

HOSPITAL DEVELOPMENT IN AMERICA

The growth of hospitals in colonial America was slow. In the one hundred and fifty years before the American Revolution (1776–1784), approximately five hospitals were founded outside of Canada. The earliest were not hospitals in the true sense of the word. They were usually almshouses that included infirmaries where the sick poor were attended by inmates. Regarded by some as the first hospitals in the English colonies, they later evolved into separate municipal hospitals.

Several hospitals claim to have been the first established in America. This discrepancy is directly related to the definition of *hospital* and the specific focus of the institution. As indicated previously, many of these early hospitals were developed as poorhouses; the care of the sick was incidental. However, the earliest hospital on record was established in New Amsterdam by the Dutch West India Company in 1658. Located on Manhattan Island, it served to care for sick soldiers and slaves coming into port as cargo on company ships.

The Philadelphia Almshouse, which was erected in 1731, cared for the sick, the indigent, the insane, the infirm, prisoners, and orphans. In 1919 the hospital was separated from the almshouse. From 1835 to 1902 it was called Philadelphia Hospital. In 1902 the name was changed to the Philadelphia General Hospital. Servants, criminals, and paupers cared for the sick. This institution is usually designated as the "oldest hospital in continuous service" and was affectionately known as "Old Blockley." It offered the typical picture of the almshouse of the late eighteenth and early nineteenth centuries. The treatment of the insane was particularly disheartening. The female lunatics were under the supervision of a male keeper who was assisted by two male paupers. These men slept among the insane and entirely managed the violent cases, even bathing and dressing the women. "Some of the patients, even in their madness, shrunk from this rude handling and raved with the increased fury at their indecent exposure. Revolting to decency as this practice was, it was not without difficulty, and only by degrees, abandoned" (Nutting and Dock, vol. 2, 1907, p. 333). In addition, it was the custom to permit the public to visit these insane wards to stare, laugh, and jeer at the inmates.

The nursing in this institution was as crude and indifferent as anything that had taken place in London. During a cholera outbreak in 1832, for example, the attendants were found to be continuously intoxicated. In their drunken state, they fought over the beds of the sick or lay in a stupor beside dead bodies.

> Nurses became clamorous for an increase in wages, which was granted. Those between terror and want of moral sense were seized with a kind of mad infatuation. They drank the stimulants provided for the sick, and in one ward where the pestilence raged in its most fearful forms, and where between the dead and the dying the sight was most appalling, these furies were seen lying drunk upon or fighting over the dead victims of the disease. In this state of disorder, application was made to Bishop Kendrick for Sisters of Charity. The request was granted, and these devoted ministers of mercy at once entered upon their mission of danger, restoring order and diffusing hope by the calm and self-possessed manner with which they moved among the diseased. These Sisters remained at their post until the 20th of May 1833.
>
> — *Bush, 1890*

Following pages, Dean Cornwell, *Osler at Old Blockley.* Canvas. *(Courtesy of Wyeth-Ayerst Laboratories, Philadelphia, Pennsylvania.)*

The situation improved with the introduction of the Sisters of Charity of Emmitsburg, who undertook the task of reform. This transpired after investigations in 1793 and 1832, which brought the shocking conditions to light. After the sisters departed, unsatisfactory conditions returned and remained for a long time. Finally, Alice Fisher, a Nightingale nurse, arrived in 1884 and proceeded to upgrade the quality of nursing care.

Bellevue Hospital had its beginnings in the small hospital established by the West India Company in 1658. It was sold in 1680 and a better building was provided. In 1736 another new building was added to serve as a "Publick Workhouse and House of Correction of New York." This building became the immediate predecessor of Bellevue and stood where New York's city hall presently stands. It was rebuilt and enlarged several times. Buildings changed according to societal needs, and the city eventually assumed a share of the expense of charity. In time, the present Bellevue Hospital was concentrated on the bank of the East River. The building was originally (1794) used as a pesthouse to serve victims of yellow fever and for several years was used only when yellow fever broke out in the city. In 1811 more ground around the hospital was bought, and a new almshouse was built and dedicated on July 29, 1811. Officially opened in 1816, this institution contained the almshouse, a penitentiary, wards for the sick and the insane, and rooms for the resident physician, warden, and attendants. The sick were cared for by paupers or prisoners, political graft flourished, and epidemics were frequent. For many years Bellevue was a "house of horrors."

Unidentified Artist, *Bellevue Hospital,* east of First Avenue between 26th and 28th Streets, New York City, c. 1885. *(Collection of the New York Historical Society, New York.)*

The location of Bellevue Hospital changed several times before it was built at its present site. It originally combined the functions of almshouse, penitentiary, and hospital. Frequently rebuilt and enlarged in accordance with societal needs, it continued as an almshouse and hospital until 1848, when it became specifically a hospital.

Hospitals were as a rule in a disgraceful state of degradation. They were dirty and ill ventilated, they reeked with infection, so that patients who came in suffering from one disease, or from a wound, caught another disease or some virulent infection. The death rate was fearfully high, sometimes actually more than 50 per cent. In the days before Lister, hospital surgery was extremely discouraging. The only nurses that could be obtained for hospitals were women who did the menial work besides caring for the patients.

— *Walsh, 1929*

A committee was designated in 1837 to investigate the deplorable state of the hospital. According to Carlisle (1893), the prevailing conditions cited by the committee included filth, no ventilation, overcrowded wards, no clothing or supplies, patients with high fever lying naked in bed, putrefaction, and vermin. In addition, it was stated that the resident physician—with his students, the matron, and the nurses—had left the building. As a result, the pesthouse, the prison, and later the psychiatric wards were removed to Blackwell's Island. A new era began with the creation of a medical board in 1847. The almshouse and hospital, however, remained together until 1848, when Bellevue began its ensuing career as a hospital.

Bellevue was probably the first institution to establish an ambulance service (1869). Provisions were made for emergency treatment:

Beneath the driver's seat was a box containing a quart flask of brandy, two tourniquets, a half-dozen bandages, a half-dozen small sponges, some splint material, pieces of old blankets for padding, strips of various lengths with buckles, and a two-ounce vial of persulphate of iron.

Kane, 1934, p. 332

Charity Hospital of New Orleans was founded with funds left by a sailor, Jean Louis, in 1737. This money, designated to be used for the establishment of a hospital for the care of the sick, included funds to purchase equipment. It served as both a hospital and an asylum for the poor. Several catastrophes occurred, and the hospital was rebuilt in 1832. The Sisters of Charity were placed in control of the institution in 1834.

Sick Woman in Ward Overrun by Rats in Bellevue Hospital. Engraving, *Harper's Weekly*, 1860. *(Museum of the City of New York, New York.)*

This illustration appeared with the following quote:

We give herewith a picture of the beds in Bellevue Hospital in this city, in one of which the newborn child of Mary Connor was eaten by rats on Monday morning, April 23 . . . the building's swarming with rats, as many as 40 having been found in the bathtub one evening, and Mary Connor herself mentions that in her agony, she felt them running over her body.

P.T. Goist, *View of Pennsylvania Hospital in the Early Twentieth Century.* Engraving. *(Courtesy of Pennsylvania Hospital, Philadelphia.)*

Cornerstone of Pennsylvania Hospital, 1755, with an inscription written by Benjamin Franklin. (Courtesy of Pennsylvania Hospital, Philadelphia.)

Pennsylvania Hospital was founded at the suggestion of Benjamin Franklin. It became the first hospital in the United States that was designed solely for the curative care of the sick. Its seal is that of the Good Samaritan: "Take care of him and I will repay thee."

IN THE YEAR OF CHRIST
· MDCCLV.
GEORGE THE SECOND HAPPILY REIGNING
(FOR HE SOUGHT THE HAPPINESS OF HIS PEOPLE)
PHILADELPHIA FLOURISHING
(FOR ITS INHABITANTS WERE PUBLICK SPIRITED)
THIS BUILDING
BY THE BOUNTY OF THE GOVERNMENT,
AND OF MANY PRIVATE PERSONS,
WAS PIOUSLY FOUNDED
FOR THE RELIEF OF THE SICK AND MISERABLE;
MAY THE GOD OF MERCIES
BLESS THIS UNDERTAKING.

INSCRIPTION ON CORNER STONE OF EAST WING
LAID MAY 28, 1755.
as written by Benjamin Franklin

In 1751 the first *hospital,* in the truest sense of the word, was founded in Philadelphia through the efforts of Dr. Thomas Bond and other Philadelphia physicians. This group proposed that a general hospital be established there and worked to obtain contributions. With the assistance of Benjamin Franklin, they were able to secure funds from the Province (State) of Pennsylvania and from private donors. The Pennsylvania Hospital became the first hospital in the United States that was designed solely for the curative care of the sick. The insane, too, were placed in the category of those who were ill and needed treatment. After careful selection, servant-nurses were employed. The seal of this institution is that of the Good Samaritan: "Take care of him and I will repay thee." The hospital's medical library was the best in the area for a long time. The most renowned physician of colonial times, Dr. Benjamin Rush (1745–1813), served the mentally ill in Pennsylvania Hospital. His most famous work, *Medical Inquiries and Observations Upon Diseases of the Mind,* was published in 1812 and contained a foresighted approach to care. A separate department for the mentally ill was developed in 1841, and it was referred to as "Kirkbride," after Dr. Thomas Kirkbride, who was in charge of the service for forty-two years. Before this time, lunatics had been caged in the basement of the general hospital.

The New York Hospital received its charter granted by King George III in 1771. According to Nutting and Dock (1907), however, it did not receive patients until January 1791. The original building burned to the ground. The hospital was used by British and Hessian soldiers as a barrack, and it suffered the disorganizations of war. It was backed by the most prominent and cultured citizens, and its attendants were probably superior to those of Bellevue and Blockley. The care offered to patients was also better than that given in the almshouses. Dr. Valentine Seaman gave the nurses a series of lectures that focused on anatomy, physiology, maternal nursing, and the care of children. The latter lectures were published in *The Midwife's Monitor and Mother's Mirror* in 1800. Dr. Seaman regarded midwives as indispensable; he believed that they should be thoroughly and carefully taught. He did not seem to make a clear differentiation between midwivery and nursing.

In addition to the Pennsylvania Hospital (Philadelphia) and the New York Hospital, Massachusetts General Hospital (1807) was also located in a large city. All of these hospitals had excellent buildings (block-type) for the period and tended to follow the British models. Massachusetts General was a private enterprise and was established by a group of prominent physicians. It subsequently began to build pavilion wards with the idea that patients needed to be segregated and provided with increased light, air, and space. It eventually acquired a reputation for cleanliness and good nursing care.

Other hospitals that still carry on public service, along with several dispensaries, originated before 1860. In 1786 the Quakers established the Philadelphia Dispensary to care for the sick in their homes. It was independent of any hospital, and finances were taken care of through appeals to public sympathy. The concept that large numbers of people needing treatment were not sick enough to be hospitalized was a relatively new one. As a result of this idea, the expense of hospital care became unnecessary. Medical, surgical, and obstetrical services were offered under the supervision of Dr. Joseph Warrington. Physicians treated individuals without charge and made home visits when necessary. The dispensary was a success, and the idea spread to other cities. The New York Dispensary was opened in 1791; the Boston Dispensary, in 1796. The latter had the first dental, lung, and evening pay clinic for working people in the nation; in addition, it housed the first food clinic in the world. The dispensaries sank into neglect and almost obscurity when public and professional interest turned to hospitals. Services dwindled until a first-aid service and the issuance of free medicines were the only remaining functions.

MEDICINE IN THE COLONIES

Bleeding Bowl, c. 1760. Porcelain, Strasburg. *(Private Collection/The Bridgeman Art Library, London.)*

Medicine could offer little help against rampant disease and sickness in colonial America. Medieval methods were used in diagnosis, and treatments generally were not scientifically based. Emetics, purgatives, and bleeding continued to be the chief methods employed in the care of the sick. Brandy and whiskey became favorite remedies for febrile illnesses and continued to be so for a number of years. By the middle of the nineteenth century, however, the contributions to scientific knowledge made by Pasteur, Lister, Koch, and others began the modern era of medicine and surgery. The science of bacteriology provided the foundation. The introduction of ether and chloroform as general anesthetics facilitated surgical practice. These advances altered the course of medical history to the point that concepts of illness, treatments, and hygienic practices at the end of the century bore little resemblance to what they had been in the beginning. "Looking back, one may say that medicine was groping in the dark but was seeking light with growing anticipation. New concepts as well as further knowledge were essential if light was to be found" (Shryock, 1959, p. 195).

Serious health problems were brought to the New World with the migrants who left Europe. Scarlet fever, diphtheria, influenza, typhoid, typhus, tuberculosis, yellow fever, and other infectious diseases produced epidemics that were a constant nightmare. Scurvy and pellagra were the prevalent nutritional diseases and indicated a lack of proper food, particularly among the poorer classes. One in five individuals was afflicted with smallpox, which proved to be a formidable and dreaded disease. Fear became so great that experiments with inoculation were undertaken. Nearly all physicians opposed it, but the prominent clergy supported it. The opposition was apparently because of the risk factor involved with inoculation (occasionally deaths followed). The process of inoculation represented the beginnings of preventive medicine or, more specifically, immunology. A modified form called vaccination replaced the use of smallpox inoculation. Developed and reported in 1798 by Edward Jenner, it employed the use of the cowpox "virus," which proved to be safer and equally effective.

The true nature of disease remained an enigma. In addition, few persons understood how the prevailing practices used with disease and illness worked. They were ignorant of the action within the body that brought about the observed effects. In many instances it was enough just to know that it worked. "Learned men" gave advice on care of the sick and surgical care. Many laypersons thus functioned as physicians without ever receiving a formal medical degree. Colonial physicians were generally poorly educated. According to some sources, the title *doctor* was not even used in the colonies before 1769. It was an age of few doctors and of many profiteering quacks.

> Of medicine the Puritans knew little and practiced less. They swallowed doses of weird and repelling concoctions, wore charms and amulets, found comfort and relief in internal and external remedies that could have had no possible influence upon the cause of the trouble, and when all else failed they fell back upon the mercy and will of God. Surgery was a matter of tooth-pulling and bone-setting, and though post-mortems were performed, we have no knowledge of the skill of the practitioner. The healing art, as well as nursing and midwifery, was frequently in the hands of women. . . . The men who practiced physic were generally homebred, making the greater part of their living at farming or agriculture. Some were ministers as well as physicians. . . . There were a number of regularly trained doctors—though not a physician had more than a smattering of medicine.
>
> — *Andrews, vol. 6, p. 82*

Individuals who could afford the expense went to Europe to study in the medical schools of Edinburgh or Vienna. Otherwise, young students of medicine were apprenticed to a practicing physician, to whom they paid a fee (usually one hundred dollars) and rendered services about the house and stables. They were permitted to observe their master treat patients and upon completing the duration of the apprenticeship would receive the textbooks and instruments essential for their practice. The learning techniques comprised observation, reading, and practice. The average time spent in this process was approximately one hundred and forty-four weeks or close to three years. The preceptors ultimately became a powerful force that prevented progress in medical education and care.

As the colonies continued to develop, the issue of medical education increased in importance. Yet the medical departments did not find a place in colleges or universities until Harvard, the first American university (founded in 1636) was more than one hundred years old. They were then organized rapidly and included the Medical College of Philadelphia in 1765 (later a part of the University of Pennsylvania); King's College in New York City in 1767; Harvard in 1783; and Dartmouth in 1798. Other programs developed in the next century and included those established at Yale in 1810 and Johns Hopkins University in 1893.

> When the nineteenth century dawned, America had only four small medical schools to supply physicians for its burgeoning population, compelling most doctors to acquire their training by apprenticeship. In 1807 the University of Maryland Medical School was organized by a small group of Baltimore physicians as a private venture, and in succeeding years dozens of these proprietary medical schools came into existence. Three or four physicians would apply for a state charter, rent or buy a building, and begin advertising for students. The school year ordinarily lasted from eight to fourteen weeks, and the course work consisted exclusively of listening to lectures. Many proprietary schools granted degrees after one academic year, although they usually required the student to have served a one- or two-year apprenticeship prior to admission. Since these schools were dependent upon student fees for income, few applicants were ever turned down and even fewer failed to graduate.
>
> — *Lyons, 1978, p. 534*

Approximately four hundred medical schools were established before 1860, and many of them graduated poorly educated physicians. The quality of instruction was poor, libraries were inadequate, there were no laboratories, and dissection opportunities were limited. Little had been done to regulate these programs. The formation of the American Medical Association in 1847 finally led to the reform and advancement of medicine. This organization advocated the improvement of medical education, the establishment of a code of ethics, and the promotion of public health measures. The advent of this association moved American medicine toward professionalization. The AMA created a permanent committee on education in 1904, and it became the AMA Council on Medical Education in 1906. This council persuaded the Carnegie Foundation for the Advancement of Teaching to evaluate medical schools according to the ability of their graduates to pass licensing board examinations. Abraham Flexner was employed by the foundation to survey the field. His report, commonly referred to as the Flexner Report, was published in 1910 as *Medical Education in the United States and Canada*. It was a damning indictment of medical education and brought foundation money to the higher-quality schools; the weaker schools were forced out of business. The council, in turn, classified the schools on an A, B, C basis, which played a primary role in the standardization of medical education.

Thomas Eakins, *The Agnew Clinic,* 1889.
Canvas, 331.5 × 179.1 cm. *(Courtesy of the
University of Pennsylvania School of Medicine,
Philadelphia.)*

The Agnew Clinic depicts a striking contrast to Eakins' earlier work, *The Gross
Clinic.* Here significant reforms and
advancements in surgical techniques and
procedures in the operating room are
apparent. Surgeons wear gowns, instruments are sterilized, ether is used, and the
patient is covered. An operating room
nurse is a prominent member of the team.

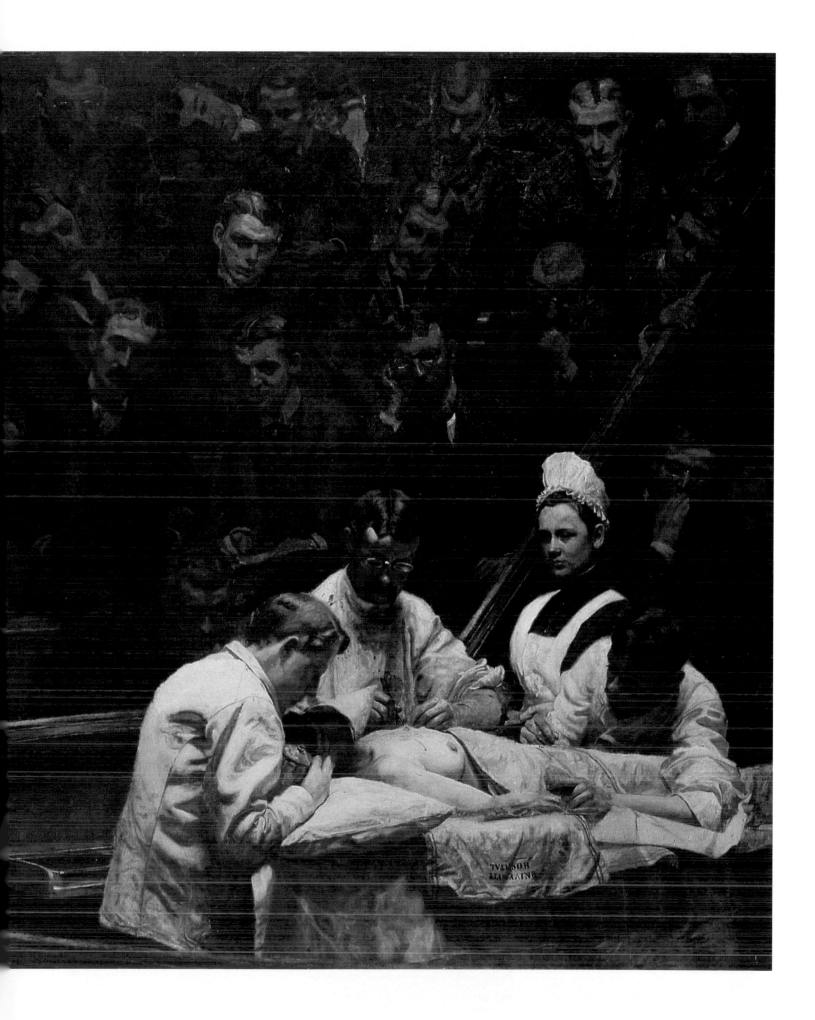

The remarkable progress that was finally achieved in the scientific basis of patient care was illustrated by Thomas Eakins (1844–1916). This American artist left two paintings that vividly present a "before-and-after" look at the medical scene. His celebrated painting, *The Gross Clinic* (1875), depicts grand rounds in which Dr. Samuel Gross explains the surgical operation being performed to medical students. It appears that he is totally unaware of the patient and oblivious to the horror of the patient's mother, who sits to his right. *The Agnew Clinic* (1889) depicts a distinct change and a striking contrast to the earlier work. The surgeons wear gowns, instruments are sterilized, the patient is covered, and ether is being used. The operation being performed is a mastectomy for breast cancer. This painting also depicts an operating room nurse (nursing schools had finally opened) as a prominent member of the operating team. The needed reforms had begun to occur.

RELIGIOUS NURSING ORDERS IN AMERICA

Many priests and nuns came to America with the French and Spanish settlers and supplied at least a minimum of nursing care to the Catholic communities. The Augustinian Nuns, Ursuline Nuns, and Sisters of Charity are most often mentioned in the history of nursing service in the hospitals of North and South America. Religious orders of women also contributed greatly to

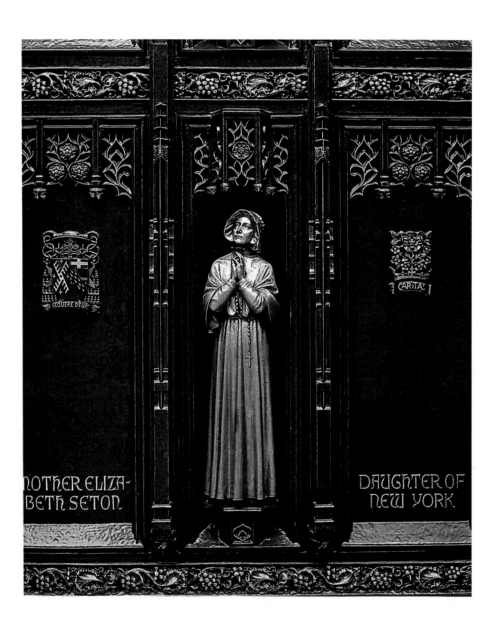

"St. Elizabeth Ann Seton," detail from *The Great Bronze Doors. (St. Patrick's Cathedral, New York.)*

nursing care during the Civil War. Their organization and motivation provided a distinct advantage over the so-called lay nurses of the day. The members of these orders had some education and had been carefully instructed. Those recruited to these orders were usually refined, intelligent women with a sincere interest in the care of the sick.

Among the earliest religious communities that took part in the care of the sick in hospitals and homes in the United States was the Sisters of Charity of Emmitsburg, Maryland. This order was founded by Mother Seton (1774–1821) in 1809. Elizabeth Ann Bayley Seton became the first native-born North American to be canonized (in 1976) for her charitable works. Her original community was known as the Sisters of Charity of St. Joseph's, but in 1850 the members united with the worldwide community of the Daughters of Charity of St. Vincent de Paul. A habit of blue with a large linen headdress (cornette) was chosen at this time in lieu of the original dress of the community. (The founding group wore a habit that resembled Elizabeth Seton's widow's dress.) Eventually numerous orders or different branches of orders in the Roman Catholic Church bore the name of Sisters of Charity: the Sisters of Charity of New York (Black Cap Sisters of Charity); the Sisters of Charity of Greensburg, Pennsylvania; of New Jersey of Cincinnati; of Halifax, Nova Scotia; and the Sisters of Charity of Nazareth, Kentucky. The latter community was founded by Mother Catherine Spalding; its members used horses for travel to the homes of patients. These various orders were also called by other names: Grey Sisters or Grey Nuns, Daughters of Charity, and Sisters of St. Vincent de Paul. Opportunities were provided in nursing education, the delivery of nursing service, and parochial education.

Elizabeth Seton was the daughter of Richard Bayley, an eminent American physician who was the first professor of anatomy at King's College (now Columbia University). Elizabeth Seton and other society matrons established the Society for Relief of Poor Widows with Small Children (1797) in New York to raise money for poor widows, to visit them in their homes, and to nurse and comfort them. Upon her husband's early death in 1803, she was left with five children and no financial support. Her conversion to Catholicism alienated friends who otherwise might have assisted her. She turned to teaching and opened a school for girls in Baltimore. A piece of land in Emmitsburg was chosen for the school, and it was not long before other young women joined her and became sisters in this teaching order. This event was the beginning of parochial education in the United States.

These Sisters of Charity became well known for their remarkable work in hospital nursing and nursing during epidemics. They were asked to manage a number of hospitals, including the Baltimore Infirmary, the Mullanphy Hospital in St. Louis, and the Charity Hospital of New Orleans. Nursing thus became an important branch of their work. The members were also instrumental in founding several hospitals and mental and foundling asylums.

Demands for nursing care by the religious orders increased as the settlements of the new country progressed. The various Catholic nursing orders responded rapidly and developed extensive networks throughout the country. The Sisters of Mercy, the Sisters of the Holy Cross, the Irish Sisters of Mercy (who came to America in 1843), the Dominicans, the Sisters of the Poor of St. Francis, and other communities worked in hospitals and homes and in all types of settings. The majority of them also nursed under fire on the battlefields. They founded hospitals everywhere and provided the highest standards of nursing of the times. Many of the first hospitals in America were named Mercy Hospitals, such as those in Pittsburgh, Chicago, and San Francisco. These were the better hospitals that were available at the time of the Civil War.

Sisterhoods of the Protestant church also contributed to the nursing effort in America. The Episcopal Sisterhood of the Holy Communion was founded in New York in 1845 by Pastor Muhlenberg at what is currently St. Luke's Hospital. The work of the English Lutheran Church began with four dea-

Filicchi, *Portrait of St. Elizabeth Ann Seton*, c. 1804, Oil on canvas. *(Courtesy of Daughters of Charity, St. Joseph's Provincial House, Emmitsburg, Maryland.)*

241

Foundling Hospital of the Sisters of Charity of St. Vincent de Paul of New York, "Washing the Babies," 1869. Engraving. (The Bettmann Archive, New York.)

The New York Foundling Asylum was one of the most important foundations of the Sisters of Charity in New York. Foundling children received at the almshouse or cared for at Bellevue almost invariably died. If they survived, their upbringing was minimal at best. The Foundling Hospital's system of caring for children became a prototype for similar organizations in countries around the world.

conesses who were brought to Passavant's Hospital in Pittsburgh by Pastor Fliednor in 1849. In Baltimore there was a branch of the English All Saints Sisters. The English Sisterhood of St. Margaret's (Episcopal) was brought to Boston about 1869, the beginning of its forty-some years of service to the Children's Hospital of that city. Many deaconess hospitals were established, particularly in the Midwest. Protestant religious nursing groups also gave nursing care to the sick and the wounded during the time of the Civil War.

THE REVOLUTIONARY WAR

Colonial wars were fought from 1607 until the Revolution. These wars involved American Indians, emigrants, loyalists, and patriots, and colonist against colonist. The desire for independence grew stronger and stronger as the colonists became more self-sufficient. Yet until 1774 they considered themselves Britons. In that year Patrick Henry made his famous statement: "The distinctions between Virginians, Pennsylvanians, New Yorkers, and New Englanders are no more. I am not a Virginian but an American." The inevitable conflict between the British Crown and the colonies terminated in the Revolutionary War.

The American Revolution involved all the English colonies along the Atlantic coast. The colonies were, however, ill prepared for the burdens, the expense, and the organization necessary to wage war on their own. The hastily mobilized army had no medical corps, no Red Cross, and no trained nurses. The nuns of the Catholic Church placed themselves and their hospitals at

John Edward Svenson, *Sisters of Providence,* installed 1980. Mahogany, 1.8 meters wide × 2.4 meters high. *(Providence Alaska Medical Center, Anchorage, Alaska.)*

The sculpture was formally dedicated in February 1980. The artist commented during the dedication, "I want this sculpture to be understood by all. If a man of eighty and his grandson of eight years look at it together, there are people and animals and scenes that both would understand and appreciate."

The sculpture contains nine different scenes, with the lighting designed to flow down to create the proper visual effect: Alaska today . . . and tomorrow, sisters first arrive in Alaska; the Chena River floods; new Alaskans arrive at Providence; Captain Cook; an Aleut; Alaska's wildlife; Providence survives the earthquake; and modern technologies. The Sisters of Providence have served in Alaska since 1902.

the disposal of the military authorities, since they were the only organized groups with some knowledge of nursing. Goodnow quotes a colonial writer who vividly depicted this state of affairs:

> At the start of the war the tale of the medical department was a sorry one. There was practically no organization nor discipline. Surgical instruments were few. Drugs were few and bad; opium and quinine were scarce and ether was then unknown. Trained nurses and scientific nursing did not exist. Blundering assistants called 'mates' were the only help the surgeons had.
>
> — *Goodnow, 1942, p. 182*

Several private homes in Cambridge were made into hospitals after the Battle of Bunker Hill, and Dr. John Warren was placed in charge. These are regarded as the first military hospitals. Other hospitals were established in Boston, where the nurses were mostly men. Women made no attempt at organized nursing, although meager records indicate that a few women were actually employed as nurses to care for the soldiers. According to a congressional resolution of July 17, 1775, there would be one nurse to every ten patients in the personnel for military hospitals (Hahn, 1927). These women were to be paid one fifteenth of a dollar per day, the equivalent of two dollars per month (Stimson, 1925).

The government authorities were not indifferent to the condition of the military hospitals; however, they were involved with the general burdens of a revolution. Finally, in 1777 General Washington ordered that women be obtained to nurse the soldiers. Many women were subsequently employed, but they did little more than cook and serve meals. Often women followed their husbands to the battlefield and nursed them under the greatest of obstacles. Little surgery was performed because there were no anesthetics; the main type of surgery was amputation. There were frequent epidemics of scarlet fever, dysentery, and smallpox. Food rations were meager, and shoes and clothing rapidly wore out. An interesting commentary about the aftermath of the war was rendered by Robinson:

> War, with its sudden collections of sick, wounded, and maimed, stimulates the progress of medicine: 'The War of the Revolution was the making of medicine in this country.' In the change from colonial to national medicine, the casualty was woman: woman was not ignored, she was expelled. The female practitioner, denied the opportunity and instruction of the new time, ceased to exist. Trained male obstetricians, invading the lying-in chamber, thrust out the immemorial midwife. As later expressed by a Boston physician (1820): 'It was one of the first and happiest fruits of improved medical education in America, that females were excluded from practice; and this has only been effected by the united and persevering efforts of some of the most distinguished individuals of the profession.' In the male monopoly of medicine, there was no room for the trained nurse: any grandmother, any destitute old woman who could be hired, was requisitioned as nurse, and none other was desired.
>
> — *Robinson, 1946, p. 139*

NURSING IN THE CIVIL WAR (1861–1865)

Winslow Homer, *Our Women and the War.* Engraving, approx. 34.3 × 52.1 cm. *Harper's Weekly,* September 6, 1862. *(National Library of Medicine, Bethesda, Maryland.)*

At the outbreak of the Civil War, the Union had no army nurse corps, ambulance service, field hospital service, or organized medical corps. There was still no group of trained nurses in the country, but after the first battles the need for nurses became imperative. Many religious orders volunteered and offered

THE SISTER OF CHARITY · HOME TIDINGS

HEROES AND HEROINES OF THE WAR.

ENSIGN & BRIDGMAN,   156 WILLIAM STREET, N.Y.

Thomas Nast, *Heroes and Heroines of the War,* Civil War, nineteenth century. Engraving. *(Chicago Historical Society, Chicago, Illinois.)*

Represented in this print are the many diverse activities of the United States Sanitary Commission, which provided nurses both on and off the battlefield, as well as helping to make supplies and raise money to support health care.

Cared For. Wood engraving. *Harper's Weekly,* January 21, 1871. *(National Library of Medicine, Bethesda, Maryland.)*

their services. They provided nursing care in their own hospitals, in army hospitals, and on the battlefield. Approximately six hundred Sisters from twelve orders participated during this critical period in history. They were given permission by President Abraham Lincoln to purchase any supplies needed for their work. Lincoln knew that most "good nursing" was being done by these religious sisterhoods, that they had helped in epidemics, that they were already organized and were accustomed to discipline and obedience to authority. He therefore supported their efforts to the fullest. There were not, however, enough sisters to care for the large number of sick and wounded. Hundreds of other women and men simply appeared in the camps and offered their services. With and without experience, they assisted with nursing care in whatever way they were able. The majority were volunteers, although some received compensation. It is estimated that between two and ten thou-

Eleven Vignettes of Scenes in the U.S. Army's Citizens Volunteer Hospital, c. 1860. Lithograph. *(National Library of Medicine, Bethesda, Maryland.)*

These scenes depict the Army's Citizens Volunteer Hospital in Philadelphia during the Civil War, where volunteer nurses served in the wards.

sand women or more were engaged in nursing and hospital administration during the Civil War. (The large range is a result of the variance in citations in reference materials.) The most famous of these were Dorothea Lynde Dix, Clara Barton, Louisa May Alcott, Mary Ann "Mother" Bickerdyke, and Walt Whitman.

The total number of men lost either from battle injuries or from disease during the American Civil War was 618,000; 360,000 men were Union soldiers and 258,000, Confederates. Many of these died on the battlefield. Those with less serious wounds faced inadequate sanitary conditions and a generally awkward and unorganized medical corps. Septicemia, erysipelas, gangrene, and tetanus were common complications among the wounded. Almost any type of building became a military hospital; base hospitals were located in hotels, churches, warehouses, schools, farmhouses, and other public buildings.

Allyn Cox, *Rotunda as a Hospital During the Civil War,* 1862, corridor, House Wing. *(Library of Congress, Washington, D.C.)*

In addition, structures were hastily erected or tents were pitched. Even the Capitol was used, with four hundred soldiers nursed in the Senate and House and three hundred in the Rotunda. Ward masters and orderlies were available in many of the hospitals to do as much nursing as possible. Women nurses gave medicines, tended to the diets, and dressed wounds.

The sick and injured were originally removed from the battlefield in hand-carried litters. Later a medical transport service was organized with horse-drawn covered wagons used as ambulances. These springless wagons often inflicted much pain on the wounded as they bumped for hours over badly kept roads. Hospital trains were furnished by the railroads. Vessels along the eastern seaboard and the Mississippi water route were used to evacuate patients and as "floating hospitals." The first navy hospital ship, the steamer *Red Rover,* was put into service. Captured from the Confederates, this steamer was converted into a floating hospital and then added to the federal fleet of ships. The Catholic Sisters of Mercy volunteered to do the nursing on board and can be considered the first navy nurses. A description of the *Red Rover* was provided in a letter to Flag Officer A.H. Foote:

> I wish that you could see our hospital boat, the *Red Rover,* with all her comforts for the sick and disabled seamen. She is decided to be the most complete thing of her kind that ever floated, and is in every way a decided success. The Western Sanitary Commission gave us, in cost of articles, $3,500. The icebox of the steamer holds 300 tons. She has bathrooms, laundry, elevator for the sick from the lower to the upper deck, operating room, nine different water closets, gauze blinds to the windows to keep the cinders and smoke from annoying the sick, two separate kitchens for sick and well, a regular corps of nurses, and two water closets on every deck.

— Roddis, 1935, p. 92

"The Sister."   Convalescent Ward.

The Sister and Convalescent Ward on the Naval Ship Red Rover. Wood engraving. Harper's Weekly, May 9, 1863. (National Library of Medicine, Bethesda, Maryland.)

Theodore R. Davis, *The Ward*. Drawing, *Harper's Weekly*, 1863. (National Archives and Records Service, Washington, D.C.)

Scene from one of the wards on the *Red Rover* Hospital Ship during the Civil War.

249

United States Sanitary Commission

Within a month after Lincoln's initial request for soldiers, Elizabeth Blackwell, America's first woman physician, organized the Women's Central Association for Relief in New York City. Louisa Lee Schuyler was elected president. Through the efforts of this group and similar ones, the Rev. Dr. Henry W. Bellows and four physicians were persuaded to go to Washington to plead for the establishment of a sanitary commission. This commission would act as advisor to the medical department of the army and would investigate the health conditions of the Union army. After both governmental and military opposition was overcome, the United States Sanitary Commission was established by order of President Lincoln on June 3, 1861. Its aim was stated as "a simple desire and resolute determination to secure for the men who have enlisted in this war, that care which it is the duty of the nation to give them" (Boardman, 1915, p. 53). A sum of five million dollars in cash and fifteen million dollars worth of supplies was raised. This organization has been called the forerunner of the American Red Cross.

The Women's Central Association for Relief became a branch of the Sanitary Commission. Where branches did not exist, it stimulated the formation of new ones. It coordinated all the relief organizations throughout the country and sent nurses to areas where they were needed most. Preparatory programs were planned for the nurses at New York Hospital, Bellevue Hospital, and several Boston hospitals. The nurses received one month's observation and work experience. The Western Sanitary Commission was distinct from the eastern one but cooperated with it. It operated hospital steamers on the Ohio and Mississippi Rivers in addition to a hospital train. The Confederacy had no such organization, but a number of women's groups rendered valuable service to the cause of the war.

William Groth, *U.S. General Hospital During the Civil War,* Mound City, Illinois. *(National Archives and Record Service, Washington, D.C.)*

This hospital served as the staffing base for the USS *Red Rover.*

The Sanitary Commission wished to secure the most healthful conditions in the military camps, hospitals, and on transports. It first inspected the army camps in the vicinity of Washington and found these to be lacking in a variety of areas, including sanitation and hygiene, rations, and space. The report revealed that fifteen percent of the Northern regiment physicians were poorly qualified or totally incompetent. Soon after, the Northern forces suffered defeat at the Battle of Bull Run, and an inquiry showed that the defeat lay in those conditions identified by the commission. In general, the soldiers had entered battle in an unfit condition.

The Interior of a Sanitary Steamer. Engraving, *Harper's Weekly,* 1862. *(National Archives and Records Service, Washington, D.C.)*

The Interior of a Sanitary Steamer.

After the Battle, 1881. Engraving. *(The Bettmann Archive, New York.)*

251

After the first battles of the war, the wounded had practically no care. 'Common soldiers, untrained, lazy, and indifferent or brutal, were cooks and nurses for the war hospitals, the largest of which had 40 beds. There were no medicines, no stores, nor ambulances. The camps were dirty and unsanitary.' When they (the Sanitary Commission) first offered supplies and service, the Government Medical Bureau looked upon the proposal with suspicion; but its dire need soon forced it to accept. The Commission collected and distributed supplies of all sorts, planned camps and attended to their sanitation, tended the wounded on the field and in hospitals; in short, undertook a large share of the health work for the army. It provided such things as green vegetables, given by the farmers for the soldiers, thus preventing scurvy, the great army scourge.

— *Goodnow, 1942, pp. 190–191*

Dorothea Lynde Dix

On June 10, 1861, Dorothea Lynde Dix was appointed Superintendent of the Female Nurses of the Union Army by the Secretary of War, Simon Cameron. This action provided for a corps of volunteer women nurses to be organized under her direction. Dix was given the power to organize hospitals for the care of all wounded and sick soldiers, to appoint nurses, and to oversee and regulate specially donated supplies for distribution to the troops. Dix was past the age of sixty when she received her appointment. She was not granted military rank, nor were the members of her corps. Although she did not have preparation in nursing, she possessed the necessary organizational skills from

Portrait of Dorothea Dix. (National Library of Medicine, Bethesda, Maryland.)

Dorothea Lynde Dix became well known for her crusades to reform insane asylums. She traveled thousands of miles to inspect the existing mental institutions. Armed with evidence of shocking mistreatment, she appealed to state legislatures for improved treatment and improved facilities.

252

her previous humanitarian efforts in the area of mental health. Circular No. 7 of the surgeon general's office in the War Department read:

> In order to give greater utility to the acts of Miss Dorothy L. Dix as superintendent of women nurses in general hospitals, and to make the employment of such nurses conform more closely to existing laws . . . Miss Dix has been entrusted by the War Department with the duty of selecting women nurses and assigning them to general or permanent military hospitals. Women nurses are not to be employed in such hospitals without her sanction and approval except in case of urgent need. . . . Women wishing employment as nurses must apply to Miss Dix or to her authorised agents. Army regulations allow one nurse to every ten patients (beds).

Dix's requirements for candidates were specified in Circular No. 8, dated July 24, 1862. No candidate for a nurse position would be considered unless she was between the ages of thirty-five and fifty. Matronly and plain-looking persons of experience, of superior education, and of serious disposition were to have preference.

The following is the actual wording of the circular:

CIRCULAR NO. 8

Washington, July 24, 1862

No candidate for service in the Women's Department for nursing in the Military Hospitals of the United States, will be received below the age of thirty-five years, nor above fifty.

Only women of strong health, not subjects of chronic disease, nor liable to sudden illnesses, need apply. The duties of the station make large and continued demands on strength.

Matronly persons of experience, good conduct, or superior education and serious disposition, will always have preference; habits of neatness, order, sobriety, and industry are prerequisites.

All applicants must present certificates of qualification and good character from at least two persons of trust, testifying to morality, integrity, seriousness, and capacity for care of the sick.

Obedience to rules of the service, and conformity to special regulations, will be required and enforced.

Compensation, as regulated by Act of Congress, forty cents a day and subsistence. Transportation furnished to and from the place of service.

Amount of luggage limited within small compass.

Dress plain (colors brown, grey, or black), and, while connected with the service, without ornaments of any sort.

No applicants accepted for less than three months' service; those for longer periods always have preference.

— D. L. Dix

Approved:
William A. Hammond,
Surgeon-General

Many women who were unable to meet the requirements ignored them and nursed during the war without official recognition or compensation. At the close of hostilities the office of the superintendent was abolished, and Dorothea Dix returned to her civilian life of reformative work in public institutions.

Mary A. Livermore (1820–1905) served as a nurse with the United States Sanitary Commission. She believed that the more accomplished and refined a volunteer was, the better nurse she would be. After the Civil War she became a leader in the suffrage movement and advocated for education for women. She would later address the sixth annual convention of the Nurses' Associated Alumnae in 1903 and acknowledge nursing as a new profession arising in part from the Civil War experiences.

CHRISTIAN HERALD

AND SIGNS OF OUR TIMES

OFFICES: BIBLE HOUSE NEW YORK.

Rev. T. De Witt Talmage, D.D., Editor.

COPYRIGHT 1898, BY LOUIS KLOPSCH.

NEW YORK, MARCH 9, 1898.

VOLUME 21.—NUMBER 10.

PRICE FIVE CENTS.

"I AM WITH THE WOUNDED."—Clara Barton's Cable Message from Havana to "The Christian Herald."

"I am with the wounded," flashed along the wire
 From the isle of Cuba, swept with sword and fire.
Angel sweet of mercy, may your cross of red
 Cheer the wounded living: bless the wounded dead.

"I am with the starving," let the message run
 From the stricken island, when this task is done;
Food and money plenty wait at your command.
 Give in generous measure: fill each outstretched hand.

"I am with the happy," this we long to hear
 From the isle of Cuba, trembling now in fear.
May the great disaster touch the hearts of men,
 And, in God's great mercy, bring back peace again.

—JAMES CLARENCE HARVEY.

"I Am With the Wounded." Clara Barton's
cable message from Havana, from the
cover of the *Christian Herald,* March 9,
1898. *(The Christian Herald Association,
Chappaqua, New York.)*

Clara Barton

During the Civil War, Clara Barton (1821–1912) became known as the "little lone lady in black silk." Nearly all war nurses were under the supervision of Dorothea Dix; the relief workers were associated with relief or aid societies, the Sanitary Commission, or religious organizations. Clara Barton, however, could not take orders or share authority and relied on her own initiative. She independently operated a large-scale war relief operation in which she arranged for huge quantities of supplies to be furnished to the army and the hospitals. She also personally nursed in federal hospitals and with the armies on the battlefield and cared for the wounded of the Confederate armies. Her impartiality was expressed in the nursing care she extended to both whites and blacks, Northerners and Southerners. She frequently used her own resources to furnish such necessities as medical supplies, proper clothing, food, and bedding. On more than one occasion, bullets made holes in her dress and the men she was nursing were shot in her arms. Barton eventually became one of the most prominent figures among the lay nurses of the Civil War. Her work embodied the ideals now characteristic of the Red Cross and became the foundation for her later success in the development of the American Red Cross.

Clara Barton (Clarissa Harlowe) was born in North Oxford, Massachusetts. A former New England schoolteacher, she was appointed to a clerkship in the Patent Office in Washington, D.C., in 1854. This may have been the first time a woman held a government position. Barton was, however, dismissed from this position because of her outspoken opinions on slavery. She seemed to have a flair for being the first to arrive on a scene and the first to leave when others appeared. She was already in Washington giving aid to the Sixth Massachusetts Regiment when Dorothea Dix arrived. When peace was

Clara Barton is well known for her service as a nurse during the Civil War and the Franco-Prussian War. The American Red Cross was established in 1881 as a result of her perseverance. Barton's portrait is depicted in an oval on the stamp; to the right of the portrait is a Red Cross symbol with the wording "Founder of the American Red Cross." Barton coordinated relief work during all types of natural disasters, including floods, famine, and epidemics. This stamp was placed on sale September 7, 1948, in Oxford, Massachusetts, Barton's birthplace. *(Stamp courtesy of Medical Economics Publishing, New Jersey.)*

This Red Cross commemorative stamp was placed on sale May 21, 1931, at Washington, D.C., location of the national headquarters, and at Dansville, New York, location of the first local chapter. The central design of the stamp is the figure of a Red Cross nurse kneeling with outstretched hands before the globe. The scene is reproduced from a 1930 poster entitled "The Greatest Mother." The Greek cross with five equal squares, the emblem of the organization, is printed in red and located at the upper left of the stamp. *(Stamp courtesy of Medical Economics Publishing, New Jersey.)*

Left, Two Nursing Nuns and a Red Cross Nurse Tend Casualties During the Franco-Prussian War. Wood engraving. From *La Mode Illustrée,* c. 1870. *(National Library of Medicine, Bethesda, Maryland.)*

Judy Waid, *Nursing: A Tradition of Caring*, 1992. *(Copyright Judy Waid and District Three, Ohio Nurses Association, Youngstown, Ohio.)*

This third edition medallion depicts a historical perspective of the nursing profession. Clara Barton, founder of the American Red Cross, nursed the soldiers on the battlefields of the Civil War and distributed supplies to the wounded. She is remembered for her contributions as a teacher, nurse, social and political reformist, journalist, and humanitarian.

finally made, Clara Barton conducted a prolonged search at her own expense for eighty thousand missing men of the army. She also delivered three hundred lectures about the battlefields of the Civil War and established the first national cemetery on the Andersonville grounds. Barton was overcome by nervous prostration, a condition that had surfaced earlier, and was directed by physicians to go to Europe, where she remained for four years. A month after arriving in Europe, she learned about the International Red Cross.

Clara Barton served with the Red Cross in 1870 during the Franco-Prussian War. On the battlefields and in the ravaged cities of France, she repeated her American Civil War performance. She also observed the systematic organization and remarkable effectiveness of the Red Cross and promised that America would join. She was subsequently decorated with the Iron Cross by the kaiser. After a four-year absence, Barton returned to the United States and began her crusade for the establishment of the American Red Cross. A Red Cross Committee was finally formed in 1881, but it took until 1882 for the U.S. government to ratify the Geneva Convention and give the committee official standing. Clara Barton became its first president and held this office until 1904. Her home in Glen Echo, Maryland, served as the national headquarters. According to the official charter, the Red Cross was dedicated

> to continue and carry on a system of national and international relief in time of peace and to apply the same in mitigating the sufferings caused by pestilence, famine, fire, floods, and other national calamities, and to devise and carry measure for preventing the same.

> — *Pilcher, 1907*

W.A. Rogers, *The Scene at the Bridge*, 1889. *(American Red Cross, Washington, D.C.)*

In this picture, the artist depicts the tremendous devastation wrought by the raging flood that swept through Johnstown, Pennsylvania, on May 31, 1889. On the bank of the Conemaugh River, a nurse symbolically offers succor to the victims. Five days after the flood, on the first train to get through, Clara Barton and some fifty Red Cross workers arrived to start a relief and rehabilitation program that was to extend for five months.

Assistance was first given in the United States during a yellow fever epidemic in Florida in 1888 and during the Johnstown flood of 1889. Red Cross nurses thereafter rendered service in numerous disasters that included tornadoes, hurricanes, cyclones, floods, and fires. In 1909 the American Red Cross was reorganized under Jane Delano. At that time plans were made for a Red Cross Nursing Service to be staffed by a reserve corps of graduate nurses with specified qualifications. This pool of nurses acted as a supplement to the regular army and navy nurses as the occasion warranted.

Volunteer Nurses

A large number of lay men and women volunteered as nurses during the Civil War. Many of them emerged as leaders and greatly influenced nursing during this period. All of them gave devoted service to the soldiers in time of need. They brought hope to the abandoned and gave faith to those who despaired. They nursed the sick and the wounded and comforted the dying. Most were amateurs, but their efforts had a positive effect on the troops.

> The Civil War is America's greatest tragedy, whose wounds have not healed with the balm of a century, yet it is a tragedy brightened by noble names in the North and in the South. America will lose a precious heritage if ever it permits these names to be forgotten. New ways and new names claim our attention, crowding out the old. From time to time, green leaves should be entwined with the sear laurels of the nurses of the Civil War.
>
> — *Robinson, 1946, p. 207*

Mother Bickerdyke (Mary Ann Ball, 1817–1901) belonged to this saga of America. Her blanket-shawl, calico dress, and Shaker bonnet were indicative of her pioneer ways, which have passed with a period of American history. She was given the name *Mother* by the soldiers, as an affectionate term that expressed their gratitude. Mother Bickerdyke had been a widow from Galesburg, Illinois, with a moderate education and two small sons when she answered the call to help with the war effort. Her minister, Henry Ward Beecher, had issued a plea for some women of his congregation to proceed to government hospitals and battlefields to care for the sick and the wounded. She had taken a short course in homeopathy from Dr. Samuel Hahnemann and received a degree of doctor of botanic medicine (Baker, 1952).

Mother Bickerdyke served under fire in nineteen battles from Fort Donelson in Tennessee to Savannah, Georgia. She organized diet kitchens, laundries, and an ambulance service. She supervised the nursing staff and distributed supplies. At night she often walked through the abandoned battlefields, afraid that someone who was still alive would be left. She became known as one of the greatest nurse heroines of the Civil War, and numerous tales were told about her exploits.

> Looking from his tent at midnight, an officer observed a faint light flitting hither and thither on the abandoned battlefield, and, after puzzling over it for some time, sent his servant to ascertain the cause. It was Mother Bickerdyke, with a lantern. Stooping down (among the dead) and turning their cold faces towards her, she scrutinized them searchingly, uneasy lest some might be left to die uncared for. She could not rest while she thought any were overlooked who were yet living.
>
> — *Baker, 1952, p. 11*

Mary Ann Bickerdyke was indeed the soldier's friend. She fought particularly hard for the rights and comforts of the common soldier. General Ulysses S. Grant and General William T. Sherman were among her powerful friends (Davis, 1886). Her accomplishments were recognized by the government at the launching of the hospital ship, the SS *Mary A. Bickerdyke* in 1943 at Richmond, California.

The Soldiers' Quarters at Georgetown, D.C., During the War 1861–1865. From *Leslie's Weekly,* July 6, 1861. *(Culver Pictures, Inc., New York.)*

Volunteer nurses attended the sick and the wounded at the U.S. General Hospital at Georgetown during the Civil War.

Louisa May Alcott (1832–1888) longed for a wider field of activity than that permitted a New England minister's daughter. She was a prominent advocate of women's rights, and at times this got in the way of her ambitions. Alcott is best known for her books *Little Women* and *Little Men,* and her poems and short stories were published in the *Atlantic Monthly.* This American novelist and writer of children's books served as a nurse at the Union Hospital at Georgetown (Washington, D.C.) for six weeks from 1862 to 1863 (Austin, 1957). This improvised hospital accommodated approximately three hundred patients who were in various stages of injury and disease. Alcott was placed in charge of a forty-bed ward, where she performed a variety of functions in her role of nurse. She dressed wounds, read novels to soldiers, wrote letters, made night rounds, and gave medicines. Her daily schedule was hectic, as portrayed in her journal:

> Up at six, dress by gaslight, run through my ward and throw up the windows, though the men grumble and shiver. But the air is bad enough to breed a pestilence, and as no notice is taken of our frequent appeals for better ventilation, I must do what I can . . . for a more perfect pestilence box than this house I never saw—cold, damp, dirty, full of vile odors from wounds, kitchens, washrooms, stables. Till noon I trot, trot, trot, giving out rations, cutting up food for helpless 'boys,' washing faces, teaching my attendants how beds are made or floors are swept, dressing wounds, dusting tables, sewing bandages, keeping my tray tidy, rushing up and down after pillows, bed linens, sponges, and directions until it seems as if I would joyfully pay down all I possess for fifteen minutes rest. At twelve comes dinner for the patients and afterward there is letter writing for them or reading aloud. Supper at five sets everyone running that can run . . . evening amusements . . . then, for such as need them, the final doses for the night.
>
> — *Alcott, 1863, p. 74.*

Alcott described the work done by the volunteer nurses in Civil War hospitals in letters that were published in 1863 in a book entitled *Hospital Sketches.* This is considered to be her first famous work. This small book of little more than a hundred pages is narrated by Nurse Tribulation Periwinkle, who vividly and at times humorously recounts the nursing experiences of these volunteers.

Another writer, Walt Whitman (1819–1892), left a record of the care of the sick during the Civil War. This was done in a collection of poems, *Drum-Taps,* and in a diary, *Specimen Days and Collect,* which described his experiences as a hospital nurse in Washington. Walt Whitman was described by the Danish scholar Frederick Schyberg as a "natural and inevitable product of the tendencies, the struggles, the crises of America in 1860." Accounts of his ministrations to the wounded and his varied responses to the war were dispersed in dozens of notebooks, newspaper dispatches, letters, and other types of published and unpublished works. These were compiled, edited, and then published for the first time in *Walt Whitman's Civil War* in 1960. Whitman carefully recorded each wounded soldier's simple request, noted his patients' names and addresses, wrote letters for soldiers who could not write, and drew a cross by the name of each patient who died. (In January 1995, four notebooks that contained these contents and had been missing from the Library of Congress were discovered by Sotheby's auction house in New York while making an evaluation for a client).

Whitman was self-educated and learned the printer's trade in his boyhood. He subsequently worked at various jobs and was the editor of different newspapers. In 1862 he left his odd jobs to visit the Civil War front. Upon his return to Washington, he spent the rest of the war period as a volunteer nurse and companion to wounded soldiers. He did this while earning a modest living as a government clerk, a position from which he was fired in 1865 because of official disapproval of the sexual terminology in *Leaves of Grass.* Whitman spent his final years of life (1873–1892) as an invalid in Camden, New Jersey. Of all his Civil War poetry, Whitman's perceptions of the sufferings of the men and his efforts on their behalf are best described in "The Wound-Dresser":

> Bearing the bandages, water and sponge,
> Straight and swift to my wounded I go,
> Where they lie on the ground after the battle brought in,
> Where their priceless blood reddens the grass, the ground,
> Or to the rows of the hospital tent, or under the roof'd hospital,
> To the long rows of cots up and down each side I return,
> To each and all one after another I draw near, not one do I miss,
> An attendant follows holding a tray, he carries a refuse pail,
> Soon to be fill'd with clotted rags and blood, emptied, and fill'd again.
>
> I onward go, I stop,
> With hinged knees and steady hand to dress wounds,
> I am firm with each, the pangs are sharp yet unavoidable,
> One turns to me his appealing eyes—poor boy! I never knew you,
> Yet I think I could not refuse this moment to die for you, if that would save you.
> On, on I go, (open doors of time! open hospital doors!)
> The crush'd head I dress, (poor crazed hand tear not the bandage away,)
> The neck of the cavalry-man with the bullet through and through I examine,
> Hard the breathing rattles, quite glazed already the eye, yet life struggles hard,
> (Come sweet death! be persuaded O beautiful death! In mercy come quickly.)
>
> From the stump of the arm, the amputated hand,
> I undo the clotted lint, remove the slough,
> wash off the matter and blood,
> Back on his pillow the soldier bends with
> curv'd neck and side falling head,
> His eyes are closed, his face is pale, he
> dares not look on the bloody stump,
> And has not yet look'd on it.

— *Whitman, 1961, pp. 44–45*

Louisa May Alcott is known primarily as an American author and writer of children's books, most notably *Little Women.* Less well known is her service as a Civil War nurse. Born in Germantown, Pennsylvania, in 1832, she was remembered in the U.S. "Famous Americans" series of stamps issued in 1940. *(Courtesy of Howard B. Hurley.)*

During the Civil War Walt Whitman worked as a volunteer hospital nurse in Washington, D.C., where he penned poetry about the conflict and wrote two of his most famous poems about President Abraham Lincoln, "When Lilacs Last in the Dooryard Bloom'd" and "O Captain! My Captain!" The United States stamp in his honor in the "Famous Americans" series was issued in February 1940 at Camden, New Jersey. *(Courtesy of Howard B. Hurley.)*

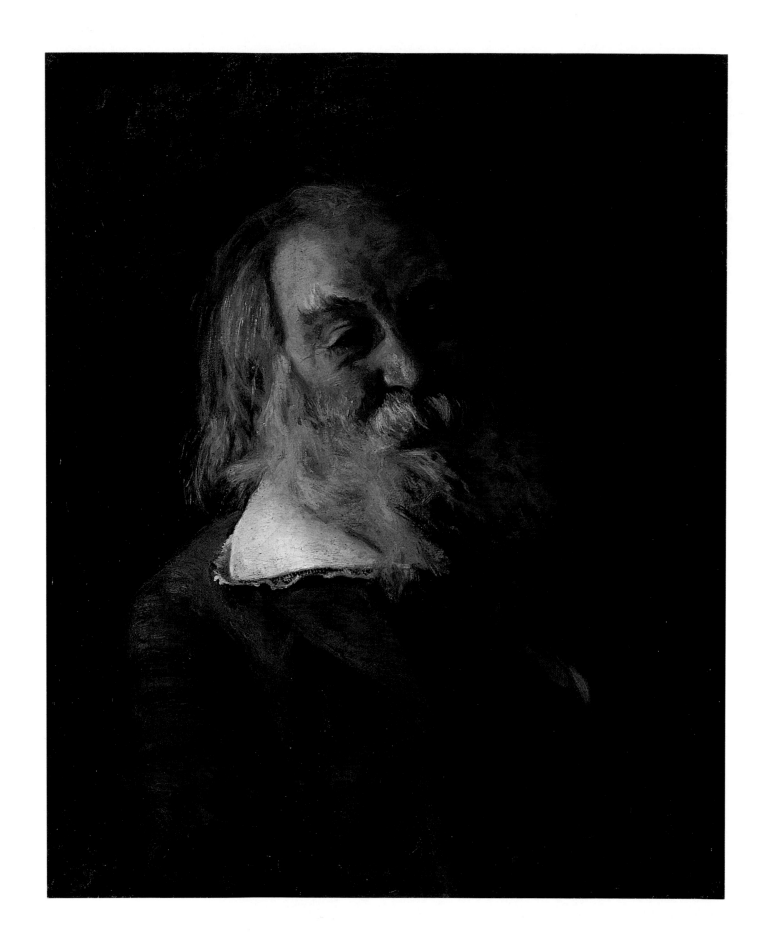

Thomas Eakins, *Walt Whitman,* 1888. Oil
on canvas. 76.5 × 61.6 cm. *(Courtesy of the
Pennsylvania Academy of the Fine Arts,
Philadelphia, General Fund Purchase.)*

Walt Whitman did not approve of women nursing in military hospitals. Even with his liberal views, he did not believe that it was a proper activity for respectable women. Yet many of the women who served as nurses in the Civil War were women from socially prestigious families who possessed strong political beliefs and educational backgrounds. Among them were the Woolsey sisters (Jane Stuart, Georgeanna, Eliza Howland), Margaret Breckinridge, Harriet Foote Hawley, Ella Louise Wolcott, and Louisa Lee Schuyler.

The women of the Confederacy also gave heroic service during the Civil War. Religious sisters and lay women volunteered to function as nurses. They opened their homes to sick and wounded soldiers to be used as hospitals and convalescent centers. Some, as in the North, followed their husbands to war and to the battlefield, where they assisted in every way possible. The list included Kate Cumming, Ella King Newsom, Annie Johns, Betsy Sullivan, and a host of others. However, one individual in particular stands out. The Confederate army did not appoint a director of nursing, but President Jefferson Davis granted the rank of captain to Sally Louisa Tompkins (1833–1916). She was the only woman to hold a commission in the army of the Confederacy. Miss Tompkins was the daughter of a wealthy Virginian and had been active in the charitable works of her church. She established a private hospital in Richmond and maintained it entirely at her own expense. Tompkins needed the rank in order to requisition supplies, but she refused to accept compensation for her work. The most serious and critical cases were brought to her independent institution because of its reputation. Yet the mortality rate was low: only 73 of 1333 patients died.

L. Daniel, *Walt Whitman as Nurse*. From *Selections From "Leaves of Grass" by Walt Whitman*, introduction by Walter Lowenfels, 1961. *(Crown Publishers Inc., New York.)*

Walt Whitman was a volunteer nurse in the truest sense of the word. He cared for wounded soldiers in various hospitals; he talked to them, read to them, wrote letters, and gave them gifts. A number of his poems reflect his thoughts and feelings during his service in the Civil War.

Winslow Homer, *Campaign Sketches: The Letter From Home*, 1863. Lithograph. *(Print Collection, The New York Public Library, New York. Astor, Lenox and Tilden Foundations.)*

Nurses Behind the Lines During the Civil War, c. 1860. Wood engraving. *(National Library of Medicine, Bethesda, Maryland.)*

Sojourner Truth, a nurse in the Civil War. *(Courtesy of W. B. Saunders Company, Philadelphia, Pennsylvania.)*

Sojourner Truth was one of the first people to identify the similarity between the problems of blacks and those of women. A former slave and an abolitionist, she lectured throughout the country and assisted newly freed slaves with finding jobs. After she was freed, she took her own name and eventually published her autobiography. Truth was a significant symbol of the struggle of black women to overcome the oppression not only of their race but also of their sex.

Kate Cumming (1828–1909) chronicled her work as a volunteer nurse in a diary, *Journal of Hospital Life in the Confederate Army of Tennessee from the Battle of Shiloh to the End of the War: With Sketches of Life and Character and Brief Notices of Current Events during That Period* (1866). She describes the care and lack of care of the sick and wounded in hospitals and battlefields. She identifies numerous problems that occur relative to food, transportation, clothing, and so forth, as well as diseases that are fatal. Although not prepared for nursing work, she volunteered her services, stating that "I had never been inside of a hospital, and was wholly ignorant of what I should be called upon to do, but I knew that what one woman (Florence Nightingale) had done another could." Her valor and that of other Southern women is revealed through the writings in this journal.

Black women also made significant contributions to Civil War nursing. Some were volunteers; others were employed under the general orders of the War Department at a salary of ten dollars per month. There has been, however, a paucity of published works relating to the specific and general contributions of blacks in nursing, which still makes it difficult to render a fair and comprehensive portrayal of their work. Several of them competently cared for wounded soldiers in the Union army. Harriet Tubman (1820–1913) was called the "Moses of her people" (Bradford, 1961) and is credited with making nineteen trips to the South to assist more than three hundred slaves in their quest for freedom (Miller, 1968). She was an abolitionist who became active with the Underground Railroad movement after her own escape to the North. At the onset of the Civil War, Harriet Tubman turned her energies to the care of those who needed her ministrations. She rendered her services in the Sea Islands off the coast of South Carolina (Hine, 1989). She was a highly respected, fearless, and courageous individual who served the sick and suffering of her own race. According to Bradford (1961), Tubman held the position of "nurse or matron" at the Colored Hospital in Fort Monroe, Virginia.

Sojourner Truth (1797–1881) could be regarded as an early feminist. She was an ardent supporter of the women's movement and actively participated in the cause. She was one of the first women to expose the similarity between problems of blacks and problems of women. She, too, competently assisted with the care of wounded soldiers for the Union army as an unpaid volunteer in Washington, D.C. After the Civil War she lectured and published her autobiography. In addition, she helped newly freed slaves find jobs.

Susie King (1848–1912) was the wife of Sergeant Edward King of the 33rd W.S. Colored Infantry. She was a volunteer nurse during the Civil War for more than four years. Susie King was welcomed and respected by both physicians and soldiers and frequently accompanied Clara Barton on her rounds (Elmore, 1976). Her care went beyond the physical aspects; she read letters to the soldiers, offered comfort in whatever way possible, and even began to teach some of the soldiers to read and write. Her knowledge of curative properties of various flora served her well as she treated black soldiers in Camp Saxton, South Carolina (Hine, 1989).

Large numbers of men and women served as nurses in a variety of capacities during the Civil War. They were volunteers, members of the army, persons from religious nursing orders, members of relief societies, or independent individuals who took it upon themselves to assist with the care for the sick and the wounded. These nurses represented all levels of society and consti-

Judy Chicago, "Sojourner Truth," plate from *The Dinner Party*, 1979. China-painted porcelain, 35.6 cm diameter. *(Copyright Judy Chicago, 1979. Photo copyright Donald Woodman. Through the Flower, Albuquerque, New Mexico.)*

Ambulance Train Returning From the Trenches With Wounded During the Campaign at Charleston Harbor. Engraving. *(Harper's Weekly,* September 12, 1863. *(National Library of Medicine, Bethesda, Maryland.)*

tuted much intelligence, diplomacy, daring, and experience. Overall, they demonstrated a courageous spirit.

> The ordeal of the Civil War matured America; by that time America had made many contributions of first rank in medicine and surgery, but not a single contribution to nursing. . . . A century elapsed from the date of the Boston Tea Party (1773) to the opening of America's first Nightingale school for nurses (1873), and many believed that, of the two experiments, the latter was the more daring.
>
> — *Robinson, 1946, pp. 145–146*

THE EVOLUTION OF SCHOOLS OF NURSING

The experiences of the Civil War emphasized the inadequate preparation of the majority of nurses who participated. Public interest in nursing was thus aroused, and awareness of the need to develop training programs for nurses increased. This movement was assisted by the large number of women from socially prominent families who had served. Their involvement and support lent a certain measure of respectability to the image of nursing. Two specific documents clearly indicated this rising interest in the potential development of nursing education. The first was written by a group of physicians; the second appeared as an editorial in a prominent women's magazine.

In 1868 Samuel D. Gross (1804–1884), president of the American Medical Association, voiced support for the training of nurses:

> I am not aware that the education of nurses has received any attention from this body; a circumstance the more surprising when we consider the great importance of the subject. It seems to me to be just as necessary to have well trained, well instructed nurses as to have intelligent and skillful physicians. I have long been of the opinion that there ought to be in all the principal towns and cities of the Union institutions for the education of men and women whose duty it is to take care of the sick and to carry out the injunctions of the medical attendant. There is hardly one nurse, of either sex, in twenty who has a perfect appreciation of the requirements of the sick room, or who is capable of affording the aid and comfort so necessary to a patient when oppressed by disease or injury. It does not matter what may be the skill of the medical practitioner, how assiduous or faithful he may be in the discharge of his functions as guardian of health and life, his efforts can be of comparatively little avail unless they are seconded by an intelligent and devoted nurse. Myriads of human beings perish annually in the so called civilized world for the want of good nursing.
>
> — *Committee on the Training of Nurses, American Medical Association, 1869*

The following year at the New Orleans meeting of the American Medical Association (1869), Samuel Gross, chairman of the Committee on the Training of Nurses, presented a report. This committee had been appointed to investigate the best possible method to organize and manage institutions for the training of nurses. The strange neglect of nursing in the United States was identified and the need for good nursing emphasized. Early American efforts toward hospital reform were mentioned, and the vast extent of volunteer nursing in the Civil War was stressed. The committee made the following proposals:

I. That every large and well-organised hospital should have a school for the training of nurses, not only for the supply of its own necessities, but for private families; the teaching to be furnished by its own medical staff, assisted by the resident physicians.

II. That, while it is not at all essential to combine religious exercises with nursing, it is believed that such a union would be eminently conducive to the welfare of the sick in all public institutions, and the committee therefore earnestly recommend the establishment of nurses' homes, to be placed under the immediate supervision and direction of Deaconesses or lady superintendents.

III. That, in order to give thorough scope and efficiency to this scheme, district schools should be formed and placed under the guardianship of the county medical societies of every State and Territory in the Union, the members of which should make it their business to impart instruction in the art and science of nursing.

— *Proceedings of the American Medical Association, 1869, pp. 339, 351*

Further suggestions related to the importance of forming societies of nurses, the qualities necessary for the nurse to possess, and the sending of copies of the report to medical societies all over the country. It is particularly interesting that in November of that same year Rudolf Virchow presented similar recommendations to a women's association in Berlin, Germany.

Fifty Years, 1838 to 1888. Two figures from the supplement to the *Nursing Record,* December 20, 1888. *(Courtesy of Croom Helm Ltd. Publishers, Kent, England.)*

The *Godey's Lady's Book and Magazine,* popular in the late nineteenth century, strongly influenced women's fashions and manners. It had been founded by Louis A. Godey, who appointed Sarah Josepha Hale as editor in 1837. Hale's interest in the education of nurses was illustrated by an editorial, entitled "Lady Nurses," that appeared in the February 1871 issue:

> Much has been lately said of the benefits that would follow if the calling of sick nurse were elevated to a profession which an educated lady might adopt without a sense of degradation, either on her own part or in the estimation of others. . . . There can be no doubt that the duties of sick nurse, to be properly performed, require an education and training little, if at all, inferior to those possessed by members of the medical profession. To leave these duties to untaught and ill-trained persons is as great a mistake as it was to allow the office of surgeon to be held by one whose proper calling was that of a mechanic of the humblest class. The manner in which a reform may be effected is easily pointed out. Every medical college should have a course of study and training especially adapted for ladies who desire to qualify themselves for the profession of nurse; and those who had gone through the course, and passed the requisite examination, should receive a degree and a diploma, which would at once establish their position in society. The "graduate nurse" would in general estimation be as much above the ordinary nurse of the present day as the professional surgeon of our times is above the barber-surgeon of the last century.
>
> When once the value of the "graduate nurses" became known, there is no doubt that the demand for them would be very great. Every village of a thousand inhabitants would, with the country about it, give occupation for two or three, at least. In any case of severe and protracted illness, their services would be called for as a matter of course, when the circumstances of the family allowed it.
>
> — *Hale, 1871, pp. 188–189*

The need for nurses was great. According to Hale, however, this need also involved a well-planned educational program that would generate "professional nurses." Her advice was not followed, and "training schools" for nurses eventually were established and proliferated.

A Trained Nurse, a cartoon from the Rush Medical College yearbook, *Pulse,* 1895 (published by the sophomore class, p. 134). *(Rush-Presbyterian-St. Luke's Medical Center, Chicago, Illinois.)*

This cartoon had the same historical validity as the other jokes under the "Medical Terms Illustrated" in this yearbook. The word "trained" comes from the name of the nursing schools. In those days every nursing school was called a "training school."

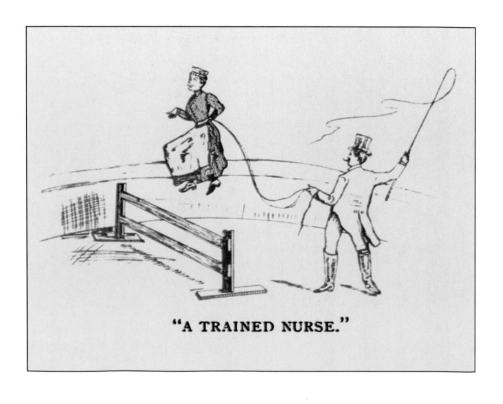

"A TRAINED NURSE."

First Instruction for Nurses

Until the inception of the first formal training schools for nurses, individuals who were involved with the care of the sick and midwives received intermittent lectures from physicians in the eastern cities of the United States. This was in no way, however, an organized course of instruction. Most information was gleaned simply by doing nursing, such as it was. The only organized preparation available was offered in Catholic sisterhoods, and it was restricted to members of the order.

It is difficult to determine who should receive the distinction of having the first trained nurses in America. There were a number of individuals whose foresight led them to appreciate the need for training nurses. These pioneers attempted to rectify the situation. Valentine Seaman, a medical chief at the New York Hospital, is usually credited with initiating the first system of instruction for nurses on the North American continent. Below his portrait in the original hospital building is an inscription that praises his achievement: "In 1798 he organized in the New York Hospital the first regular training school for nurses, from which other schools have since been established and extended their blessings throughout the Community" (Nutting and Dock, vol. 2, 1907, p. 339). Seaman's lectures were described earlier in this unit.

Almost a generation later, the next attempt was made to train women for obstetrical nursing. This movement was initiated by Joseph Warrington, a physician in obstetrics to the Philadelphia Dispensary for the Medical Relief of the Poor. (He formed another institution in 1832, the Philadelphia Lying-in Charity for Attending Indigent Females in Their Own Homes.) As a result of his efforts, a society was formed on March 5, 1839. The basic purpose of

Lecture on Bandaging at the Blockley Training School for Nurses in Philadelphia, 1886. (The Bettmann Archive, New York.)

The Home Nurse. (The Bettmann Archive, New York.)

the Nurse Society of Philadelphia was to provide an organization of women who would supply a maternity service in homes. Under the Quaker influence a combined Home and School were opened in 1850; in time, service was extended to include medical and surgical patients. The women followed a plan of instruction that included lectures given by Warrington, demonstrations, and practice on a mannequin. They received certificates and were eligible for calls after satisfactorily serving six cases. Accepted candidates, who were referred to as "probationers," had been thoroughly screened. The constitution of the society stated:

> Whereas, in our widely extended and densely populated city a large number of poor females are subject to great suffering and risk of life, during and shortly after the period of parturition, for want of competent nurses to guard them and their helpless offspring . . . the undersigned, impressed with the importance of this subject, do associate for the purpose of providing, sustaining, and causing to be instructed as far as possible, pious and prudent women for this purpose, and do adopt the following regulations:
>
> I. The Association shall be called the Nurse Society of Philadelphia.
> II. The Board of Managers shall consist of twelve females, who are, or have been, heads of families.
>
> — *Nutting and Dock, vol. 2, 1907, pp. 341–342*

Early reports refer to this structure as the "First Nurse Training School founded in America" and the "First School in America established to Train Women as Nurses." In 1897 the plan of instruction was extended to one year.

Woman's Hospital of Philadelphia opened a training school in 1861. However, it progressed slowly until 1872, when it received an endowment. (This institution can be called the first endowed school of nursing in America.) This school was organized and conducted by two women physicians, Ann Preston and Emmelin Horton Cleveland. It was unique in the sense that it had been planned specifically with the education of student nurses, rather than the care of patients, as its primary objective. In 1863 Preston wrote a pamphlet, *Nursing the Sick and the Training of Nurses,* which described the ideal nurse as having "the patience of hope [and] the faith of love. The good nurse is an artist!" The course of instruction lasted six months and covered content in surgery, medicine, obstetrics, poultice and plaster preparation, dietetic principles, and methods of cooking.

Similar developments were transpiring in Boston. As early as 1860, the *New England Hospital for Women and Children* had attempted the teaching of nurses. This institution, staffed by women physicians, took the first step toward the development of a school of nursing with the arrival of Dr. Marie Zakrzewska in 1859. Upon her advice, the hospital charter issued in 1863

W.L. Taylor, *Nurse Administering Medicine to Ailing Girl.* Woodcut. *(The Bettmann Archive, New York.)*

included a nursing school. The first bylaws were adopted on June 5, 1863, and declared the objectives of the institution to be:

I. To provide for women medical aid by competent physicians of their own sex.

II. To assist educated women in the practical study of medicine.

III. To train nurses for the care of the sick.

Students were required to attend the entire six-months course, which included practice at the bedside of the patient. The first month was a probationary period. Few women applied, and only six were trained over the next two years. In 1872 the hospital moved to new quarters at Roxbury, Massachusetts, and admitted a class of five students to its newly formed training school. The specific plan of the school has been described in the following way:

> Young women of suitable requirements and character will be admitted to the Hospital as school nurses, for one year. This year will be divided into four periods; three months will be given respectively to the practical study of nursing in the Medical, Surgical, and Maternity Wards, and night nursing. Here the pupil will aid the head nurse in all the care and work of the wards under the direction of the Attending and Resident Physicians and Medical Students.
>
> In order to enable women entirely dependent upon their work for support to obtain a thorough training, the nurses will be paid for their work from one to four dollars per week after the first fortnight, according to the actual value of their service to the Hospital.
>
> A course of lectures will be given to nurses at the Hospital by the physicians connected with the Institution beginning January 21. . . . Certificates will be given to such nurses as have satisfactorily passed a year in practical training in the Hospital.
>
> — *Munson, 1948, p. 552*

This school was under the direction of Dr. Susan Dimock. The students worked from 5:30 AM until 9:00 PM and slept in rooms near the ward in order that they might be immediately available if necessary. Their uniform consisted of a simple calico dress and felt slippers. Dr. Zakrzewska taught the simple details of nursing. There were no head nurses and no superintendent. The growth of the school continued, and in 1882 the course was extended to sixteen months. By this time the school had two head nurses and a superintendent of the training school. The program was lengthened to two years in 1893 and finally, in 1901, to three years.

One student graduated at the end of the first year, on October 1, 1873. Melinda Ann (Linda) Richards (1841–1930) received her certificate and became known as the "first trained nurse in the United States" or "America's first trained nurse." She was overwhelmed with job offers upon her graduation but finally decided to accept the position of night superintendent at Bellevue Hospital. A variety of experiences awaited her there, some of which were particularly appalling. During her stay at Bellevue, Richards made three significant contributions: she insisted on light at night (the gas had been turned so low that a lighted candle was necessary, but only two candles per week were allowed each ward); she instituted written case histories instead of verbal reports; and she exposed the mortality rate from puerperal fever, which thus led to the removal of mothers to Blackwell's Island (Robinson, 1946). After a year, Richards went to the Boston Training School (Massachusetts General Hospital) as its superintendent. There she gave actual patient care, as well as performing the required administrative duties.

Linda Richards went to England in 1877 to study nursing methods and became acquainted with Florence Nightingale. Richards went to Japan as a missionary and nurse, remained there for five years (1885–1890), and organized the earliest training school in the islands of the Orient. Richards eventually returned to her alma mater and became the superintendent of the New England Hospital for Women and Children. Her later efforts, in collaboration with Edward Cowles, were directed toward the nursing of the insane. It is to her credit that for more than half a century she was an avid, active supporter of adequate education for nurses.

Mary Eliza Mahoney (1845–1926) completed the sixteen-month course of training at the New England Hospital for Women and Children on August 1, 1879. She is thus considered to be America's first black professional nurse, the first black nurse to graduate from a school of nursing. Mahoney gave the welcoming address in 1909 at the first convention of the National Association of Colored Graduate Nurses. Throughout her life she primarily engaged in private-duty nursing and worked for the acceptance of blacks in nursing. (As in most Northern schools, racial quotas had been established at the New England Hospital; the charter of the nursing school allowed for only *one* Negro and *one* Jewish student to be accepted each year.) After her death the National Association of Colored Graduate Nurses established an award in her honor that was presented for the first time in 1936. The Mary Mahoney Medal is presented at the American Nurses' Association convention to an individual who has been instrumental in promoting equal opportunities to minority persons in nursing.

Separate schools for educating black nurses eventually arose. They became a necessity in order that blacks, who were banned from many schools, could receive training in nursing. The first of these was established at Spelman Seminary in Atlanta, Georgia, in 1886. Two similar institutions began in 1891, Hampton Institute in Virginia and Provident Hospital in Chicago. A school of nursing was also started at Tuskegee Institute in Alabama in 1892; it, however, was developed primarily to provide service rather than education. These schools experienced difficulties similar to those of the early white schools, but also suffered from societal prejudice toward blacks.

Portrait of Mary Mahoney. (Schomburg Center for Research in Black Culture, The New York Public Library, New York.)

Mary E. P. Mahoney was the first black nursing school graduate. She attended the New England Hospital for Women and Children in Boston. She constantly worked for the acceptance of blacks in nursing and for the promotion of equal opportunities.

First Convention of the National Association of Colored Graduate Nurses. (Schomburg Center for Research in Black Culture, The New York Public Library, New York.)

The National Association of Colored Graduate Nurses (NACGN) made valuable contributions to nursing until its dissolution. It brought the concerns of blacks in America to the attention of both nurses and the general public. The founding of the organization was an important landmark in the development of black nursing.

J. Reinhart, *Colored Nurses*, 1866. *(Schomburg Center for Research in Black Culture, The New York Public Library, New York.)*

Work was also begun in Canada to provide training for nurses. Around 1864 the community of St. Catharine's, Ontario, started a hospital with a little house, one nurse, a steward, and ideas for the teaching of nurses. Under the direction of Theophilus Mack, a physician at the hospital and president of the board, the hospital grew steadily and definite teaching for nurses emerged in 1873. He was certain that the prejudice of many sick people against going into public hospitals would be overcome by a profession of trained lay nurses. At Mack's direction, a woman named Money was sent to England to bring back two trained nurses and five or six probationers. A system of training was in effect by 1874. The hospital was named St. Catharine's General and Marine Hospital. The nurses were required to stay for three years. For the first six months they were probationers without pay. They then received a stipend, board, and uniforms. The first annual report, dated July 1, 1875, illustrated the value of trained nurses:

> The vocation of nursing goes hand in hand with that of the physician and surgeon, and they are absolutely indispensable one to the other. Incompetency on the part of a nurse renders negatory the best efforts of the doctor in the most critical moments, and has frequently resulted in loss of life. All the most brilliant achievements of modern surgery are dependent, to a great extent, upon careful and intelligent nursing, and the obstetrician knows only too well how fearful may be the consequences of ignorance and negligence on the part of attendants in the chamber of accouchement. The skilled nurse, by minutely watching the temperature, conditions of skin, pulse, respiration, and the various functions of all the organs, and reporting faithfully to the attending physician, must increase the chances of recovery two-fold.
>
> — *Gibbon and Mathewson, 1947, p. 145*

The Nightingale Plan in American Schools

Improvement in the care of the sick in both hospitals and homes rested with the development of a system of training nurses. The time was finally ripe for the organization of schools of nursing. Following the Civil War, interest in nursing education was high and culminated in the almost simultaneous appearance of three important schools. In 1873 the famous trio of schools that encouraged the steady progress of nursing evolved: Bellevue Training School in New York City on May 1, the Connecticut Training School in New Haven on October 1, and the Boston Training School (later the Massachusetts General Hospital Training School for Nurses) on November 1. These schools were initially based on the Nightingale model, but they were soon forced to deviate and follow a somewhat different path. The alterations that occurred greatly influenced the direction of nursing in America.

The earliest schools were created independent of hospitals by committees or boards that had the power to develop the schools. They were soon absorbed, however, into the hospitals to which they were attached because of a lack of endowment. This factor proved to be the greatest weakness in the system, since many hospitals soon discovered that schools could be created to serve their needs and a valuable source of almost free labor could be obtained.

> In the absence of public or private support, the schools from the time of their inception faced financial problems of major proportions. An agreement by the school to give nursing service for the hospitals providing clinical experience was the primary means of overcoming this difficulty. This type of apprenticeship agreement was the factor promoting hospitals to establish schools on their own initiative. Having a school of nursing became accepted as the most popular and least expensive means of providing nursing care. The hospital was the master and the student nurse was the apprentice, with the latter giving free labor to the former in return for informal training in the traditional manner.
>
> — *Ashley, 1976, p. 9*

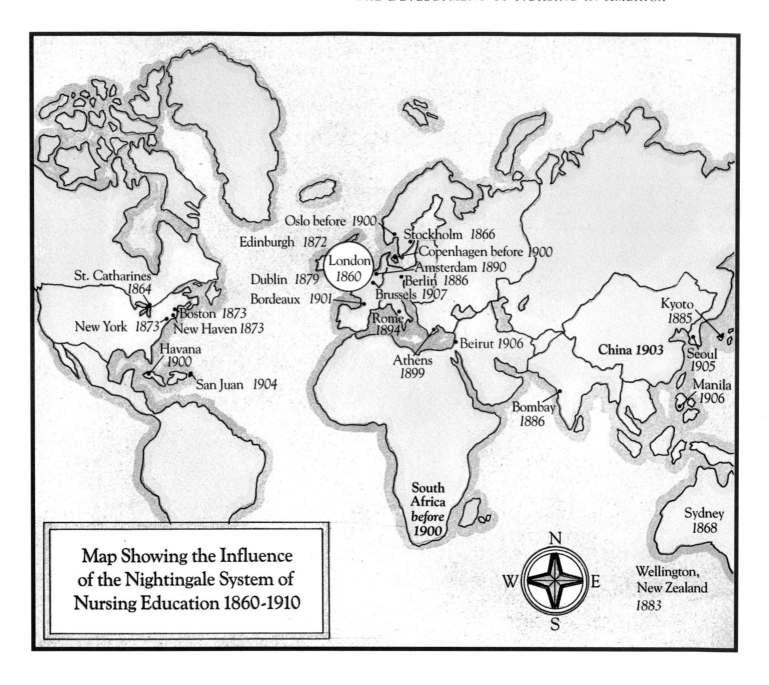

Oslo before 1900
Edinburgh 1872
Stockholm 1866
Copenhagen before 1900
London 1860
Amsterdam 1890
St. Catharines 1864
Dublin 1879
Berlin 1886
Bordeaux 1901
Brussels 1907
Boston 1873
New York 1873
New Haven 1873
Rome 1894
Kyoto 1885
Havana 1900
Beirut 1906
China 1903
Seoul 1905
San Juan 1904
Athens 1899
Manila 1906
Bombay 1886
South Africa before 1900
Sydney 1868
Wellington, New Zealand 1883

Map Showing the Influence of the Nightingale System of Nursing Education 1860-1910

Map showing the influence of the Nightingale system of nursing education between 1860 and 1910. The dates indicate the approximate year of the first school of nursing in each country.

Nursing care became the major product dispensed by hospitals. The real function of the school of nursing became *not education,* but *service.* In addition, no policy for control of the numbers of nursing schools or the standards for admission and graduation was established or accepted. Consequently a proliferation of nursing schools occurred. The first decade of the twentieth century demonstrated a period of phenomenal growth, with the establishment of close to seven hundred new schools. All school functions were ultimately placed under the control and general direction of hospital authorities.

Bellevue Hospital Training School. Women involved in the reform movement following the Civil War turned their endeavors toward the improvement of hospitals. Louisa Lee Schuyler and other women who had been prominent during the war effort and the U.S. Sanitary Commission founded the New York State Charities Aid Association in 1872. This voluntary body was concerned with the care of paupers, orphans, and the sick and regularly visited charitable institutions. Their intent was to evaluate for needed reforms. Some very prominent women—Mrs. Joseph Hobson, Mrs. William H. Osborn, Julia Gould, and Euphemia and B. Van Rensselaer constituted one of its committees (Kalisch and Kalisch, 1995). This particular committee, with Mrs. Joseph Hobson as its chair, inspected Bellevue Hospital and found it in a deplorable state of affairs. The nursing care was given primarily by women who were ex-convicts; fees were collected from the patients for the inadequate services they received; drunkenness and foul language were prominent; supplies such as soap, linens, and dishes were unavailable; and conditions were particularly bad at night, when three night watchmen made periodic rounds of the wards. On the basis of the shocking report that was presented to the association, it was determined that the improvement of nursing was one of the essential ingredients for hospital reform.

A resolution passed in April 1872 and addressed to the Commissioners of Charity begged this group to consider a plan for establishing a training school for nurses. The commissioners, in turn, referred the plan to the medical board, which remained silent on the subject for a time. However, Dr. Gill Wylie of the hospital staff voluntarily visited England to study schools established under Florence Nightingale, who had identified the essentials of a good training school. The following is a sample of some of those essentials:

A year's practical and technical training in hospital wards, under trained head-nurses who themselves have been trained to train.

The training of probationers should be as much a part of the duty of the head-nurse as directing the under-nurses or seeing to the patients.

To tell the training, you require weekly records . . . kept by the head-nurses of the progress of each probationer in her ward-work, and in the moral qualities necessary in her ward-work; a monthly record by the matron of the results of the weekly records; and a quarterly statement by her as to how each head-nurse has performed her duty to each probationer. The whole to be examined periodically by the governing body.

Clinical lectures from the hospital professors . . . elementary instruction in chemistry . . . physiology . . . and general instruction on medical and surgical topics; examinations, written and oral, at least four of each in the year, all adapted to nurses; as also lectures and demonstrations with anatomical, chemical and other illustrations, adapted especially to nurses. . . .

A good nurses' library of professional books, not for the probationers to skip and dip in at random, but to be made careful use of, under the medical instructor and class-mistress. . . .

The authority and discipline over all the women of a trained lady-superintendent . . . who is herself the best nurse in the hospital, the example and leader of her nurses in all that she wishes her nurses to be. . . .

An organization not only to give this training systematically, and to test it by current tests and examinations, but also to give the probationers, by proper help in the wards, time to do their work as pupils as well as assistant-nurses, and above all to make it a real moral as well as nursing probation—for nursing is a probation as well as a mission.

Accommodation for sleeping, classes, and meals; arrangements for time and teaching and work; surroundings of a moral and religious, and hard-working and sober, yet cheerful tone and atmosphere, such as to make the training-school and hospital a "home" which no good young woman of any class need fear by entering to lose anything of health of body or mind; with moral and spiritual helps, and an elevating and motherly influence over all, such as to make the whole place which will train really good women, who can withstand temptation and do real work, and neither be "romantic" nor "menial."

— *Florence Nightingale, 1883, pp. 1039–1041*

Although Wylie was unable to personally confer with Nightingale, he received a letter from her upon his return home. This letter offered support and encouragement along with valuable information regarding the mechanics of a nursing school. In addition, it reiterated Nightingale's position that the nurse and the physician have different aspects of service and render different kinds of care. Finally, opposition was overcome, although somewhat reluctantly, and the commissioners agreed to the use of six wards in Bellevue for the training of nurses. Funds were raised and a house was rented for the nurs-

Nurses' Training, c. 1900. White Caps of Bellevue Hospital, New York, during instruction in a bacteriological lab. *(The Bettmann Archive, New York.)*

es' home. The purpose of the program was "to train nurses for the care of the sick in order that women shall find a school for their education and the public shall reap the advantage of skilled and educated labor" (Dock, 1901, p. 90). Sister Helen Bowden of the Sisterhood of All Saints was selected to direct the program. She was familiar with the Nightingale system and equated the conditions in Bellevue to those in the English workhouses. Therefore Sister Helen Bowden adopted a system similar to that of St. Thomas's School. The Nightingale system became known in America as the "Bellevue System," since it was introduced in that institution.

The Bellevue Hospital Training School for Nurses was founded in May 1873, and five students enrolled in the first class. The program was for one year, but the students were required to remain a second year in service. The students received only occasional lectures; the majority of time was spent in practical work through which they gained experience. They received ten dollars per month after completing a probationary period of one month. Initially the students wore no uniforms, but after the first year the training school committee decided that a standard uniform should be adopted. (No nurse in America had ever worn a uniform.) This created a stir among the nurses, who were reluctant to wear uniforms. The committee astutely granted Euphemia Van Rensselaer—one of the students with a distinctive family name, social position, and personal beauty—a two-day leave of absence from Bellevue. She returned in a uniform, apron, and cap that had been made especially for her. Her tailored uniform consisted of a long blue seersucker dress with white

A Critical Case—A Bedside Consultation for the Benefit of Students and Nurses at Bellevue Hospital, 1890. Engraving. *(The Bettmann Archive, New York.)*

apron, collar and cuffs, and a white cap. Within a week every nurse was wearing the uniform, which eventually became the mark of a Bellevue nurse. A pin designed by Tiffany and Company in 1880 also distinguished the graduates of Bellevue.

The Bellevue school flourished and became one of the leading nursing schools in the country. In October 1874, Linda Richards became the night superintendent. A *Manual of Nursing* was published in 1876. Many brilliant leaders emerged from this program, including Isabel Adams Hampton Robb, Lavinia Lloyd Dock, Mary Agnes Snively (a Canadian who fostered the progress of the training school at the Toronto General Hospital and the Canadian Nursing Association), and Jane A. Delano.

Connecticut Training School. The Connecticut Training School in New Haven was established through the efforts of Georgeanna Woolsey Bacon, her husband Dr. Francis Bacon, and a wealthy philanthropist, Charles Thompson. Georgeanna Bacon and her two sisters had served as nurses in the Civil War and remained actively involved in nursing. The training school, established as an organization separate from the hospital, opened in October 1873 with four students. It was controlled by a board of directors who contracted an exchange with the hospital whereby nursing service would be provided for educational services. Physicians supported the school from the very beginning. Miss Bayard, who had been trained at the Women's Hospital of Philadelphia, became the head of the school, and it grew rapidly. By the end of the second year of operation, the first graduates were sent out to private families. By the fourth year the school was able to furnish superintendents of nursing to other hospitals. The school remained independent until 1906, when the hospital assumed control.

In 1879 the *New Haven Manual of Nursing,* created by a committee of both nurses and doctors, was published by the Connecticut Training School. It was a comprehensive text that found widespread acceptance among the nursing schools in the country. The school was one of the first to obtain a university affiliation (1924, Yale University) and an endowment of one million dollars from the Rockefeller Foundation. The Yale School of Nursing was the first in the world that was established as a separate university department with an independent budget and its own dean, Annie W. Goodrich.

Boston Training School. The Massachusetts General Hospital of Boston was the last of the three institutions to open a school for nurses. The idea was initiated by the Woman's Educational Association, which called a meeting to consider the subject. A training school committee was established

to decide upon a plan, to ask for cooperation of the physicians, to raise funds, and to seek permission from the trustees of Massachusetts General to develop a school in connection with that hospital. The school of nursing began operation as the Boston Training School and opened its doors in November 1873 with a superintendent, two head nurses, and six pupils to take charge of two wards. Mrs. Billings, who had experience as a hospital nurse in the Civil War, was the first superintendent.

From the very beginning, the medical staff had not favored or supported the school. Under the new arrangement the wards did not run smoothly, and the school was identified as the source of the difficulties. The training school committee was given another year's trial only after assuring the trustees that a graduate nurse would be placed in charge of the school; at the end of that time, a decision would be made to either close or continue the school. Linda Richards was placed in charge in November 1874, an event that marked a steady march of progress and success for the floundering program. She reorganized the school, conducted classes, and personally cared for patients. Because of the high quality of her nursing, Richards proved to be an excellent example for students to follow. The training committee administered the school until 1896, when control reverted to Massachusetts General Hospital because of financial problems.

These early schools soon proved their value, and by 1879 there were eleven training schools in the United States. By the turn of the century there were no less than 432 schools, and most of these had expanded their programs to two or three years. The standards, however, varied greatly among the schools. Active renovation in hospitals and the creation of new ones occurred between 1873 and 1895. One of these was Johns Hopkins Hospital (Balti-

Facing page, top, Harry Fenn, *The Massachusetts General Hospital in Boston.* Drawing. *(The Bettmann Archive, New York.)*

Facing page, below, View of Johns Hopkins Hospital, 1889. *(Special Collections, Milbank Memorial Library, Teachers College, Columbia University, New York.)*

Johns Hopkins University was financed by Johns Hopkins, who had willed his fortune to establish a hospital and university. A medical school was also to be organized. John Shaw Billings, an advisor to the board of trustees, included plans for a school of nursing as he developed arrangements for hospital management and other programs. The school of nursing opened in 1889.

View of a Ward at Johns Hopkins Hospital, turn of the century. *(Special Collections, Milbank Memorial Library, Teachers College, Columbia University, New York.)*

more), whose training school opened in 1889 under Isabel Adams Hampton (Robb). The function of the hospitals slowly changed from refuges of the destitute to institutions for the care of the sick and injured. The value of trained nurses had finally been proven, and this resulted in a growing demand for trained nurses.

CANADIAN SCHOOLS

Canada had one of the earliest schools patterned after the Nightingale schools, the one located at the General and Marine Hospital in St. Catharine's (1874). The bylaws for nurses were laid down in the regulations for the training school (later called the Mack Training School) and were influenced by the Nightingale principles. The first of these bylaws stated:

> The nurses in the daily discharge of their duties must observe the strictest secrecy, and carefully avoid "gossip," their demeanour should be kind and respectful on all occasions, and when on duty at private houses, they are expected, in addition to taking the complete charge of their patients, to avoid giving unnecessary trouble, to wait upon themselves, and to pay the closest attention to the preparation of aliments for the sick, as well as to cheerfully assist in many matters not strictly within their duty—to faithfully carry out the physician's directions, and in the event of emergencies, to report any instance when the execution of his orders have been exceeded or omitted. To evince no bias to any favourite medical practitioner. To attend scrupulously to the special duties to the patient with the gentleness and exactitude taught by their superiors, and never to interfere with or criticize the treatment.
>
> — *Gibbon and Mathewson, 1947 pp. 144–145*

Excerpts from "The First Annual Report of The St. Catharine Training School and Nurses' Home," dated July 1, 1875, are particularly enlightening:

> Every possible opportunity is seized to impart instruction of a practical nature in the art of nursing, while teaching will be given in chemistry, sanitary science, popular physiology and anatomy, hygiene and all such branches of the healing art as a nurse ought to be familiarized with. . . . The vocation of nursing goes hand in hand with that of the physician and surgeon, and they are absolutely indispensable one to the other. . . . By observing the known principles of hygiene, she will co-operate intelligently with him, also in placing the sufferer from disease in the best relation to the ground he is above, the surrounding heat, light, air, aliments he is sustained by, and the liquids he drinks. She will, likewise, by the proper precautions well recognized in hygiene, avert the evils of contagion or infection, and the spread of disease by noxious miasma. . . . Finally, she will inspire confidence, allay terror, soothe anxiety, and often quiet the mental state while taking care of the physical, and prevent injurious interference from officious bystanders.
>
> — *Gibbon and Mathewson, 1947 p. 145*

The second Canadian hospital to consider the idea of a training school for nurses was Montreal General (1821). In 1875 the hospital board sought the assistance of Florence Nightingale in establishing a school. Five nurses were sent from St. Thomas's Hospital, but they were appalled by the environment and eventually resigned; one of the original five died of typhoid fever. The conditions in the Montreal General Hospital were much like those of Bellevue. Filth was the primary feature, with armies of rats scurrying about the wards and sometimes attacking patients. Other attempts were made to start the school, but they also proved unsuccessful. Finally, Nora Gertrude Livingstone, a graduate of the New York Hospital, succeeded in establishing a school in 1890. Under her direction the nursing school had its real beginning.

The founder of modern nursing is the nurse most frequently remembered on stamps. Florence Nightingale is portrayed by the Republic of China with a student nurse holding her candle. This 1964 stamp was issued to observe Nurses' Day, May 12. *(Courtesy of Howard B. Hurley.)*

The history of the Toronto General Hospital was similar to that of Montreal General. From 1877, attempts were made to establish a training school, but it was not until 1884 that the real fame of the school began. At this time Mary Agnes Snively, a graduate of Bellevue Hospital, became the superintendent. She reorganized the school and developed a modern plan of work and study. During her tenure the school became well known throughout the nursing world as embodying the highest ideals in nursing. Snively remained until 1910 and greatly elevated the standards of the Toronto school.

Other schools soon followed in Canada: the Children's Hospital at Toronto in 1886; the Winnipeg General (1887), which claims to have been the first hospital in western Canada to start a training school for nurses; St. Boniface General in Winnipeg (1890); the Royal Jubilee at Victoria (1890); Victoria General in Halifax (1892); and the Royal Victoria at Montreal (1894). Snively reported that by June 1909 there were seventy schools for nurses; of these, ten offered a two-year course, three had a program of two and one-half years; and fifty-seven required a three-year course (Gibbon and Mathewson, 1947). The introduction of training schools for nurses became almost automatic for progressive Canadian hospitals after 1890. Trained nurses began to emerge in Canada almost simultaneously with those in the United States.

NURSING IN THE SPANISH-AMERICAN WAR

The war with Spain provided American nurses with their first experience in army nursing. The Spanish-American War also graphically illustrated American deficiencies, such as the lack of a Red Cross nursing service, the need for an army nurse corps, and the lack of emergency reserves. The U.S. Army Medical Department was made up of 983 members, but it had very little prestige. Certainly, the number of members was not adequate to care for the

Nurses on Screened Bed Ward at Walter Reed Hospital in Washington, D.C. (National Library of Medicine, Bethesda, Maryland.)

Nurses on Deck of the Hospital Ship Relief *Near Cuba.* The Red Cross during the Spanish–American War, c. 1898. *(National Library of Medicine, Bethesda, Maryland.)*

twenty-eight thousand members of the regular army. American battle casualties were small during this war, but hastily constructed army camps were devastated by typhoid fever, malaria, dysentery, and food poisoning. Epidemic diseases caused ten times more deaths than did bullets. Nurses were desperately needed. The Nurses' Associated Alumnae of the United States and Canada (renamed the American Nurses' Association in 1911) offered assistance, but the army rejected it. The primary objection to the organization was that it had been in existence for a relatively short time and was not recognized as the representative body for nurses. The offer had also come one day too late. The Daughters of the American Revolution had already volunteered, and Anita Newcomb McGee (1864–1940), their vice-president and a physician with no previous administrative experience, had been appointed in charge of the Army Nursing Service. McGee was given the position of acting assistant surgeon in the U.S. Army.

Congress authorized the employment of women nurses on a contract basis, which provided thirty dollars per month plus room and meals. The contract, however, did not provide for personal care if the nurses became ill. McGee preferred graduate nurses with proper endorsements from their own schools and suggested that all applicants be examined and cleared through the Daughters of the American Revolution. Nearly eight thousand volunteer nurses were placed under contract and in essence represented the beginning of the current Army Nursing Corps. Nearly sixteen hundred graduate nurses served; members of Catholic orders also served in large numbers, particularly the Daughters of Charity. The first nurses were appointed in May 1898, and they were stationed in army hospitals in the United States, Puerto Rico, Cuba, Hawaii, and the Philippine Islands. In addition, they served on the hospital ship, the USS *Relief.* This ship carried supplies of medicines and dressings and enough equipment to outfit a 750-bed hospital for six months. Six women nurses were aboard when it left Tampa harbor.

The army hospitals had been tended by hospital corpsmen who lacked training and experience. These men were recruits who were often the dregs of the units and were totally unqualified to care for the sick. They were guilty of unsanitary practices, such as using the same bucket for food and excrement, which helped spread disease throughout the camps. Consequently conditions of the worst type met the nurses when they arrived. The nurses often worked day and night with inadequate supplies and shelter. They eventually won respect and recognition, not only from the servicemen but also from the surgeons, who initially had been prejudiced against them. Thirteen nurses died while rendering nursing care during this war.

The army was continually exposed to typhoid and yellow fever during the Spanish-American conflict. Therefore research was begun to investigate the cause and spread of typhoid fever. A committee headed by Major Walter Reed determined that flies and unclean practices were the obvious sources of the illness. Yellow fever had also been particularly virulent and the cause of many fatalities. A team of physicians, including James Carroll, Aristides Agramonte, Jesse W. Lazear, and Major Walter Reed, was sent to Cuba by the U.S. government to find some method of control for this problem. Reed and Agramonte consulted with Carlos Finlay, a physician in Havana, regarding his theory (of nineteen years) that yellow fever was caused by a common house mosquito. They then proceeded to conduct experiments requiring that human volunteers be bitten by mosquitoes under controlled conditions so that reactions could be studied. The first volunteers were physicians; some survived, others died. These experiments proved that the mosquito now called *Aedes aegypti* was the yellow fever carrier, and they led the way to conquest of the disease.

W.A. Rogers, *A Message From Home.* A hospital scene during the Spanish-American War. *(The Bettmann Archive, New York.)*

Dean Cornwell, *Conquerors of Yellow Fever.* *(Courtesy of Wyeth-Ayerst Laboratories, Philadelphia, Pennsylvania.)*

Drs. Jesse Lazear, James Carroll, Carlos Finlay, and Major Walter Reed investigate the mosquito-borne disease in Cuba following the Spanish-American War, August 27, 1900.

Group of Three Nurses at Yellow Fever Hospital, Franklin, Louisiana, c. 1898. *(National Library of Medicine, Bethesda, Maryland.)*

Graduate nurses were employed by the government on a contractual basis during the Spanish-American War. Nearly sixteen hundred nurses functioned in a subtropical climate without adequate resources and in horrible conditions. Thirteen nurses died; approximately ten percent of all the nurses serving the government on this basis succumbed to a variety of diseases.

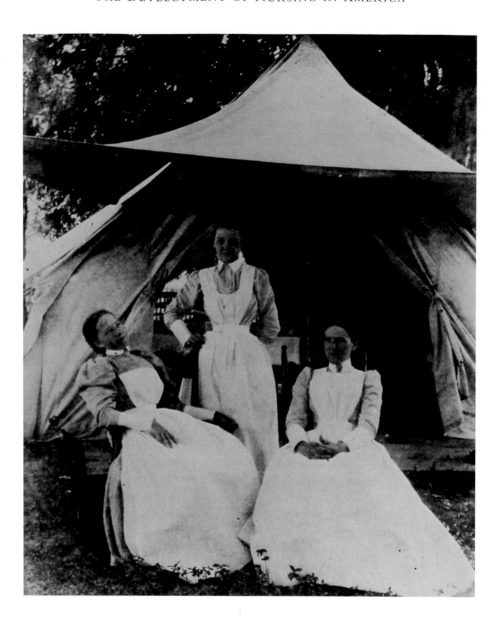

The last person to be used for the yellow fever experiment was a nurse who gave her life. She was remembered by the medical officer in charge of the hospital where her death occurred:

> On many occasions during the Spanish-American War the nurses showed heroism and devotion to duty equal to that of any soldier or sailor in battle. The majority of those with me at Las Animos Hospital, Havana, had not had yellow fever, yet they all unflinchingly nursed the malignant cases of that disease, staying by those who died, to the very last, trying to alleviate the suffering and save life, their clothing, hands, and sometimes their faces smeared with blood and black vomit. One of those Las Animos [sic] nurses, Miss Clara Maass, gave up her young life from a high sense of duty. She thought she would be more useful in Cuba as a nurse after having had yellow fever, and requested to be bitten by infected mosquitos in order to contract the disease and become immune. I tried to dissuade her from the step, telling her that her life was too valuable to be exposed to such great risk. . . . Nevertheless, she insisted, and the fatal mosquitos were applied to her arm. Three or four days later, she developed a malignant, hemorrhagic case of yellow fever, from which she died in about a week.
>
> — *Quoted in Frank, 1953, p. 259*

Clara Louise Maass (1876–1901) graduated from the Christina Trefz Training School for Nurses of the Newark German Hospital in 1895. This hospital has since been renamed the Clara Maass Memorial Hospital. Maass was one of the first five students to graduate from the two-year program. She remained on the staff and three years later became a head nurse. She volunteered to become a contract nurse with the U.S. Army during the Spanish-American War and served in Florida, Georgia, Cuba, and the Philippines. After her term of service was complete, Clara Louise Maass volunteered in response to Major William C. Gorgas's call for nurses in Havana, where experiments on yellow fever were being conducted. She nursed the victims of this disease through the spring of 1901. On June 4, 1901, she allowed herself to be bitten by a mosquito. She suffered a mild attack of yellow fever, recovered, and was bitten again on August 14. She had seriously doubted that the slight fever had given her immunity to the disease. The second attack proved fatal, and she died ten days later at the age of twenty-five.

Maass was the only American and the only woman to die during the experiments. After her death the experiments were discontinued, and the disease was ultimately conquered. Maass's body was sent to Fairmount Cemetery in Newark for burial with full military honors. In 1951 a commemorative stamp was issued in her honor by Cuba. In 1976 the United States issued a commemorative stamp in honor of her service to humanity. This was the first U.S. stamp to honor an individual nurse. In addition, a special medal commemorating the one-hundredth anniversary of Clara Maass's birth was struck by the Franklin Mint.

In 1976, the United States honored the first individual American nurse, Clara Maass, with a commemorative thirteen-cent stamp for her contribution to the nursing profession and to humanity. The issuance marked the hundredth anniversary of her birth. *(Courtesy of Howard B. Hurley.)*

Clara Louise Maass. (Author's Collection.)

The hundredth anniversary of the birth of Clara Maass was celebrated with the issuance of an official first day cover sponsored by *RN* magazine and the Clara Maass Memorial Hospital in 1976. Clara Maass was a heroic nurse who gave her life for the advancement of yellow fever research.

The war experience definitely proved the superiority of the trained nurse over the untrained volunteer and led to the initiation of a permanent nurse corps. Immediately following the war, both the Associated Alumnae, with the backing of influential citizens, and Anita McGee proposed bills for the establishment of a nursing corps that would have the sanction and permanence of law. These bills were not passed. Finally, in 1900, after a number of surgeons had spoken positively to Congress about the work done by the nurses, the Army Reorganization Bill was presented. It provided a permanent Nurse Corps as part of the Medical Department of the army; the corps would be composed of fully trained nurses (hospital school graduates) under an able director. An amendment stating that the superintendent of the Nurse Corps had to be a hospital school graduate was added before the bill was passed on February 2, 1901. The bill stated that the U.S. Army nurse's salary would be forty dollars per month for duty in the United States and fifty dollars per month for duty elsewhere. In 1918 the name was changed to the Army Nurse Corps (ANC). Its motto has been "Where go the United States troops, there go the Army Nurses."

Since she was not a nurse, Anita McGee was forced to resign when the Army Nurse Corps was established. She was succeeded by Dita H. Kinney, head nurse of the United States Army Hospital at Fort Baynard, New Mexico. The status of the army nurse has shown slow but consistent improvement. Several events have assisted this process: army nurses were accorded relative rank in 1920; they became eligible for retirement benefits in 1926; in 1947, army nurses became part of the regular army with full commission, pay, and other benefits as granted to male officers. A succession of leaders served in the position of superintendent, including Jane Delano, Isabel McIssac, and Dora Thompson, the first to have served in the military. In 1908 the U.S. Navy Nurse Corps was founded as an integral unit of the Navy.

EDUCATIONAL ADVANCEMENT FOR GRADUATE NURSES

By the end of the nineteenth century new educational opportunities became available for graduate nurses attending Teachers College, Columbia University. The Teachers College program was founded as a direct result of the efforts of the American Society of Superintendents of Training Schools for Nurses (renamed in 1912 the National League of Nursing Education and reorganized in 1952 under the present National League for Nursing). A special committee of the society, with Isabel Hampton Robb as its head, was created to investigate a means to better prepare nurses for leadership in schools of nursing. According to one source, "It was useless to look to our own institutions for the solution of this problem, and the ordinary normal school or college was equally incapable of adjusting its facilities to our peculiar needs" (Stewart, 1909, p. 1). Teachers College, which had opened ten years earlier for the training of teachers, seemed the logical choice. The program was originally designed to prepare administrators of nursing service and nursing education. It was established as an eight-month course in hospital economics in 1899.

> The original course for nurses in hospital economics at Teachers College was at first rather heavily weighted with technical subjects in the household arts with some recognition of the sciences also present. Pedagogical subjects such as psychology and the philosophy of education were soon identified as valuable in the study of the problems of nursing education and were incorporated within the program. Additional lectures by leaders in the Society shared nursing experiences gained through accumulated years of practical service in hospitals and training-school work. In 1906, a new department of institutional administration was established in the college, the course in hospital economics becoming incorporated within its structure. From this time forward there was no longer any ques-

Facing page, Armour's Army and Navy Art Calendar, 1899. (Author's Collection.)

Modern nursing movements followed the Spanish-American War, the first war in which graduate nurses served the armed forces.

tion as to the place of nursing in the general scheme of university education. The department continued to grow, broaden its educational program, emphasize the social and educational phases of the nurse's work, and include nursing specialties such as teaching and supervision, public health nursing, school nursing, and other related branches. Eventually, the name was changed to the Department of Nursing Education.

— *Donahue, 1981, pp. 41–42*

Mary Adelaide Nutting, former superintendent of nurses and principal of the Training School for Nurses at Johns Hopkins Hospital, came to Teachers College in 1907 and became the first nursing professor in the world. She was thus the first nurse to occupy a chair on a university faculty. Under her direction the department progressed and became a pioneer in education for nurses. The school became known as the "motherhouse" of collegiate education because it fostered the initial movements toward undergraduate and graduate degrees for nurses.

The Visiting Nurse

U N I T   7

Advancing Toward New Frontiers

here is probably no ten-year span in nursing's history during which so many important events occurred or so many fateful decisions were made than in the period between 1890 and 1900. It was a time of unprecedented growth in American nursing, a period of emergence of several of our most important nursing leaders, an era of tremendous proliferation of schools of nursing, and the decade of the greatest organizational strides for the fledgling profession.

— TERESA E. CHRISTY

P. Buckley Moss, *The Visiting Nurse,* 1993, Offset lithograph from watercolor, image size: 29.69 × 29.54 cm; paper size, 42.39 × 42.24 cm. *(The Moss Portfolio, Mathews, Virginia, copyright P. Buckley Moss.)*

The titles and job descriptions of nurses who have functioned in community-based roles have frequently changed. Titles have included visiting nurse, public health nurse, community health nurse, and home health nurse. These transitions have been consistent with the political, economic, and sociological changes in society that have affected the delivery of nursing and health care. Direct patient care and health teaching have been vital components of community nursing.

	1850	1865	1880	1895

DAILY LIFE

1864 Geneva Convention establishes neutrality of battlefield medical facilities

1876 Korea becomes an independent nation

1877 Edison invents the telephone

1878 Electric street lighting installed

1880 The game of Bingo is devised

1883 First skyscraper built in Chicago

1890 Global influenza epidemic

1900 First trial flight of Zeppelin

1900 Cake Walk most fashionable dance

1901 Oil drilling begins in Persia

SCIENCE AND TECHNOLOGY

1873 Color photographs first developed

1894 Röentgen discovers X-rays

THE VISUAL ARTS

1853–1890 Vincent Van Gogh, Dutch painter

1863–1944 Edvard Munch, Norwegian painter

1874 First impressionist exhibition in Paris

1881–1973 Pablo Picasso, Spanish painter

1889 Alexander Gustave Eiffel designs the Eiffel Tower

1895 Art Nouveau style predominates

MEDICINE AND HEALTH CARE

1871 Leprosy bacillus discovered

1878 Iodoform used as antiseptic

1887 Phenacetin, analgesic drug, discovered

1889 Von Mehring and Minkowski prove that pancreas secretes insulin

1890 Rubber gloves used for first time in surgery at Johns Hopkins

NURSING

1885 First American nursing text published, *A Textbook of Nursing for the Use of Training Schools, Families and Private Students* by Clara Weeks Shaw

1887 British nurses begin campaign for nurse registration

1888 British Nurses Association established

1888 *The Trained Nurse and Hospital Review* (renamed *The Nursing World*) published

1889 Queen Victoria Jubilee Institute for Nurses established

1891 First registration law in Cape Colony, South Africa, part of medical act

1893 Henry Street Settlement established

1893 American Society of Superintendents of Training Schools of Nursing formed

1896 Nurses' Associated Alumnae of the United States and Canada formed

1899 International Council of Nurses founded

1900 *American Journal of Nursing* published

1901 First nurse registration act passed in New Zealand

1908 Fountain pens become popular
1908 Model T Ford produced
1918 Worldwide influenza epidemic strikes nearly twenty-two million people

1929 Term "apartheid" used for first time
1934 Refrigeration process for meat cargoes is devised
1939 Nylon stockings introduced
1950s Years of the "Cold War"
1957 Russian Sputnik launched

1903 Electrocardiograph developed by Wilhelm Einthoven
1905 Albert Einstein, physicist, formulates specific theory of relativity
1919 First experiments with short-wave radio
1922 Self-winding watch invented
1927 Iron lung developed

1951 J. Andre-Thomas invents heart-lung machine

1903 Gustav Klimt paints ceiling at Vienna University
1910 Frank Lloyd Wright becomes well-known architect

1926 Academy of Motion Picture Arts and Sciences founded

1904 W.C. Gorgas eradicates yellow fever in Panama Canal Zone
1909 Ehrlich prepares salvarsan for cure of syphilis

1928 Alexander Fleming discovers penicillin
1937 Insulin used to control diabetes
1939 Rh factor in blood discovered by Levine and Stetson
1948 First World Health Assembly meets in Geneva
1955 Salk develops polio vaccine

1903 First nurse practice acts passed in North Carolina, New Jersey, New York, and Virginia

1907 Canadian Society of Superintendents of Training Schools established

1907 M. Adelaide Nutting named first professor of nursing at Teachers College

1908 Canadian National Association of Trained Nurses formed

1908 National Association of Colored Graduate Nurses established

1912 National Organization for Public Health Nursing established

1922 Sigma Theta Tau founded at Indiana University

1937 *A Curriculum Guide for Schools of Nursing* published

1952 *Nursing Research* published

1952 Associate degree nursing programs developed in community colleges y the turn of the century, the trial period was over. The training school as well as the trained nurse were recognized and accepted by hospitals, medicine, and the general public. This revolution in nursing, combined with new developments in surgery and sanitary science, led to a tremendous expansion in hospitals. It was nursing that would ultimately make the application of these discoveries possible. Hospitals of all types sprang up, multiplied at an astonishing rate, and became independent entities because there was no regulating body of any type to set and enforce controls. It soon became apparent that a school of nursing was almost indispensable to the running of a hospital. Not only did nursing students improve the nursing service to patients, but also the cost of the improved service to the hospital was less. The students worked long hours and did hard physical labor in payment for the training they received. Most hospitals, therefore, set up their own schools or assumed control over schools that had been developed on an independent basis. The right of the hospital to set up a school was not questioned; nor was there any interference with the manner in which the school was run. In some instances hospitals had schools of nursing for the sole purpose of using the service contributed by students for the care of patients. The wide diversity among these schools and the exploitation of student nurses thus became important issues as the United States approached the twentieth century.

New frontiers beckoned to women and to nursing. Although still wanting to be useful, greater numbers of women also wished to be independent and free and find the means of demonstrating their intelligence and capabilities and proving their value as citizens: they wanted to have widening opportunities for respectable positions in the social order of the times. A number of individuals envisioned nursing as an area in which this could be accomplished. However, a change in the system of nursing education and practice was necessary to achieve this goal. Consequently, nursing leaders began to organize for the control of their own educational standards and for the improvement of nursing practice. They were beginning to see that their educational difficulties could not be solved by an isolated effort, that the united energies of all nurses and all schools would be needed in any serious attempt to attack the chaos that had been created in educational standards and ideals. According to Stewart (1943, p. 129), "nursing leaders banded together to support educational standards, to set up some legal controls to prevent the spread of poor schools, and to prevent unlimited expansion."

THE TURN OF THE CENTURY

The twentieth century has been referred to as "the century of social consciousness." The beginnings of social endeavors in the nineteenth century finally became reality with the development of a variety of social agencies. The states had begun to assume at least partial responsibility for the relief of the poor early in the nineteenth century. In 1863 Massachusetts, for example, had appointed a State Board of Charities that was charged with the care of the nonresident poor and with general supervision of state institutions. New York and Ohio created similar boards in 1867. By 1930 forty-one states had created boards for the supervision of relief. This movement for social reform brought about many changes that influenced health care and nursing.

Attention began to be focused on specific dependents, such as the blind and the aged, but the provisions were totally inadequate for their maintenance. Child health received particular emphasis with the initiation of the first White House Conference on Child Welfare in 1910. Within two years the Children's Bureau was established (1912) by an act of Congress and placed within the Department of Labor. Its function was to investigate and report all matters that pertained to the welfare of children and child life among all classes of people. Studies of infant mortality, care available to mothers and infants in rural communities, and methods of instruction in hygiene were undertaken by this agency. Finally, federal aid for the reduction of infant mortality was suggested by Julia Lathrop, chief of the Children's Bureau, in 1917. Her proposals were incorporated in the Sheppard–Towner Act of 1921, which authorized appropriations to provide grants-in-aid to states that would set up services for the welfare and hygiene of mothers and children.

Hundreds of nurses were employed to make home visits and supply health education and health screening of mothers and infants. These monies continued for seven years and stimulated the establishment of prenatal, infant, and preschool child health centers. By the end of the act, child health agencies had been established in forty-five states and Hawaii. The impact of the Sheppard–Towner Act on the decrease in the infant death rate was well documented. Efforts were made to renew the Sheppard–Towner Act, but they were unsuccessful in the face of conservative forces. The continuation of this act was opposed by the American Medical Association:

> Resolved that the House of Delegates condemns as unsound in policy, wasteful and extravagant, unproductive of results and tending to promote communism, the federal subsidy system established by the Sheppard–Towner Maternity and Infancy Act and protests against a renewal of the system in any form.
>
> — *American Medical Association, 1930*

Public health nurses, on the other hand, supported a renewal and watched with deep concern. When the federal aid ceased, the majority of the states continued to provide funds, although in decreased amounts.

Thomas Webster, *Sickness and Health*, 1843. *(Copyright The Board of Trustees of the Victoria and Albert Museum, London, England.)*

Nursing of the sick has never been the sole concern of nurses throughout its history. Attention to all the needs of human beings in all types of circumstances has been a vital concern. Prevention of illness and maintenance of health have always been important aspects of the nurse's practice.

297

This 1936 postage stamp is one of a set of four issued by Germany in connection with the Sixth International Community Congress. It shows the nurse as symbol of community service. *(Courtesy of Howard B. Hurley.)*

The dove of peace is held high in the hand of a nurse in this stamp issued by Czechoslovakia in 1952. A prominent red cross appears in the background. *(Stamp courtesy of Medical Economics Publishing, New Jersey.)*

The Settlement House Movement also became a popular cause. A "settlement house" frequently developed as a branch of the university, where intellectuals investigated the distressful conditions of the poor. The movement was started through the efforts of Arnold Toynbee, whose interest in the poor led him to establish university settlement projects. After his death, Oxford University students at Toynbee Hall (1875) in East London continued to study ways to alleviate community problems. Through their efforts the very poor had the opportunity to enrich their lives educationally, socially, and culturally. Every aspect of neighborhood and community welfare was aided by social workers who lived among the people they served. The primary purpose of settlement work was to teach and assist wage earners to develop their potential in order to provide security and comfort for their families. Philanthropists who lived among the lower classes thus became their role models.

The first American settlement was developed on the Lower East Side of New York by Stanton Coit in 1886. Originally known as the "Neighborhood Guild," it was later called the "University Settlement." In 1889 Hull House was founded in Chicago by Jane Addams (1860–1935). This settlement came to be typical of ones that developed in other parts of America. The beginning of Hull House was a big old house that had been purchased by Jane Addams and a friend, Ellen Gates. The doors were opened to the neighborhood, which comprised representatives of over thirty nationalities. Help of all types was offered for any situation. Addams's neighbors clung to their customs, yet they wanted an education for their children and all the opportunities that America had to offer. Eventually, a day nursery, a kindergarten, and a library became essential components of Hull House. The community came to rely on Jane Addams, who also fought for suffrage and was the joint recipient of the 1931 Nobel Peace Prize (with Nicholas Murray Butler). By 1900 there were 103 settlement houses in the United States.

Before the Civil War, another social agency was extended from England to America. The Young Men's Christian Association (YMCA) was established in London in 1844 and in the United States in 1851. Its initial function dealt with the spiritual, social, physical, and intellectual well-being of men, but it gradually expanded to include relief work, visiting of the sick, and employment assistance. The YMCA also provided specialized services in wartime. Several branches joined to form the United States Christian Commission to assist with the welfare of soldiers during the Civil War. Later, this commission cared for prisoners and provided recreation for soldiers in World War I. In World War II it cooperated with other agencies to form the United Service Organization (USO) for planned recreational programs for members of the armed forces. Corresponding with the development of the YMCA was a movement among women that resulted in the formation of the Young Women's Christian Association (YWCA).

The Salvation Army (1878), founded by William Booth (1829–1912), was originally organized as a mission for the poor in London. Booth and his associates eventually became known as the "Salvation Army," which was set up with a military structure from that time on. By 1893 this agency had spread to a large portion of the world. It, too, was interested in the physical and spiritual welfare of the individual. Christian living was practiced through the giving of food, clothing, and shelter to the poor. Those who were miserable could find a certain amount of protection through the organization.

Social services had no boundaries, and missionaries helped to establish hospitals, schools of nursing, and dispensaries wherever they were needed. Nurses helped with these reforms by traveling to lands wherever people were in need of care. The work of Sir Wilfred Grenfell (1865–1940) is just one example of the remarkable achievements. Sir Wilfred was an English medical missionary who went to Labrador in 1892 and built a chain of hospital centers. Physicians, nurses, and college students volunteered at this mission, which ultimately developed into a complete health service to cover both physical and spiritual needs.

Visiting Nurse. Puerto de Tierra–Home Visiting. *(Schomburg Center for Research in Black Culture, The New York Public Library, New York.)*

Visiting Nursing

The apostolic deaconesses are considered to be the ancestors of the current visiting nurses. Early nursing orders, too, particularly the Sisters of Charity, visited the sick in their homes and became well known for their efforts. During specific periods in history, home visits were the primary activity of nursing, until modern municipal hospitals were fully developed. The Protestant Sisters of Charity— organized by Elizabeth Fry—St. John's Home, the Order of St. Margaret, and other groups were initiated for this purpose. In addition, the deaconesses at Kaiserswerth received part of their nurses' training out in the community.

A formal structure for visiting nursing was established in Great Britain through the endeavors of William Rathbone, a wealthy citizen of Liverpool. His wife had died in 1859 after a long and painful illness during which she was cared for by a competent trained nurse. Rathbone pondered the fact that his wife, a woman who had everything that money could buy, had received relief from skilled nursing care. He concluded that the poor, whose illnesses were compounded by a lack of wealth and by inadequate surroundings, would be helped even more. Nurses, therefore, should be sent to the homes of the needy sick. Rathbone employed Mary Robinson, the nurse who had cared for his wife, for a trial period of three months to give nursing care and comfort to the poor of Liverpool. His plan was opposed on the basis of the unsanitary conditions often found in the homes of the poor. According to Rathbone, a contemporary physician made this statement:

> It is evident that the essential conditions of rational and successful sick nursing such as good air, light, warmth, bedding, good food, etc., are altogether wanting in the homes of the poor. Of what use are the gratuitous supply and regular giving of medicines, if every necessity is wanting for ordinary healthy living? It is not that the nurse shrinks from the privations and injurious influences existing in the cottages and hovels, but it is the impossibility of being useful under such circumstances that renders home nursing unattainable for the poor. One can comfort them in their cottages, and give them food and medicine, but to nurse and heal them there with any prospect of success cannot be done.
>
> — *Rathbone, 1890, p. 7*

The general feeling was that if the poor were seriously ill, they should go to a hospital. However, Rathbone disagreed on the basis that many patients with serious illnesses were refused admission to general hospitals, that there would never be enough hospitals to take care of all serious illnesses among the poor, and that care given by the visiting nurse was less costly than that offered in the hospital. He soon hired additional nurses and began to train them at the school he founded at the Liverpool Royal Infirmary. His persistence resulted in the firm establishment of visiting nursing in Liverpool, which grew into a powerful organization. This experiment was soon followed by the emergence of other visiting nurses societies.

Visiting nursing received a boost in 1887, when Queen Victoria celebrated her fifty-year jubilee. Of the £76,000 raised by the women of England, the Queen donated £70,000 to the cause of visiting nurses. This sum was augmented by other sources to establish the Queen Victoria Jubilee Institute for Nurses, which received its royal charter in 1889. Nurses in this organization were called the "Jubilee Institute Nurses," but they were also referred to as the "Queen's Nurses." Their example was followed by similar groups in Canada with the King Edward VII Order; the Bush Nursing Association in South Africa; and the Plunket Nurses in New Zealand.

Although organized attempts at the development of visiting nursing occurred quite early in the history of the United States, the momentum needed for its progression was slow in coming. The earliest visiting nurse services were connected with denominational groups participating in religious and charitable works. Nondenominational societies were established in 1877 in New York (the Women's Branch of the New York City Mission), in 1886 in Boston and Philadelphia, and in 1889 in Chicago. These visiting nurse associations (VNA), which employed trained nurses chiefly for the care of the sick in their homes, were often called "Instructive District Nursing Associations." Teaching, as the name indicates, was also a vital function of the home care of the sick; principles of hygiene and sanitation were taught, in addition to specific aspects of health and illness. Isabel Hampton commented on the association name in an address to the International Congress of Nurses in 1893:

> In District Nursing we are confronted with conditions which require the highest order of work, but the actual nursing of the patient is the least part of what her work and influence should be among the class which the nurse will meet with. To this branch of nursing no more appropriate name can be given than "Instructive Nursing," for educational in the best sense of the word it should be.

The number of organizations continued to grow; by 1890, visiting nursing in the United States was occurring through the efforts of twenty-one organizations.

Nurses of the Instructive Visiting Nurse Association stand on the steps of the IVNA building, c. 1920s. *(Courtesy of the Visiting Nurse Association of Maryland.)*

The Henry Street Settlement

The "nursing settlement" was one of the factors that assisted with the expansion of the scope of visiting nursing into the larger field of public health nursing. However, it approached social problems from the point of view of nursing. The work environment, low wages, the neighborhood environment, the cultures and customs of the people, and other variables were examined and evaluated for their particular influence on health. The first of these was the world-famous Henry Street Settlement, which was opened as a cooperative and partially self-supporting neighborhood service in 1893. Its history is vividly described in two books authored by Lillian Wald, *The House on Henry Street* (1915) and *Windows on Henry Street* (1934).

Lillian D. Wald (1867–1940), a wealthy young woman of high ideals, became interested in the need for nursing and social services among the poor soon after she graduated from the New York Hospital School of Nursing in 1891. Born in Cincinnati and raised in Rochester, New York, she was of Polish–German–Jewish stock. Lillian Wald was educated at Miss Crittenden's English and French Boarding and Day School for Young Ladies and Little Girls. Influenced by her physician relatives, however, she left to become a nurse. After her graduation she spent a year nursing at the New York Juvenile Asylum, but then she entered Woman's Medical College in New York. During her medical school days Wald was asked to go to New York's Lower East Side to instruct immigrant mothers on the care of the sick. She was profoundly shocked by what she found there.

Abraham Phillips, *The House on Henry Street, Exterior of Henry Street Settlement,* Etching. *(Collection of The New-York Historical Society, New York.)*

The Nurses' Settlement House was set up on Jefferson Street by Lillian Wald and Mary Brewster. Within two years, the need for expansion was apparent. Larger accommodations were acquired at 265 Henry Street, which became fondly known as "The House on Henry Street." The services of the Henry Street Settlement House were available to all those who needed them. No distinction for service was made on the basis of economics, race, culture, or religion. Those in need had direct access to nursing care.

William Valentine Schevill, *Lillian Wald*, 1919. Oil on cardboard, 71.7 × 71.7 cm., feigned circle. *(National Portrait Gallery, Smithsonian Institution, Washington, D.C. Gift of the Visiting Nurse Service of New York.)*

Those nurses requesting information about this portrait may be surprised to find Lillian Wald listed in the category of "Social Worker" by the National Portrait Gallery. This is understandable in view of the fact that her contributions to society included not only nursing but also those activities aligned with settlement houses. In addition, the activities of early nurses were frequently a combination of social work and nursing.

At the turn of the century the Lower East Side of New York was a wilderness of overcrowded tenements where the sick lay unattended. Groups of immigrants of different nationalities filtered into the neighborhood and lived under great physical hardships. Death and morbidity rates were extremely high, and those who were fortunate moved to better neighborhoods before they succumbed to the health hazards of the slum. Lillian Wald soon personally experienced these dreadful conditions when a child approached her for help as she was teaching a group of mothers. She described this turning point in her life in the following way:

> From the schoolroom where I had been giving a lesson in bed-making, a little girl led me one drizzling March morning. She had told me of her sick mother, and gathering from her incoherent account that a child had been born, I caught up the paraphernalia of the bed-making lesson and carried it with me.
>
> The child led me over broken roadways . . . between tall, reeking houses . . . past odorous fish-stands for the streets were a market-place, unregulated, unsupervised, unclean, past evil-smelling, uncovered garbage cans, and perhaps worst of all, where so many little children played. . . .
>
> The child led me on through a tenement hallway, across a court where open and unscreened closets were promiscuously used by men and women, up into a rear tenement, by slimy steps whose accumulated dirt was augmented that day by the mud of the streets, and finally into the sickroom.
>
> All the maladjustments of our social and economic relations seemed epitomized in this brief journey and what was found at the end of it. The family to which the child led me was neither criminal nor vicious . . . and although the sick woman lay on a wretched, unclean bed, soiled with a hemorrhage two days old, they were not degraded human beings. . . .

Visiting nurse standing at the door with little boy on crutches, c. 1920s. *(Courtesy of the Visiting Nurse Association of Maryland.)*

It would have been some solace if by any conviction of the moral unworthiness of the family I could have defended myself as a part of society which permitted such conditions to exist . . . miserable as their state was, they were not without ideals for the family life, and for society, of which they were so unloved and unlovely a part.

That morning's experience was a baptism of fire. Deserted were the laboratory and the academic work of the college. I never returned to them. . . . To my inexperience it seemed certain that conditions such as these were allowed because people did not *know,* and for me there was a challenge to know and tell. When early morning found me still awake, my naive conviction remained that, if people knew things—and "things" meant everything implied in the condition of this family—such horrors would cease to exist, and I rejoiced that I had a training in the care of the sick that in itself would give me an organic relationship to the neighborhood in which this awakening had come.

— *Wald, 1915, pp. 4–8*

In 1893 Wald persuaded a classmate, Mary Brewster, to go into the tenement district with her to live and work. The two nurses rented the top floor of a tenement house on Jefferson Street and began to carry on whatever nursing and social work fell their way. As their workload increased, the house at 265 Henry Street was acquired with the help of Jacob H. Schiff, a banker and philanthropist, and others. This "House on Henry Street" became the Henry Street Visiting Nurse Service and eventually encompassed nursing service, social work, and an organized program of social, cultural, and educational activities. The scope of the settlement went far beyond the care of the sick and the prevention of disease. It aimed at rectifying those causes that were responsible for the poverty and misery itself. In keeping with this aim, Lillian Wald battled for legislative reforms that would ensure some measure of justice for the "unfortunates." Her initiative and skill in securing support for new ideas and new plans made her one of the most influential health workers of her day (Stewart and Austin, 1962).

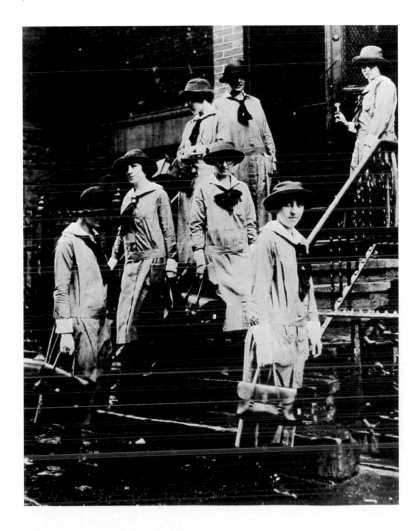

Henry Street Settlement House. (The Bettmann Archive, New York.)

Nurses leave the headquarters of the Henry Street Settlement to help the poor and the needy in lower Manhattan in the early 1900s.

School Nurse

Lillian Wald is regarded as the founder of what is now called public health or community nursing. She coined the phrase "public health nursing" and transformed the stereotyped visiting nursing of her time into the community movements that ultimately widened the horizons of modern nursing (Robinson, 1946). She created a system whereby patients had direct access to nurses and nurses had direct access to patients. Wald insisted that the nurses should be at the call of people who needed them, without the intervention of a medical man (Woolf, 1937). When warranted, however, a patient would be referred to a physician at one of the free dispensaries. No distinction was made between those who could pay and those who could not; services were available to all who sought them.

Lillian Wald's contributions to nursing and society at large were numerous and included the following:

1893   Supplied sputum cups and disinfectants to pioneer tuberculosis nurses.

1895   Made adjoining backyards into a neighborhood playground (Bunker Hill of Playgrounds).

1897–1909   Investigated unemployment, cases of dispossessed tenants, New York midwives, children out of school because of physical defects, working fourteen-year-old children, labor and construction camps in New York, and working conditions of girls in department stores, factories, and canneries.

1899   Assisted with the development of lectures on public health nursing at Teachers' College, Columbia University. By 1913 she and Mary Adelaide Nutting had established an educational program in public health nursing in which nurses would receive theoretical coursework at Teachers' College and practical experience at the Henry Street Settlement.

1902   Initiated public school nursing in America. (Started as a one-month experiment with Lina L. Rogers, a Henry Street nurse providing care to school children. The New York Board of Health eventually appointed numerous school nurses to function in New York City.)

1905   Served on the mayor's Pushcart Commission.

1908   Served on the State Immigration Commission.

1909   Initiated nursing service for industrial policyholders of the Metropolitan Life Insurance Company. (The Henry Street Settlement visiting nurses furnished services to policyholders in a limited section of Manhattan for a three-month period; services were then extended to other parts of the city. This arrangement was so successful that it was expanded to care in other cities where either local visiting nurses or nurses hired by the company provided care.)

1912   The United States Children's Bureau was created by act of Congress as part of the Department of Commerce and Labor. Wald is credited with the idea for this federal bureau.

1912   Established the Rural Nursing Service of the American Red Cross. (The name was changed in the following year to the Town and Country Nursing Service.)

1912   Became the first president of the National Organization for Public Health Nursing.

Lillian D. Wald's achievements and leadership were recognized through numerous citations and awards, including the degree of doctor of laws from Mount Holyoke College (1912), the medal of the National Institute of Social Sciences (1913), and the Certificate for Distinguished Service to the City of New York (1937). She received one of the most esteemed awards when she was named to the *Hall of Fame for Great Americans* (1971). With the death of Lillian D. Wald the nation had truly lost a unique citizen. Throughout her life she had opposed political and social corruption and supported those measures that would improve the health, welfare, and happiness of humanity.

Facing page, P. Buckley Moss, *The School Nurse,* 1994, Offset lithograph from watercolor, image size: 15.72 × 16.35 cm; paper size: 24.76 × 25.08 cm. *(The Moss Portfolio, Mathews, Virginia, copyright P. Buckley Moss.)*

The first school nurse began as an experiment in the New York schools through the efforts of Lillian Wald. Before the development of the school nurse, children who appeared to be unfit to mingle with others were sent home by physicians and teachers. Many were sent home with conditions that were easily resolved. Wald offered the services of a Henry Street nurse to demonstrate what could be done. The experiment was a success, resulting in a marked decrease in dismissals from school. Dozens of school nurses were soon appointed to assist with the effort.

Judy Waid, *Nursing: A Tradition of Caring,* 1993. *(Copyright Judy Waid and District Three, Ohio Nurses Association, Youngstown, Ohio.)*

This fourth edition medallion depicts an historical perspective of the nursing profession in 1893. In celebration of the Hundredth Anniversary of Community Health Nursing, Lillian Wald, a native Ohioan, is remembered for her establishment of a free-standing nursing care service center. The House on Henry Street, formerly located on the lower east side of New York City, addressed the needs of tenement dwellers.

She had stirred the melting-pot on her adopted block, and it became a community undertaking. In the amalgamation of the multitudes that came to these shores, in the eternal warfare against prejudice, she was a steadfast guide. Amid the darkness of ignorance and poverty, she pointed the path to the light. An American who devoted her life to those of foreign birth, this descendant of immigrants walked the ways of democracy. Her work was an international rainbow of friendship across humanity's sky. . . . Presidents, governors, senators, have paid her appropriate tribute. The credo of the Visiting Nurse Service of the Henry Street Settlement is Lillian D. Wald's finest epitaph: Response to every call for help, without regard to race or creed or color.

— *Robinson, 1946, p. 296*

The Henry Street Settlement paved the way for the foundation of nursing settlements in other American cities. The earliest among these were in Richmond, Virginia (1900), San Francisco (1900), and Orange, New Jersey (1903).

The Frontier Nursing Service

There is a striking contrast between the development of midwifery in Europe and in the United States. Midwifery was always considered an important specialty in Europe, with a two-year course usually required. Nearly all state-

Cartoon, "A Man-Mid-Wife or a Newly Discovered Animal," depicting a midwife bisected into male and female halves. (From S.W. Fores, *Man-Mid-Wifery Dissected*, London, 1793. The Wellcome Institute for Medical Science, London, England.)

THE CARELESS NURSE·

SWEET HOME SOAP.

The Careless Nurse. (The Bettmann Archive, New York.)

registered nurses in England were at one time registered midwives who had six months or more of specialized training. Yet in the United States the training of nurses in the area of midwifery had been prevented primarily by the attitudes of physicians. The physicians held the view that every woman should be assisted in delivery by a physician, an attitude that continued to be prominent into the 1930s. This opposition, which was related to the belief that nurse-midwifery represented an intrusion on the field of medical practice, ignored the high maternal death rate. A large number of untrained, ignorant midwives were practicing; and thousands of women employed incompetent midwives.

The use of midwives was customary among the foreign-born in the cities, those living in isolated communities, and among blacks, particularly those in the rural regions of the South. In many instances medical care for these women was nonexistent. Approximately thirty percent of all deliveries were attended by midwives in the United States. Although many of the midwives had practical experience that was an asset in normal deliveries, injury or death to the mother or child (or both) often occurred with abnormal or difficult deliveries. Early in the 1900s studies were undertaken that began the long march to reform in the care of mothers and babies. In addition, some nurses began to advocate the training and use of nurse-midwives in America, particularly in those areas where medical care was lacking. However, this movement lacked support from physicians, nurses, and the general public and therefore did not have a strong impact.

Several physicians aided the advance to training in the area of midwivery. Joseph Warrington, while working as an obstetrician at the Philadelphia Dispensary for the Medical Relief of the Poor, became aware of the need for trained midwives to deliver babies to poor women. In 1832 he formed the Philadelphia Lying-in Charity for Attending Indigent Females in Their Own Homes; no fee would be charged and the women would deliver in their homes. Warrington soon began to train nurses in the art of midwivery. Dr. Samuel Gregory of Boston facilitated another school for nurse-midwives in 1846. He firmly believed that midwives should be able to acquire scientific knowledge upon which their practice would be based. To that end, he published several pamphlets stressing that more and better courses of instruction should be available.

A few schools for nurse-midwives were finally developed. In 1911 Bellevue Hospital established a school of midwifery that continued until 1935. This school was specifically designed to aid the forty thousand New York women who were being assisted in delivery by untrained women. It was discontinued when the majority of women entered hospitals for delivery. The founding of centers that offered courses and granted certificates in nurse-midwifery followed. Such institutions included the Maternity Center Association (which opened the first school for nurse-midwives in the United States) in connection with the Lobenstine Clinic in New York; the Tuskegee Institute in Alabama (a short-lived school for black nurse-midwives assisted by federal funds during the war); the Frontier Nursing Service in Kentucky; and the Catholic Maternity Institute in New Mexico. Finally, certificates in nurse-midwifery were offered in conjunction with a master's degree at Yale University, Johns Hopkins University, New York Medical College, Catholic University, Columbia University, and the University of Utah (Dolan, Fitzpatrick, and Hermann, 1983).

The Frontier Nursing Service provided the first organized midwifery service in this country. It was founded in 1925 by Mary Breckinridge, the daughter of a family distinguished in American history. Although married twice, she retained her maiden name. Her only children, Breckie and Polly, died in infancy, and this was thought to be the catalyst for her interest and involvement in midwifery. Mary Breckinridge graduated from St. Luke's Hospital Training School in New York (1910) and later from the British Hospi-

Logo for the Frontier Nursing Service, a demonstration in family-centered primary health care since 1925. *(Courtesy of the Frontier Nursing Service, Hyden, Kentucky.)*

Mary Breckinridge on Horseback, c. 1938. Breckinridge was founder of the Frontier Nursing Service. *(Courtesy of the Frontier Nursing Service, Hyden, Kentucky.)*

tal for Mothers and Babies, Woolwich, London (1925), where she received her certificate in midwifery. For several years (1919 to 1923), she became occupied with public health activities in devastated France and actually organized public health nursing there.

Mary Breckinridge recognized the need for a rural midwifery service in the Appalachian Mountains of Kentucky, where for centuries both nursing and midwifery had been practiced under almost medieval conditions by the "granny women." These "midwives" were generally illiterate, had no formal training in midwifery, knew little about prenatal or postnatal care, and were often superstitious. They rarely called a physician, even when faced with serious complications. Their practices ranged from the use of soot as a medication to the placing of an axe, blade side up, under the bed as a preventive measure.

The people who settled in these hills became isolated from the rest of the country because of their location. They maintained the old customs of early marriage and large families. The Appalachian area was part of the "cradle of the nation" and had one of the highest birth rates in the United States. Mary Breckinridge, who had witnessed midwifery services firsthand in England, New Zealand, and Australia, was determined to initiate a similar plan for the care of mothers, babies, and children in these foothills. To accomplish her goal she was forced to use English-trained midwives for many years, since there were so few trained midwives in America.

A member of the Frontier Nursing Service is preparing to attend a childbirth as a youngster watches. *(The Bettmann Archive, New York.)*

The members of the Frontier Nursing Service worked in Leslie County, Kentucky, where the lack of highways necessitated travel by horse or mule. The area was divided into eight districts of approximately seventy-eight square miles each. Two nurses lived in the middle of each district and were responsible for the health of all who lived there. A primary form of health care was provided in which a family-centered approach was emphasized. Each of the "nurses on horseback" had certification as a nurse-midwife, and the nurses gave antepartal, intrapartal, and postpartal care to the women in their districts. They performed normal deliveries but called a physician in the event of a complicated case. A study of the first one thousand cases showed that the proportion of complications during pregnancy and delivery was lower among patients cared for by the service than among the general population. Child-care services were also offered; babies under one year of age were seen twice a month, preschool children (one to six years of age) once a month, and schoolchildren every two months. Mary Breckinridge and her staff had demonstrated the usefulness of such a service in areas where physicians were not readily accessible.

By 1935 a small, twelve-bed general hospital, the Hyden Hospital and Health Center, was founded and functional. The medical director not only was responsible for the hospitalized patients but also responded to the nurses in the several districts. The advent of World War II prompted the establishment of a Graduate School of Midwivery, since the British nurses wished to return home to care for their own people. This school was founded by the Frontier Nursing Service in 1939 at Hyden, Kentucky.

In recent years a growing number of nurses have begun to specialize in the practice of nurse-midwifery. It involves a definite return to or reintro-

A Nurse-Midwife Cuts the Cord of a Newborn Infant Lying Between the Legs of the Mother on the Bed, c. 1850. Colored lithograph. From Beach's Improved System of Midwifery. (National Library of Medicine, Bethesda, Maryland.)

duction of past techniques. For example, the practices of home delivery and natural childbirth, the use of the sitting position on "obstetrical chairs" or "birthing chairs," and the employment of nurse-midwives are on the rise. In some respects this has been fostered by third-party insurance reimbursement for midwifery services and the development of birthing centers in hospitals and freestanding maternity centers.

The Status of Women

The history of nursing is essentially the story of women. From primitive times nursing has been inextricably bound to the female of the species; even today the majority of nurses are still women. Robinson vividly depicts the origin of the mother-nurse in a rather simplistic summary. Yet the description serves to emphasize the close bond that occurred between the two roles:

> Biology made the female the nurse of the species. The first mother who leaned over the first cradle of leaves in the primitive forest was the first nurse—and back of this fat-hipped woman with the hanging breasts, the projecting face, and the heavy eyebrow ridges, stretched countless ages of her prehuman ancestry. In the purposeful efforts of animals to aid their young and injured are found the rudiments of medicine and nursing. The utter helplessness of the human infant, even after he has mastered the difficult art of holding his overgrown head erect, developed a prolonged connection between mother and child. Before the dawn of agriculture, the male stepped out of his cave or rock-shelter, club in hand, the hunter of all living things; the female remained behind, the nurse of the young and the sick.

> — *Robinson, 1946, p. 360*

The development of nursing, therefore, parallels and reflects the women's movement. For a long period in history, the position of women in society left much to be desired. The role of women remained passive, although statements about the equality of women with men were heard periodically. Throughout the centuries women were generally regarded as the property of men and had no legal rights or power. (Rare exceptions can be cited, such as the position of the Roman matron at the start of the Christian era.) For example, the Code of Hammurabi stated that women were the exclusive property of men. Ancient norms regarding women were enforced, particularly during the time of the Reformation. Yet some glimmers of potential for change began to surface as early as the beginning of the seventeenth century. A group of courageous and persistent women emerged to champion the cause of their sex and earn the title of "feminists." These women advocated equal rights for women that would include legal and academic privileges, marriage reform that would allow for preference rather than arrangement, and the right to vote, own property, and hold office. Although they met vehement opposition to their cause, they continued their struggle toward the emancipation of women. Through their efforts the position of women slowly began to improve.

Books, essays, and articles that dealt with women's rights began to appear. Works written by the early feminists included "The Excellencies of Women and the Errors of Men" by Lucretia Marinelli of Italy; *The Learned Maid,* a book by Anna von Schurman of Holland; "A Serious Proposal to the Ladies" by the English feminist, Mary Astell; and two volumes on *The Strictures on Female Education* by another Englishwoman, Hannah More. This movement owed much to Mary Wollstonecraft's epic book, *A Vindication of the Rights of Women,* written in 1792. The "rights" that were discussed in this work were simply human rights that should have been impartially applied to women. This author argued against the existing double standard of morality that was prevalent in the society. Mary Wollstonecraft was, indeed, a fitting example of her beliefs. She had acquired an education and entered the business world as a translator for a publisher in London. Supporters of her ideas turned them into action.

Successful and powerful novels also began to be published by women. Among these were *Evelina* by Fanny Burney; *Pride and Prejudice* by Jane Austen; *Jane Eyre* and *Wuthering Heights* by Charlotte Brontë; *The Mill on the Floss* by George Eliot; and *Uncle Tom's Cabin* by Harriet Beecher Stowe.

Women became reformers, educators, and developers—making their voices heard in any way possible. They rallied to advance their right of suffrage when they discovered that social reforms could be achieved through the power of the vote. Prominent in the American women's movement was Susan B. Anthony (1820–1906). English women later began suffrage efforts and met with comparable resistance. Even Queen Victoria voiced her protest against:

> this mad, wicked folly of Woman's Rights, with all its attendant horrors. Lady—ought to get a *good whipping.* It is a subject which makes the Queen so furious she cannot contain herself. Tennyson has some beautiful lines on the difference of men and women in *The Princess.* Woman would become the most hateful, heartless, and disgusting of human beings were she allowed to unsex herself, and where would be the protection which man was intended to give the weaker sex?
>
> — *Quoted in Robinson, 1946, p. 365*

After nearly seventy-five years of frustration and struggle, the United States Constitution was amended in 1920 to allow women to vote.

Nursing leaders were involved in women's rights as well as in human rights. Nurses were found among the marchers in the pilgrimages of the suffragettes. The most colorful and zealous suffragist was Lavinia Lloyd Dock (1858–1956), one of nursing's greatest leaders and a radical feminist. She was actively engaged in social protest, picketing and parading for women's rights,

Anonymous, *Dr. Pierce's Favorite Anuric,* c. 1918. Poster. *(Philadelphia Museum of Art, Philadelphia, Pennsylvania.)*

Judy Chicago, "Mary Wollstonecraft," plate from *The Dinner Party*, 1979. China-painted porcelain, 35.6 cm diameter. *(Copyright Judy Chicago, 1979. Photo copyright Donald Woodman. Through the Flower, Albuquerque, New Mexico.)*

Mary Wollstonecraft lived in a confining environment like most women of her time. Her life was spent working for the "rights" of women, believing that the tyranny of men needed to be crushed both politically and socially in order for women to be free. She first encountered the severe limitations of female education as a young schoolteacher.

Designed by Thomas Stothard, R.A., *Asylum for Female Orphans*, c. 1785. Engraving. *(Copyright The British Museum, London, England.)*

and protesting against war; these were not regarded as "nurselike" or "lady-like" activities. She also voiced her opinions and concerns about social issues whenever an opportunity arose. At one point "Little Dockie" was to speak about the history of nursing in Europe to a group of nursing students at Teachers College. Nutting was away, and the incident was described by Isabel Stewart:

> I was quite young and I'd never seen Miss Dock. . . . I was sure I'd know her when I met her, because she'd be tall and angular and intellectual looking. Who should turn up at the door but this small, short sort of roly-poly little person with curly hair. She'd just been at a suffrage meeting, and had "Votes for Women" across her hat and "Votes for Women" across her chest. She said, "Now what am I going to talk about?" I said . . . "you were to talk about nursing on the Continent." "Oh," she said, "very bad. It'll not be any better till they get the suffrage. I'll talk about suffrage."
>
> — *Stewart, 1961, pp. 139–140*

Stewart continued:

> This suffrage thing—it was the whole thing for her; she wanted not only to work for it but really to suffer for it. She went over to Britain to work with Mrs. Pankhurst, and she wanted above all things to go to jail. Oh, she got there all right . . . that was during the war, at the beginning of the First World War. She was a member of the advanced wing of the Suffrage Party, and they were having a meeting in Washington at the time that Wilson was beginning to think of the possibility of war. They discussed it, and a friend of mine who was there at the time tells me that Lavinia got up and seized the flag which was there and said, "Youth to the Colors!" and on she marched, out of the door, and they followed her, and she went right to the White House, and they picketed the White House!
>
> She is about this high, you know. . . . Anyway, they all went into the cooler for the night. I think it just pleased her no end.
>
> — *Stewart, 1961, p. 275*

Lavinia L. Dock, one of six children in a cultured and affluent family, was born in Harrisburg, Pennsylvania. Both of her parents were well educated and insisted upon equal education for both their sons and daughters. Lavinia was an accomplished organist and pianist, but she decided to enter Bellevue Hospital Training School for Nurses, from which she graduated in 1886. She became a night supervisor at Bellevue Hospital, where she wrote one of the first textbooks for nurses, *The Textbook on Materia Medica for Nurses* (1890). She was aware of the problems the students encountered in learning about drugs and solutions and wrote this book to aid them in the mastery of this content. Since the publisher was unwilling to make the original investment, Lavinia's father advanced the necessary amount. According to Roberts (1956), this investment paid off handsomely; over one hundred thousand copies of several editions were sold.

During her life Dock held various positions in nursing. She became an assistant to Isabel Hampton Robb at Johns Hopkins Hospital for a time. After leaving Johns Hopkins, she was appointed superintendent of nurses at the Illinois Training School in Chicago. She regarded this brief venture as a failure and left there wondering how they had put up with her. She then joined the Henry Street Settlement to work with Lillian Wald. Dock considered the work at the settlement suited to her, and she was happiest there.

Lavinia Dock was concerned with the many problems that were plaguing nursing. She questioned the serious and long-term effects of women's subjugation to men. She believed that male dominance in the health field was the major problem confronting the nursing profession. In 1903 Dock spoke of those developments that would almost ensure male dominance and, in turn,

Portrait of Lavinia L. Dock. *(Special Collections, Milbank Memorial Library, Teachers College, Columbia University, New York.)*

Lavinia Lloyd Dock was one of nursing's greatest leaders and a radical feminist. She was often to be found among the marchers in the pilgrimages of the suffragettes. "Little Dockie" actively engaged in social protest and was outspoken on the then-taboo subject of venereal disease.

315

have a major impact on the development of nursing. Her pleas for caution went unheeded, and nurses became accomplices to their own subordination.

> Nursing leaders ignored all her warnings and in the second decade of the century actually became nonvoting members of the American Hospital Association. They worked with physicians and administrators on joint committees, expecting their oppressors to help them solve nursing problems. They sought approval from men, not liberation. As a result, from the first decade of the century onward, physicians and hospital administrators have remained in positions of dominance and control over nursing and health care.
>
> — *Ashley, 1975, p. 1466*

The oppression of nurses was built into the law and the educational system through the legalization of paternalism and the institutionalization of apprenticeship. The threats became a reality as male domination progressed to a state of completion. A powerful combination of male domination and sexual discrimination surfaced and prevented the recognition of nurses as professional equals of physicians with the right to practice independently. Even at present, inequality in the health care field continues to be a serious impediment to the development of the highest potential of nursing.

Lavinia Dock served nursing in numerous elected capacities. Her keen and versatile mind was respected by her colleagues at home and abroad, who looked to her for guidance. She conducted a study of professional organization bylaws and was instrumental in the establishment of the American Society of Superintendents of Training Schools for Nurses. Dock became this organization's first secretary, as well as the first secretary of the International Council of Nurses (1899). She is regarded as the chief American influence in the organization of the nurses of the world. Lavinia Dock was active in the movement to effect passage of legislation for the control of nursing practice.

Lavinia Lloyd Dock. (The Alan Mason Chesney Medical Archives of The Johns Hopkins Medical Institutions, Baltimore, Maryland.)

This photograph of Lavinia Dock was taken at her home when she was ninety-eight years old. It is somewhat reminiscent of the photographs of Florence Nightingale with her bird. The photograph was given to Johns Hopkins by Effie Taylor.

Outspoken on the then-taboo subject of venereal disease, Dock published a book in 1910, *Hygiene and Morality,* which shocked some people. The world of nursing profited by her numerous articles that appeared in the early issues of the *American Journal of Nursing.* The four-volume *History of Nursing* (vols. 1 and 2, 1907; vols. 3 and 4, 1912), written in collaboration with M. Adelaide Nutting, became the classic text on nursing history. The condensed version, *A Short History of Nursing,* was co-authored with Isabel M. Stewart. The *History of American Red Cross Nursing* was a massive, comprehensive work. These studies made Dock one of the foremost of nursing historians,

> a result achieved by the vitality of her style, knowledge of languages, command of facts, international outlook, an intelligence that would not compromise with stupidity, and a character that scorned to appease evil howsoever intrenched.
>
> — *Robinson, 1946, p. 301*

At the turn of the century, some strides had indeed been made toward the achievement of equality and freedom for women. A particular milestone occurred with the readmission of women into the medical field. Elizabeth Blackwell (1821–1910) was the pioneer who was admitted to Geneva Medical College in Geneva, New York, in 1847. This occurred, however, only after being rejected by twelve other medical schools and her Geneva application being presented to the all-male student body for a vote. Her struggle to become a doctor took place during a time when options for women, although still limited, were gradually expanding. She was the first woman in America to graduate from medical school and be licensed as a physician. Unable to obtain a hospital staff appointment after graduation, she traveled to Europe, where she worked in London and Paris hospitals. Eventually, Elizabeth and her sister Emily established the New York Infirmary for Women and Children in 1857. She was also responsible for the founding of the Women's Medical College of that institution, where women physicians could get both

Judy Chicago, "Elizabeth Blackwell," plate from *The Dinner Party,* 1979. China-painted porcelain, 35.6 cm diameter. *(Copyright Judy Chicago, 1979. Photo copyright Donald Woodman. Through the Flower, Albuquerque, New Mexico.)*

Elizabeth Blackwell's struggle to become a doctor occurred during the period when women's options were still limited but sufficiently advanced to allow her to achieve her goals. She was the first American woman to graduate from medical school and become a physician. From that time on she fought to open the medical profession to women. The first hospital where female doctors could receive both training and clinical experience was the New York Infirmary for Women and Children established by Blackwell and her sister Emily.

training and clinical experience. Emily had also had difficulty in gaining admission to medical school. She was refused admission at Elizabeth's alma mater and several other medical schools but finally was accepted at the Medical Department of Western Reserve University.

The women's movement continues today, and it experiences periodic defeats as well as intermittent successes. The ideal embodied in the efforts of these early nursing leaders has yet to be achieved. The nursing movement mirrors this journey.

THE RISE OF ORGANIZED NURSING

Modern nursing was still very young when a few farsighted leaders spurred the movement toward organizational developments. These leaders realized that a group was stronger than an individual, that an organization could accomplish things an individual could not, and that from unity came strength. They believed nursing's real power and potential could be realized through the united efforts of individual members striving to promote its interests. Their commitment to organized nursing was fostered by serious conditions that jeopardized both the recipients and the providers of nursing care. The primary concern of these leaders was, therefore, twofold: protection of the public from poorly trained nurses and the lack of standardization in nurse training.

Lack of endowments had placed the training schools under the control of medicine and hospital administration. The schools provided cheap service to the hospitals and thus became profitable enterprises for the institutions. The education of the students was incidental; the students' chief responsibility was to provide care for the hospital, to provide service. The exploitation of nurses occurred as hospitals relied on the inexpensive student labor force to staff the units. With no standards or controls, training schools proliferated at an alarming rate. Consequently, inferior schools also developed and no standards of practice existed to protect the public from unsafe care. The biggest problems facing nursing at the beginning of the twentieth century were those dealing with the setting of standards. These conditions were depicted graphically in a history of nursing in Kansas:

> Lacking a model, the majority of the hospital founders conceived of the trained hospital nurse as a substitute for the competent mother or neighbor who cares for the sick in the home. Primarily she should be a "good housekeeper" of the neighborly type. Since the average housewife of Kansas was still scrubbing her own floors and doing the family washing, it was assumed that these and similar chores were part of the work of a nurse. Even after it became apparent that there was much waste in using educated women for such labors, hospitals continued to spend every available cent to add to their number of student nurses . . . the students, promised an education, would work for little or for nothing except room and board. . . . Humanitarians, quite as much as the physicians who founded hospitals as money-making ventures, shared in the exploitation. . . . It simply did not occur to them that they were perpetuating one wrong in correcting another.
>
> — *Kansas State Nurses Association, 1942, p. 93*

Organizations for Nurses

Conditions had reached a critical point by the end of the nineteenth century, and an organizational structure was viewed as the one mechanism whereby changes could be attained in nursing education and nursing practice. The first attempt to establish an organization of nurses took place in England. Mrs. Bedford Fenwick, an internationally prominent leader from London, began a campaign in 1887 for nurse registration. This idea was not well accepted, even though the quality of nursing care was inconsistent and frequently inferior in Britain. Mrs. Fenwick was, however, convinced that standards were necessary to improve nursing, and she founded the British Nurses' Association in 1888 to achieve legal sanction. This association was the first of its type anywhere in the world. It grew rapidly, and its members numbered a thousand by the end of one year. Membership was not limited to graduate nurses but included some physicians. (A few were honorary officers!) Although there was opposition to this organization, eventually it obtained a royal charter in 1892 under the title of The Royal British Nurses' Association. Similar societies developed in other countries as the advantages from such a united endeavor were demonstrated. The overall aim of each of the organizations was similar—to improve the education and status of nurses and to secure for them state recognition.

The earliest nurses' association in America, on which there is scant information, was the Philomena Society. It was started in New York in 1886 but lasted only one year. As nursing schools developed, however, alumnae associations were formed to foster fellowship and mutual support and to provide economic assistance when necessary. These groups became convenient units for amalgamation, which later proved to be beneficial when the national organization emerged. The first alumnae associations were formed at Bellevue Hospital in New York (1889), Illinois Training School of Cook County Hospital in Chicago (1891), Johns Hopkins Hospital in Baltimore (1892), Massachusetts General Hospital in Boston (1895), and Boston City Hospital (1896).

American Society of Superintendents of Training Schools for Nurses. The year 1893 marks the "debut" of American nursing and the beginning of a new era in nursing education. At the World's Fair in Chicago in that year, the International Congress of Charities, Corrections and Philanthropy was held. A part of this congress was devoted to hospitals and dispensaries. Through the encouragement of Mrs. Bedford Fenwick, Dr. John S. Billings, chairman of the congress, agreed that nursing should occupy a place on the program. The subsection on nursing was chaired by Isabel Adams Hampton, superintendent of nurses at Johns Hopkins Hospital. The meeting was attended by both American and Canadian nurses, and papers were read that reflected and frankly presented the major nursing issues and concerns. In addition, the need for a national union was urged. Florence Nightingale sent an address that was read in which she discussed the teaching of nursing and the training of a nurse. She commented that "Training is to teach the nurse to help the patient to live. Nursing the sick is an art, and an art requiring an organized, practical, and scientific training, for nursing is the skilled servant of medicine, surgery and hygiene." Isabel Hampton spoke on the educational standards for nurses; Lavinia L. Dock discussed the relation of training schools to hospitals. The papers were eventually compiled in a publication, *Nursing of the Sick* (1893) and were viewed as a historical record of the progress made and the problems encountered in the two decades following the opening of the first training school.

The day after the nursing program had taken place, Hampton arranged for a meeting with a small group to discuss the possibilities for a nursing organization. This meeting was attended by directors of nursing schools and resulted in the formation of the American Society of Superintendents of Training Schools for Nurses as a binational organization. Membership was restricted to nurses associated with nurse training; thus, in effect, it became an accrediting agency for schools of nursing in the United States and Canada (Stewart and Austin, 1962). The first official meeting of the society was attended by forty-four superintendents in January 1894. The aim of the society was to develop high educational standards for schools of nursing through the establishment of universal requirements for admission, a sound program of theory and practice, and improved working conditions. A curriculum committee was promptly appointed, and a report was published two years later. In

1907 Canadian members formed their own independent organization, the Canadian Society of Superintendents of Training Schools, with Mary Agnes Snively as its first president. In 1912 the American society became known by a new name, the National League of Nursing Education, and still later as the National League for Nursing (1952).

The society was occupied for the first two years with the development of a national association of graduate nurses in order that the practice of all types of nursing might be represented. This effort was led by Isabel Hampton Robb, M. Adelaide Nutting, and Lavinia L. Dock, all of whom were at Johns Hopkins. Miss Dock carefully studied the laws under which professional organizations could operate and how they could be formulated. Her report to the society at the 1896 convention proposed that alumnae associations be the mode of entrance to the new organization; the development of local and state units would follow. A committee was appointed to prepare a constitution and bylaws for a national nurses' organization; it was instructed to meet with a number of delegates from the oldest alumnae associations.

Nurses Associated Alumnae of the United States and Canada. The committee of the society and the delegates of the alumnae associations met in New York in September 1896. The following year the constitution and bylaws that had been prepared by this group were accepted and a national nurses' association was established. This second organization, created for the rank and file in nursing, was called the Nurses Associated Alumnae of the United States and Canada. The original purposes of this association in 1897 were: "(1) To establish and maintain a code of ethics; (2) to elevate the standards of nursing education; (3) to promote the usefulness and honor, the financial and other interests of the nursing profession" (American Nurses Association, 1941, p. 2). A primary objective was to secure legislation to differentiate between the trained and the untrained nurse, since the title of "trained nurse" had come to mean all grades of training and all grades of women.

When the Associated Alumnae sought to incorporate, it was found that New York law prohibited foreign membership. Therefore it was necessary to eliminate the words "and Canada," which prohibited further Canadian participation. Canadian nurses withdrew from the organization as early as 1900. In 1908 the Provisional Organization of the Canadian National Association of Trained Nurses was formed. The name was changed to the Canadian Nurses Association at the 1924 convention. In the early years of the Canadian association, "the recurring problems under discussion were education of student nurses, improvement of nursing care of patients, amelioration of conditions for nurses, and the need for state registration of nurses as a safeguard to the public" (Gibbon and Mathewson, 1947, p. 348). By the time the Associated Alumnae was renamed the American Nurses Association in 1911 and chartered by the state of New York, Canadian membership had been discontinued.

The first president of the Nurses Associated Alumnae was Isabel Adams Hampton Robb (1859–1910). One author described her as "the radiant center of the magnetic force which brought the two national organizations into existence before 1900" (Roberts, 1954, p. 26). Another has called her the "architect of American nursing organizations" (Fitzpatrick, 1983). Whatever titles are used to describe her, Robb was undoubtedly one of the greatest early leaders in American nursing and perhaps the best loved. She was a forceful and farsighted individual, yet she demonstrated a gentle powerful that was considered a main characteristic of her leadership:

> With great practical ability in details, Miss Hampton had a power of seeing the future which was like that of a sibyl. She had visions of nursing growth, organization, and activities, which came first as hazy, indefinite pictures, gradually taking form until all was clear and vivid, filling her with joy and enthusiasm, eager interest, and untiring energy . . . filled with the highest belief in the mission of women as the superior moral force, and in the possibility of universal happiness.
>
> — *Nutting and Dock, vol. 3, 1912, pp. 123–124*

Logo for the Canadian Nurses Association. *(Reproduced with permission from the Canadian Nurses Association, Ottawa, Ontario.)*

Sergeant Kendall, *Isabel A. Hampton*, first Superintendent of Nurses of the Johns Hopkins Hospital Training School for Nurses, c. 1890. (*The Alan Mason Chesney Medical Archives of the Johns Hopkins Medical Institutions, Baltimore, Maryland.*)

The Nurse, Isabel A. Hampton, Bellevue Hospital, 1882. Sketched from life for *Century Magazine,* November 1882, in "A New Profession for Women." *(The Bettmann Archive, New York.)*

Isabel Adams Hampton was born in Canada (Welland, Ontario). She attended the Collegiate Institute of St. Catharine's, Ontario, after which she taught at the Merriton School for approximately three years. In 1881 she was admitted to the Bellevue Hospital Training School for Nurses and graduated in 1883. For a brief period Hampton served as a relief supervisor at Women's Hospital in New York, followed by two years as a staff nurse at St. Paul's Hospice in Rome. Upon her return to the United States, she became superintendent of nurses at Illinois Training School in Chicago, where she introduced several innovations of educational import. Hampton implemented a graded system of theory and practice, terminated the practice of students doing private duty as part of their education (she believed this practice to be an exploitation of the students, since the hospital received the fees), and originated the concept of affiliation, whereby students could gain necessary experiences not available in their home institutions. These innovations were undoubtedly influenced by her experience as a teacher and by her grounding in educational theory.

Hampton was not yet thirty when she was chosen to organize the school of nursing of Johns Hopkins Hospital. It is said that she created quite a sensation upon her arrival because of her serenity and beauty. William Osler, a fellow Canadian, supposedly stated that she entered Hopkins like "an animated Greek statue." She was likened to Venus by both men and women. Lavinia Dock expressed the overall sentiment:

> I thought I had never seen a more beautiful or majestic figure except on the pedestal of some classic sculpture. Miss Hampton's color was rich and fresh, her eyes the clearest blue, unusually large and beautifully set and opened; her voice was one of her greatest charms, being very sweet and quiet, yet with a certain thrill in it when she was in earnest. Her hands were also extremely beautiful, displaying her character and power of organization. They were perfect enough to have been modeled.

> — *Quoted in Robinson, 1946, p. 173*

More innovations were attempted. Hampton became a "principal" rather than a "superintendent," and policies for a twelve-hour day were established that included time for meals, recreation, rest, and study periods. She also recognized the need for nursing publications and wrote three influential books: *Nursing: Its Principles and Practice for Hospital and Private Use* (1894), *Nursing Ethics* (1900), and *Educational Standards for Nurses* (1907). It was at Johns Hopkins that Hampton met Hunter Robb, who had been a resident in gynecology. They were married at St. Margaret's, Westminster, London, on July 12, 1894, with the bride carrying flowers sent by Florence Nightingale. Robb was not well liked by Isabel's colleagues because they believed that he was not an equal match for her in either intellectual ability or physical appearance. The Robbs settled in Cleveland, where they eventually had two sons.

Isabel Robb continued her activities in nursing and made her greatest contributions after her marriage. She helped found the two national nursing organizations, shouldered the burden for the launching of the program for graduate nurses at Teachers College, was one of the original members of a committee to found the *American Journal of Nursing,* and was essentially the central force in the early development of professional nursing in the United States. One wonders how much more she would have accomplished had she not died prematurely in a traffic accident on April 15, 1910.

Mary Adelaide Nutting (1858–1948) was a nursing leader who was greatly influenced by Isabel Hampton Robb and, in fact, became her successor at Johns Hopkins. Nutting, too, was born in Canada (Quebec), and she received special instruction in music and art in private schools in Montreal, Boston, and Ottawa. An alumna of the first graduating class of Johns Hopkins, Nutting translated Hampton's dreams of a three-year course and an eight-hour day into reality. However, Adelaide Nutting was an innovator in her own

Cecilia Beaux, *M. Adelaide Nutting,* 1906. *(Special Collections, Milbank Memorial Library, Teachers College, Columbia University, New York.)*

right. According to Christy (1969b), she was second only to Florence Nightingale in overall contributions to nursing. "Her influence as an educational experimenter and a creative thinker went far beyond the two institutions in which her main work was done, the second being Teachers College, Columbia University" (Stewart, 1943, p. 143).

During her tenure in Baltimore, Nutting initiated and developed the preliminary course, tuition fees, and scholarships at Johns Hopkins. She helped with the organization of the Maryland State Nurses Association, served as its first president, and facilitated the efforts of the nurses in their quest for state registration. She also began collecting materials and books for a historical collection for the nursing school. These later became the basis for the first two volumes of the four-volume *A History of Nursing* (1907 and 1912) written

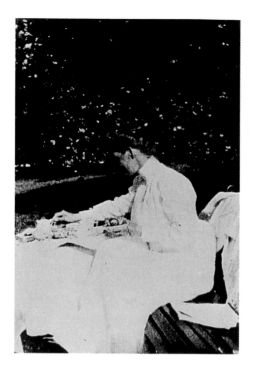

M. Adelaide Nutting, 1905. (The Alan Mason Chesney Medical Archives of the Johns Hopkins Medical Institutions, Baltimore, Maryland.)

with Lavinia Dock. Nutting wrote many articles, some of which were published as a collection in *A Sound Economic Basis for Schools of Nursing* (1926). She prepared two influential reports on nursing education that were issued through the United States Bureau of Education. Her letters, speeches, and published works demonstrated her belief in a broad education for nurses that would prepare them for great responsibilities in all life situations. Her lifelong dream was to see basic education for nurses firmly established in institutions of higher learning—in universities.

In 1907 M. Adelaide Nutting took charge of the hospital economics course at Teachers College and became the first professor of nursing in the world. Her original title was Professor of Domestic Administration, but it was changed to Professor of Nurses Education in 1910. She remained at Teachers College until her retirement in 1925. In addition to her administrative and educational responsibilities at this institution, Nutting participated in many nursing activities, including organizational work, committee work, government projects, the war effort, publications, and international endeavors. She was the prime instigator in the establishment of the Vassar Training Camp of 1918, a program that drew women who were college graduates into nursing.

Nutting received many awards in recognition of her deep, lasting commitment and service to nursing. She was granted an honorary master of arts degree from Yale in 1921, the Liberty Service Medal for humanitarian and patriotic services, and the Adelaide Nutting Medal for Leadership in Nursing Education in 1944. This medal was designed by the National League of Nursing Education. The Adelaide Nutting Historical Nursing Collection at Teachers College was dedicated to her memory and outstanding leadership. Nutting died on October 3, 1948, after a long illness. She was a visionary whose words will long be remembered as being forever relevant:

> We need to realize and to affirm anew that nursing is one of the most difficult of arts. Compassion may provide the motive, but knowledge is our only working power. Perhaps, too, we need to remember that growth in our work must be preceded by ideas, and that any conditions which suppress thought, must retard growth. Surely we will not be satisfied in perpetuating methods and traditions. Surely we shall wish to be more and more occupied with creating them.
>
> — *Nutting, 1925*

Stanislav Rembski, *M. Adelaide Nutting in Academic Robes*, c. 1932. *(Special Collections, Milbank Memorial Library, Teachers College, Columbia University, New York.)*

American Nurses Association.   The American Nurses Association (ANA) became the successor to the Nurses Associated Alumnae of the United States in 1911. The original federation of alumnae associations proved less workable as nurses became more mobile and began to move from state to state. A national organization with participation through state associations or through individual membership seemed more feasible, particularly because by 1912, thirty-nine state nurses' associations had been organized. The original body remained a federation of alumnae associations until the convention of 1916, when it was decided to establish membership through the state associations. State associations would eventually provide the means for achieving legal regulation. Unity of nurses within specific states, therefore, was essential to the passage of any licensing laws.

The ANA is *the* professional organization for registered nurses in the United States, and as such it holds membership in the International Council of Nurses. In the early years of the organization, state registration was a major concern. The purposes of the ANA have always been to foster high standards of nursing practice, to promote the welfare of nurses, and to improve the general working conditions of nurses.

International Council of Nurses.   The International Council of Nurses, established in 1899, is the oldest of all international organizations for professional workers. It was founded by Mrs. Bedford Fenwick in cooperation with nursing leaders from many countries. In 1900 the council's constitution was adopted, and the first meeting was held at the World Exposition in Buffalo, New York, in 1901. During this first meeting, Mrs. Fenwick proposed a resolution in favor of state registration:

> Whereas the nursing of the sick is a matter closely affecting all classes of the community in every land;
> Whereas to be efficient workers, nurses should be carefully educated in the important duties which are now allotted to them;
> Whereas at the present time there is no generally accepted term or standard of training nor system of education nor examination for nurses in any country;
> Whereas there is no method, except in South Africa, of enabling the public to discriminate easily between trained nurses and ignorant persons who assume that title; and
> Whereas this is a fruitful source of injury to the sick and of discredit to the nursing profession, it is the opinion of this international congress of nurses, in general meeting assembled, that it is the duty of the nursing profession of every country to work for suitable legislative enactment regulating the education of nurses and protecting the interests of the public, by securing State examinations and public registration, with the proper penalties for enforcing the same.
>
> — *Lavinia L. Dock, 1901, pp. 233*

Membership in the International Council of Nurses was open to self-governing national nurses' associations rather than to individuals. (As such, it is an association of associations.) Its established purposes were to provide a means of communication between the nurses of all nations and to offer opportunities for nurses from all parts of the world to meet and confer on questions relating to patient welfare and the nursing profession. The International Council of Nurses stands for the full development of the human being and citizen in every nurse and ever higher standards of education, professional ethics, public usefulness, and civic spirit.

National Association of Colored Graduate Nurses.   Although the nursing organizations never expressed any racial prejudice, black nurses could secure membership in the American Nurses Association after 1916 only through membership in the state nurses' associations. They were thus denied membership in sixteen southern states and the District of Columbia. Black nurses also realized they had problems of their own that would be best served by a separate organization. They needed to break down discriminatory prac-

Old and new logos for the American Nurses Association. *(Courtesy of the American Nurses Association, Inc., Washington, D.C.)*

Logo for the National Association of Colored Graduate Nurses. *(Courtesy of Schomburg Center for Research in Black Culture, The New York Public Library, New York.)*

"The Negro Nurses Stroll on the Sidewalks, Chatting in Quaint French to the Little Children," New Orleans, 1873. (Courtesy of Schomburg Center for Research in Black Culture, The New York Public Library, New York.)

Seal for the National League of Nursing Education. (Reprinted by courtesy of The National League for Nursing, New York.)

tices that occurred because of the hue of their skin and with no consideration for their nursing proficiency.

The National Association of Colored Graduate Nurses (NACGN) was established in 1908. Its founding was the direct result of the vision, wisdom, and initiative of Martha Minerva Franklin (1870–1968), a graduate of the school of the Woman's Hospital Training School for Nurses in Philadelphia. Franklin had conducted a study of the status of black nurses before sending out letters to explore interest in the formation of a national organization. A meeting was held in August 1908 in New York under the sponsorship of the alumnae of Lincoln School for Nurses and its president, Adah Belle Samuels Thoms (1870–1943). By the end of this meeting the association had been formed and its objectives determined: to achieve higher professional standards; to break down discriminatory practices facing Negro nurses in schools, in jobs, and in organizational activities; and to develop Negro nurse leadership. Franklin was named the first president of this association.

Several leaders did, indeed, emerge and make significant achievements. Adah Thoms led the campaign for the acceptance of black nurses in the Red Cross. These nurses served with the Army Nurse Corps in World War I. Thoms also founded a registry for black nurses in New York (1918) and wrote the first book on the history of the black nursing profession, *Pathfinders,* in 1929. Estelle Massey Riddle Osborne (1901–1981) was the first black nurse to serve on the ANA board of directors, was awarded the NACGN scholarship for advanced study, and was the first black nurse to earn a master of arts degree with a major in nursing from Teachers College, Columbia University. Mabel Keaton Staupers (1898-1989) served as executive officer of the NACGN from 1934 to 1949, was elected the last president of the association, and chronicled the history of the organization in *No Time for Prejudice* (1961).

The NACGN continued to make valuable contributions to nursing. It brought the concerns of blacks in America to the attention of both nurses and the general public. In 1949 the organization believed it had accomplished its purpose and voted for dissolution. The program was phased out gradually over the next two years; a press release announcing its dissolution was issued on January 26, 1951. In 1950 the ANA had committed itself to assume responsibility for the functions of the NACGN by virtue of a platform adopted by the ANA house of delegates. The platform supported "full participation of minority groups in association activities . . . and the elimination of discrimination in job opportunities, salaries, and other working conditions" (American Nurses Association, 1950). Some twenty years later, however, some black nurses would come to feel that the dissolution of the NACGN had been premature.

National League of Nursing Education. With the change of membership and scope of functions, the American Society of Superintendents of Training Schools was renamed the National League of Nursing Education (NLNE) in 1912. The membership was expanded to include individuals whose greatest interest and training were in the field of nursing education, directors of public health nursing, members of state boards of nurse examiners, and those directly concerned with teaching and supervising in nursing schools. The goal of uniform standards now was seen to be impractical, since minimum requirements for state registration varied from state to state. The league decided to assist schools of nursing to achieve professional status comparable with that of similar professional groups. Therefore special attention was given to increased financial support for nursing schools, sounder educational programs, and closer associations with institutions of higher learning. In 1932 the league became the Department of Education of the ANA, as voted upon by both organizations. Therefore it was necessary to hold membership in the ANA in order to be a member of the NLNE. The National League of Nursing Education was the organization most active in shaping educational thinking and practice in nursing for many years; its annual reports became a major asset to nursing.

The National Organization for Public Health Nursing. The third national nursing association, the National Organization for Public Health Nursing (NOPHN), was established in 1912. By this time, district and visiting nursing had expanded rapidly to keep pace with the growth of new social services. National standards were urgently needed for one of the most promising movements of modern society. In addition, the care given by the nurse in the community differed from that given by the nurse in the hospital. A joint committee of the two national organizations, with Lillian D. Wald as chair and Mary S. Gardner as secretary, was appointed. The committee arranged for representatives of agencies employing visiting nurses to attend a meeting to be held in conjunction with the ANA and NLNE convention in Chicago in 1912. As a result, this organization came into being, but it was different in the makeup of its membership:

> The name was selected with the utmost care to emphasize the fact that the new organization was not composed solely of nurses and that it would be concerned with the development of *nursing*. Three classes of membership were agreed upon: corporate (agency), individual (active public health nurses), and associate. The associate members would be non-public health nurses and lay persons, privileged to participate in discussions but with no voting power. That restriction was removed at an early date when fear of lay domination or interference with strictly professional matters had been found to be quite groundless.

> — *Roberts, 1954, p. 88*

Lillian D. Wald was destined to become the first president of the new organization. Her social vision, excellent facility in public relations, and extraordinary gift for friendship were definite assets in the overall public health movement. Wald led the members in the enormous task of establishing standards for public health nurses, arranging courses to prepare them for their work, increasing the numbers of public health nurses, and building up organized voluntary and official agencies for home and community visiting nurse services. Two other officers were equally prominent: Mary S. Gardner, a pioneer in visiting nursing and author of a book on public health nursing, and Ella Phillips Crandall, director of the first public health nursing program at Teachers College. *Public Health Nursing* was the official journal of the organization. Although the three major organizations had somewhat different functions, they also had common purposes and interests and worked closely together.

Sigma Theta Tau. Sigma Theta Tau was founded in 1922 at Indiana University through the creativity of six students who were interested in high scholarship endeavors. Their goal was to promote high standards for nursing care and to foster individual development. As the original national honor society of nursing, this organization promotes nursing research and leadership. Its members, who are selected on the basis of scholarly achievement and professional leadership, include baccalaureate degree students, graduate students in nursing programs, and community nursing leaders. Membership and chapters have increased steadily throughout the years.

The Association of Collegiate Schools of Nursing. The Association of Collegiate Schools of Nursing (ACSN) was organized in 1933 to represent schools or departments of nursing associated with universities. In 1932 a decision had been made by representatives of more than twenty schools in San Antonio, Texas, to proceed with such an organization. The following January a conference was held at Teachers College, and it was decided to form the association. The standards or purposes adopted in 1935 were:

1. To develop nursing education on a professional and collegiate level.
2. To promote and strengthen relationships between schools of nursing and institutions of higher learning.
3. To promote study and experimentation in nursing service and nursing education.

> — *ACSN, 1943, p. 30*

Seal for The National Organization for Public Health Nursing. *(Reprinted by courtesy of The National League for Nursing, New York.)*

The seal symbolically represents the public health nurse, who plants the tree of life with the hope for better health in the community. "When the desire cometh it is a Tree of Life." The National Organization for Public Health Nursing (NOPHN) was absorbed by the National League for Nursing (NLN) when the restructuring of nursing organizations occurred in 1952.

Sigma Theta Tau Logo, 1922. *(Courtesy of Sigma Theta Tau International, Indianapolis, Indiana.)*

This is the original logo of Sigma Theta Tau from when it was established in 1922 at Indiana University in Indianapolis.

Shield for the nursing honor society, Sigma Theta Tau International, established in 1922 at Indiana University in Indianapolis. *(Courtesy of Sigma Theta Tau International, Indianapolis, Indiana.)*

Membership standards were established, and membership was extended to schools that met specific criteria. The association did not originally consider itself an accrediting agency, but it visited and evaluated schools that applied for membership and thus was regarded by many as an accrediting body.

The ACSN was engaged in many activities related to higher education during its existence. It constantly emphasized the need for research in nursing and the preparation of nurse researchers. Both would be mandatory if nursing was ever to qualify on an equal basis with other departments in colleges and universities. In 1950 the association's Committee on Research recommended that the American Journal of Nursing Company be asked to publish a periodical that would focus on research in nursing. This was the beginning step toward the publication of *Nursing Research*.

When changes in organized nursing ultimately occurred, the decision was made that the responsibilities of the ACSN would be assumed by the Department of Baccalaureate and Higher Degrees of the new NLN. The association had, indeed, proven its value to nursing and nursing education in a very short time.

A NEW LOOK FOR ORGANIZED NURSING

The numerous changes that had been occurring in nursing service and education mandated changes for organized nursing. The particular challenges of the Depression and World War I had forced some modification of organized nursing's structure and activities. Increased numbers of nurses were needed to meet the World War II effort, yet no one nursing association could speak or act for nursing as a whole. A commission representing all nursing interests was thus established to facilitate the efforts of both nursing and the national defense. Originally called the Nursing Council on National Defense, it was reorganized in late 1940 and renamed the National Nursing Council for War Service. The initial voting members of the council included the ANA, NLNE, NOPHN, ACSN, NACGN, and the Red Cross Nursing Service. As soon as the American Association of Industrial Nurses (AAIN) organized in 1942, it gained membership. In addition, representatives of the Army and Navy Nurse Corps, United States Public Health Service (USPHS), Veterans Administration, Children's Bureau, Office of Indian Affairs, American Hospital Association, and the Canadian Nurses Association were ex officio members.

The representatives of these prestigious agencies were able to secure access to important sources of advice and information that greatly assisted the program. The council's preliminary work was financed by nursing. Later, beginning in 1942, the W.K. Kellogg Foundation became the council's principal source of income and contributed more than three hundred thousand dollars. (Allocations for special projects were received from other foundations and private sources.) For the duration of the war, state nurses' associations carried most of the local expenses of council-sponsored projects. The council was responsible for developing nursing programs to meet wartime needs:

1. It reviewed wartime projects in relation to the functions of the member agencies and recommended new projects to appropriate agencies.
2. It administered projects which did not fall within the scope of any one member agency.
3. Under the changing conditions of war, it outlined projects which seemed to be beyond the scope of any voluntary agency and referred them to the Government's Subcommittee.

— *Roberts, 1954, p. 358*

When the war finally ended, the council decided to continue functioning until such time as another body replaced it or another method was recommended for continued coordination among the nursing associations. Esther Lucille Brown was engaged "to direct a study of the organization, administration, and support of professional and practical nursing as a basis for influencing the quality of nursing for the public" (Fitzpatrick, 1983, p. 169). The council also appointed a committee to plan for an accrediting agency for nursing education, and the National Nursing Accrediting Service was established in 1948. The council dissolved in that same year.

The accomplishments of the council during the war and several years after it proved that unified planning could be done by nursing and that cooperative efforts could and did improve the efficiency of organized nursing. The leaders of the associations were convinced that a permanent measure was necessary to ensure continued collaboration. A special committee, the Promoting Committee for the Structure of National Professional Nursing Organizations, began its study under Amelia Grant in 1945. This resulted in a "Report on the Structure of Organized Nursing," which was delivered at the biennial convention of 1946. It was determined that the six organizations in the study—the ANA, NLNE, NACGN, NOPHN, ACSN, and AAIN—were divided on three main points: nonnurse membership, special interests, and program emphasis. Considering the import of these issues, two alternative plans for organized nursing were proposed. The first suggested a single organization, the ANA, composed of five types of membership—professional nurses, public members, allied professionals, nursing schools and service agencies, and nonnursing organizations. The second plan was a two-organization system. One organization, the ANA, would accept only nurses. The other would be a national organization for nursing service composed of nurses, lay persons, allied professionals, and agency members. Cooperation would evolve through a joint commission for common concerns and a national nursing center with representatives from both organizations on its board.

After long months of deliberation by all concerned associations and individuals, more committee work, and the development of other plans, the ANA House of Delegates cast a majority vote for a two-organization plan at the 1950 Biennial Convention. The structure called for two distinct organizations: first, a somewhat reorganized American Nurses Association (ANA), composed entirely of nurses and able to speak for the profession and, second, the National League for Nursing (NLN), composed of nurses and nonnurses, and individual and corporate members; it would represent those responsible for sound development and support of nursing services and nursing schools. Between 1950 and 1952, staffing and bylaws were developed. The new structure was adopted at the Biennial Convention in Atlantic City, New Jersey, June 15-20, 1952. That historic meeting was attended by more than nine thousand individuals. The two associations, under the direction of their newly elected presidents, Elizabeth K. Porter (ANA) and Ruth Sleeper (NLN), immediately initiated steps for the reorganization of state associations and the establishment of headquarters in New York. Several organizations were absorbed by the NLN: National League of Nursing Education, National Organization for Public Health Nursing, Association of Collegiate Schools of Nursing, Joint Committee on Practical Nurses and Auxiliary Workers in Nursing Services, Joint Committee on Careers in Nursing, National Committee for the Improvement of Nursing Services, and National Nursing Accrediting Service.

Logo for the National League for Nursing. *(Reprinted by courtesy of The National League for Nursing, New York.)*

The development of a new logo for the National League for Nursing is in process. By the time this second edition is published, it is highly likely that this logo will have been replaced by the new logo.

THE CAMPAIGN FOR LEGISLATION AND REGISTRATION

The first published words regarding licensure for nurses came from a physician, Sir Henry W. Acland, in 1860. A regius professor of medicine at Oxford University, he wrote that nurses should be centrally registered, should follow a recognized curriculum of study, and should be able to meet a minimum standard of proficiency (Mollett, 1888). British nurses, however, did not begin national norms needed to be considered. The Subcommittee on Tests of the Committee on State Board Problems of the NLNE met in 1942 and proposed that the league work closely with states to adopt machine-scored examination questions. The intent was the developement of state board examinations that would be valid and reliable. The following objectives were approved:

> To provide objective tests of nursing competency which will enable each state board of nurse examiners to discover the level of ability of each candidate and the average for each school in the state, and for the state as a whole, in comparison with the level of all other candidates tested, and the average for each other school and state.
>
> To develop improved tests of nursing ability and work towards a comprehensive test battery of high validity and reliability.
>
> To study nursing ability, as revealed in the examinations, in order to arrive at a clearer concept of the minimum level of competency as well as the average level of expectancy of professional nurses.
>
> To secure data which will be of help to the state boards of nurse examiners and the schools of nursing in improving the level of nursing preparation.
>
> To lighten the burden of busy state boards of nurse examiners by serving as their agent in preparing and scoring the licensing examinations.
>
> — *American Journal of Nursing, 1952, pp.613-615*

Individual state boards were asked to submit sample questions, which were evaluated by the Committee on Nursing Tests. Within one year after the examinations had been set up, the State Board Test Pool was operative and being used by fifteen states. The original examination contained thirteen tests: anatomy and physiology, chemistry, microbiology, nutrition and diet therapy, pharmacology and therapeutics, nursing arts, communicable disease nursing, medical nursing, nursing of children, obstetrical and gynecological nursing, psychiatric nursing, surgical nursing, and social foundations of nursing. Six tests—medical nursing, surgical nursing, communicable disease nursing, psychiatric nursing, obstetrical nursing, and nursing of children—became the norm by 1949.

Although the same examination was given by all states by 1950, the passing score varied. This created some problems with registration by reciprocity. A standard score of 350 as a minimum level of competency was recommended in 1951 and was accepted by many of the states. Ultimately, nursing became the first professional group to use the same licensing examination throughout the United States, Hawaii, and the Canadian provinces of British Columbia and Alberta.

EDUCATIONAL TRENDS AND DEVELOPMENTS

After 1900 the increasing complexity of nursing services exerted continual pressure for the improvement of nursing schools. Most schools continued under hospital control; most operated on a subprofessional level. Nursing organizations, nurses, foundations, committees, agencies, and hospital groups began to conduct surveys and studies of nurses and nursing. Consequently, recommendations began to be made relevant to educational standards and practices. The influence of newer educational viewpoints surfaced in experiments and innovations. Continued support for upgrading nursing education was being demonstrated. In *A Sound Economic Basis for Schools of Nursing*, M. Adelaide Nutting emphasized the subordination of the educational program:

> Heavy demands of the wards made it impossible for all students to attend their weekly lecture and it was always arranged that some students would choose to take very full notes and read them later to the assembled group of less fortunate. Lectures came under the category of privileges like "hours off duty" to be granted "hospital duties permitting."
>
> — *Nutting, 1926, pp. 339–340*

What must be remembered is that the progressive development in educational reforms in schools of nursing was intertwined with aspects of life in the United States at the turn of the century.

> With the frontier gone, the continent subdued, and the nation now proud of its designation as a world power, a new era of mature consolidation was at hand. The democratic political foundations upon which the nation had been established remained intact, indeed were broadened by the termination of Negro slavery. Tens of millions of Europeans of many races and peoples had been absorbed without any serious social consequences and population had increased from five to seventy-six million. The national wealth in the last half of the nineteenth century had increased from seven to eighty-eight million dollars, and the standard of living for the common man was better than almost anywhere in the world. Great strides had been made in agriculture and industry, through the utilization of limited government assistance, cheap labor, plentiful natural resources, and "clever Yankee inventions." These factors made possible the rise . . . and the upgrading of the nursing profession which accompanied it in the new era now opening.
>
> The objectives of Americans were not merely utilitarian. Free public education and freedom of religion were deeply cherished and influential ideals. In literature, the arts, and the sciences, there was tremendous enthusiasm, growing pride, and substantial achievement, and traditional reformism, aimed at removing or reducing the ills of society, remained strong and vigorous. In place of slavery and illiteracy, industrial monopoly, farm tenancy, unequal rights for women, and epidemic disease became the new targets for change.
>
> — *Christy, 1969a, pp. 3–4*

Some improvements were being made, particularly in the better schools of nursing. An early preparatory course was started in Scotland at the Glasgow Infirmary in 1893. Rebecca Strong, then superintendent, with the assistance of Dr. McEwen, who was one of Lister's students, succeeded in having nursing students enter St. Mungo's College for a short course of theoretical instruction followed by practical training in the hospital. This was the first connection of any kind that nursing students had with an institution of higher learning. The inception of preparatory or preliminary courses made these programs more like those of educational institutions rather than a strict apprenticeship system. The first such course in America was developed in 1901 through the efforts of Nutting at Johns Hopkins. This preparatory course was six months long and offered basic sciences as well as nursing principles and practice, the latter experience being on the hospital wards. The primary difference in this instance was that the clinical experience was for the purpose of education, not service.

> A number of schools adopted this plan, but many of them found it difficult to supply the theoretical and practical courses required. A few developed preparatory courses in affiliation with technical schools such as Drexel Institute, Pratt, and Simmons College.
>
> — *Dock and Stewart, 1938, p. 178*

Within ten years, approximately eighty-six schools had preparatory courses that averaged three to four months in length.

Other improvements and changes were also occurring. Terminology used to describe the individual in a nursing program was altered from "pupil nurse" to "student nurse." This change was significant because "pupil" implies intellectual immaturity and guardianship, whereas "student" describes a more mature, independent, self-directed learner. The title of Principal of the School of Nursing was being adopted to portray the nursing program as educational. Teachers and lecturers were being referred to as "nursing school faculty." A greater interest in pedagogical methods was observed. Efforts were also being made to introduce student government as a way to tone down the militaristic discipline, to treat students as adults. Other educational experiments begun at Johns Hopkins and later adopted in other schools were payment of tuition fees by pupils, payment of lecturers from university staffs, the three-year course, full-time instructors, separate nursing school announcements outlining a fully organized course of study, high school graduation as a requirement for admission, use of scholarships, and the eight-hour day (adopted by Johns Hopkins in 1895). It is clear that nurses were beginning to broaden their concept of the meaning and responsibility of the title "profession," as pointed out by Nutting in 1905:

> We claim, and I think justly, the status of a profession; we have schools and teachers, tuition fees and scholarships, systems of instruction from preparatory to postgraduate; we are allied with technical schools on one hand and here and there a university on the other; we have libraries, a literature, and fast-growing numbers of periodicals owned, edited, and published by nurses; we have societies and laws. If therefore we claim to receive the appurtenances, privileges, and standing of a profession, we must recognize professional responsibilities and obligations which we are in honor bound to respect and uphold.
>
> — *Nutting, 1905, pp. 654–655*

Nursing literature was expanding in several ways. A great increase in text and reference books, as well as other types of nursing literature, had occurred. Nurses themselves had begun to produce a large portion of this material, either individually or through their organizations. When the schools of nursing were established, textbooks were urgently needed. Clara Weeks Shaw wrote the first American nursing text in 1885, *A Textbook of Nursing for the Use of Training Schools, Families and Private Students.* She was joined by other reputable authors, including Isabel Adams Hampton, author of *Nursing: Its Principles and Practice for Hospital and Private Use* (1893); Diana Kimber, who wrote *Anatomy and Physiology* (1893); and Lavinia Dock, author of *Textbook on Materia Medica for Nurses* (1890). By 1930 there were approximately seven hundred textbooks for nurses. Most of them had been written by nurses and published in the United States.

Journals also became necessary for establishing a means of communication between nurses in various locations. The first journal, the *Nightingale,* was started in 1886; editing was done by a Bellevue graduate. The *Trained Nurse and Hospital Review* (renamed the *Nursing World*), established in 1888, was the first national nursing and hospital journal. It was eventually combined with the *Journal of Practical Nursing, Nightingale, Nurse, Nursing World,* and *Nursing Record.*

One of the first activities of the Associated Alumnae was to consider and investigate the possibility of establishing a professional journal that would be its official magazine.

On October 1, 1900, the first issue of the *American Journal of Nursing* appeared through the particular efforts of Mary E.P. Davis and Sophia E. Palmer. Individual nurses and alumnae associations had bought shares of stock to finance the original enterprise. By 1912 the ANA became the sole owner of *Journal* stock; some of it had been donated, but the majority of it had been purchased. Palmer served as editor until her death in 1920, when she was succeeded by Mary M. Roberts. The first "office" of the *American Journal of Nursing* was a trunk kept in the home of Palmer where manuscripts and other materials related to the magazine were stored. This publication became the official organ of the ANA and one of the leading professional journals in the country.

Mary Roberts was also committed to this journal's success, and she secured special preparation in journalism. Under her leadership the American Journal of Nursing Company was formed and slowly moved toward expansion in publications. Roberts, a historian in her own right (author of *American Nursing: History and Interpretation* [1954]), fostered the "story of nursing" in the pages of the *Journal.* Nell V. Beeby was appointed editor upon the

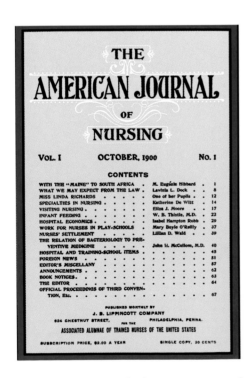

The *American Journal of Nursing,* cover of the first issue, October 1900. *(By permission of the American Journal of Nursing Company, New York.)*

retirement of Roberts in 1949. Under Beeby's administration two new journals went into production: *Nursing Outlook,* the official journal of the NLN, and *Nursing Research,* the vehicle for communication of all types of studies relating to nursing.

Affiliations between hospitals for the purpose of rounding out the students' clinical experience were also begun. These were often extended in time and set as a condition for registration, particularly for the smaller and more specialized institutions. The first formal program of affiliation was developed at the Illinois Training School in Chicago; Bellevue in New York was also a recognized leader in this regard.

A trend emerged in which university hospitals were established in various geographical locations in connection with medical departments. In a sense nursing schools thus became a part of the general university system. In most instances, however, the educational program was not classified as a university program, nor were the student nurses considered students of the university. An attempt was made to accomplish this in 1897, when the University of Texas assumed control over the John Sealy Hospital of Galveston and established it as a university hospital. The nursing school was recognized as a regular school of the medical department, and the superintendent of nurses occupied a place on the university committee of instruction. The school, however, was not required to meet the standards of the university.

In 1909, through the influence of Dr. Richard Olding Beard, the School of Nursing of the University of Minnesota became the first nursing school organized as an integral part of a university. Nursing students were admitted and registered as regular students of the university with all university requirements and privileges. "It was not an independent unit, however, since both hospital and nursing school functioned under the college of medicine and surgery. Nor did it offer at that time a college degree" (Stewart, 1943, p. 175). Ten years of pioneering effort went into the upgrading of the school before it offered a degree-granting basic program (1919). Similar schools were established in the Universities of Indiana and Cincinnati and later in several other colleges and universities.

In 1916, two five-year bachelor's degree programs were established at Teachers College, New York, in cooperation with Presbyterian Hospital and the University of Cincinnati's School of Nursing and Health. Within seven years similar programs were instituted in thirteen universities and three colleges (Committee for the Study of Nursing Education, 1923). A combined academic and professional course of five, or sometimes four, years led to both a college degree and the nursing diploma. In general, an attempt was made to mix occupational preparation with a liberal arts education.

Another significant innovation in nursing education occurred with the development of associate degree programs in community colleges. These schools exhibited a phenomenal growth, but their nursing programs evoked a great deal of controversy. It was felt that this community college connection equated nursing education with vocational training at a time when a professional status was being sought for nursing. This model of education was developed by Dr. Mildred Montag of Teachers College in 1949 as a result of planned research and eventual controlled experimentation. The original pilot project began in 1952 with seven junior and community colleges and one hospital from each of six regions of the United States. The program was administered by Teachers College, and Montag directed it. The product of this new type of program was to be the *nurse technician,* who operated somewhat below the professional nurse but above the practical nurse. The project concluded in 1957 and was followed by the rapid proliferation of community college nursing programs.

The first steps in the evolution of schools of nursing from hospitals to universities had occurred. As time went on, the superior educational opportuni-

Presbyterian Hospital, Fourth Avenue between 70th and 71st Streets, New York. Wood engraving after a photograph by Rockwood in *Harper's Weekly,* November 16, 1872. *(Collection of The New-York Historical Society, New York.)*

ties afforded by a university or a college became abundantly clear. As an integral part of the university—with its liberal education, physical facilities, resources, and level of instruction—a school of nursing would be primarily an educational undertaking.

> Hardly less valuable is the effect of the university atmosphere and surroundings on the student "morale." Ambition reacts to the atmosphere of intellectual competition; the student nurse is stimulated to do her best and take her place with credit among her fellow students of the various schools. She feels, too, a new sense of dignity and of the importance of her work through her recognition as a member of an educational institution.
>
> — *Committee for the Study of Nursing Education, 1923, p. 483*

STUDIES OF NURSING AND NURSING EDUCATION

The first comprehensive and critical survey of schools of nursing in the United States was *The Educational Status of Nursing* (1912). It was sponsored by the Federal Bureau of Education and directed by M. Adelaide Nutting, who developed the questionnaire and interpreted the data. The majority of the eleven hundred schools that responded were classified as mediocre educationally and utilitarian in purpose. It was noted in the report that the "exceptional" schools had an adequate supply of applicants; the "poor" schools complained of a continual shortage of applicants. Several recommendations were offered: that standards in nursing schools be raised; that schools of nursing secure financial independence; and that the schools become educational institutions in fact, not just in name. This study set a precedent for future investigations that soon followed.

The need for alterations in nursing and nursing education became apparent as the nation absorbed changes in its social, political, and economic structures. Rapid developments in medical science, technological advances in hospitals, and increased demands for health care highlighted this need. It was World War I, however, that particularly dramatized the indispensable role played by nursing and the need for more and better-prepared nurses. A pamphlet by Isabel M. Stewart, *Developments in Nursing Education Since 1918* (1921), summed up the impact of the war years on the nursing profession:

> Many of the old barriers of precedent and tradition were broken down, and there was a greater willingness to try new methods and to combine forces with others to conserve limited strength and other resources. Some of these war experiments . . . have been incorporated in our present system and promise to be of permanent value.
>
> Probably the greatest contribution of the war experience to nursing lies in the fact that the whole system of nursing education was shaken for a little while out of its well-worn ruts and brought out of its comparative seclusion into the light of public discussion and criticism. When so many lives hung on the supply of nurses, people were aroused to a new sense of their dependence on the products of nursing schools, and many of them learned for the first time of the hopelessly limited resources which nursing educators have had to work with in the training of these indispensable servants. Whatever the future may bring it is unlikely that nursing schools will willingly sink back again into their old isolation, or that they will accept unquestionably the financial status which the older system imposed on them.
>
> — *Stewart, 1921, p. 6*

Stewart firmly believed that the educational status of nursing schools was in some ways better at the end of the war than it had been at the beginning.

Numerous studies were initiated, but only a few exerted a profound influence on the development of nursing. These specific studies are briefly reviewed, with particular attention given to the recommendations that emerged.

Nursing and Nursing Education in the United States (The Goldmark Report of 1923)

Following World War I, attention was focused as never before on the issues of public health. In 1919 the Rockefeller Foundation invited representative men and women to a conference to consider the status of public health nursing in the United States. The consensus of opinion was that the usual program in basic schools of nursing did not adequately prepare nurses for community health practice. A committee was subsequently appointed and financed by the Rockefeller Foundation to study public health nursing education. Dr. C.A. Winslow, professor of public health at Yale, was appointed chair; Josephine Goldmark, a social worker and author, was appointed secretary and chief investigator. Six nurses were included in the committee of nineteen: Mary Beard, S. Lillian Clayton, Annie Goodrich, M. Adelaide Nutting, Lillian Wald, and Helen Wood. It soon became evident that the scope of the study was too narrow, that the subject of nursing and nursing education needed to be investigated as a whole. The work was expanded and the Committee for the Study of Nursing Education began

> to survey the entire field occupied by the nurse and other workers of related type; to form a conception of the tasks to be performed and the qualifications necessary for their execution, and on the basis of such a study of function to establish sound minimum education standards for each type of nursing service for which there appears to be a vital need.
>
> — *Committee for the Study of Nursing Education, 1923 p. 7*

Representatives of twenty-three schools of nursing and forty-nine public health agencies in various sections of the country were surveyed. After three years a preliminary report was released in 1922, followed by the final report published in 1923, commonly known as the Goldmark Report but sometimes called the Winslow-Goldmark Survey. The conclusions clearly echoed the statements that had been made by the nursing leaders of the day. Each of the ten conclusions was significant, but the following stand out:

> *Conclusion I:* . . . That as soon as may be practicable, all agencies, public or private, employing public health nurses, should require as a prerequisite for employment the basic hospital training, followed by a post-graduate course including both class work and field work, in public health nursing.
>
> *Conclusion IV:* That steps should be taken through state legislation for the definition and licensure of a subsidiary grade of nursing service, the subsidiary type of worker to serve under practicing physicians in the care of mild and chronic illness and convalescence, and possibly to assist under the direction of the trained nurse in certain phases of hospital and visiting nursing.
>
> *Conclusion VII:* Superintendents, supervisors, instructors, and public health nurses should in all cases receive special additional training beyond the basic nursing course.
>
> *Conclusion X:* That the development of nursing service adequate for the care of the sick and for the conduct of the modern public health campaign demands as an absolute prerequisite the securing of funds for the endowment of nursing education of all types; and that it is of primary importance, in this connection, to provide reasonably generous endowment for university schools of nursing.
>
> — *Committee for the Study of Nursing Education, 1923*

A direct outcome of the study was the establishment of the Yale University School of Nursing (1923), financed by the Rockefeller Foundation. Under the leadership of Annie W. Goodrich and her associate, Effie J. Taylor, who succeeded her, this school successfully demonstrated the importance of an independently endowed and professional school of nursing. Other endowed schools followed at Vanderbilt University, the University of Toronto, and Frances Payne Bolton at Western Reserve University.

Studies by the Committee on the Grading of Nursing Schools

The Committee on the Grading of Nursing Schools was composed of representatives of nursing, medical, and hospital organizations, as well as a few educational and lay members. William Darrach, a well-known surgeon, was the chairman. Dr. May Ayres Burgess, an educator, psychologist, and statistician, directed the study. The committee was officially established in November 1925 to grade and classify schools of nursing, to study the work of nurses, and to define the duties within the scope of nursing. The study was partially financed by outside sources, but nurses themselves donated $115,000 over a five-year period.

Nurses, Patients, and Pocketbooks **(1928).** The first report that focused on the supply and demand of nursing service, *Nurses, Patients, and Pocketbooks,* was published in 1928. The original purpose of the committee that wrote this report, the grading of nursing schools, was postponed because it was determined that grading needed to be based on and accompanied by careful inquiry into nursing education and employment. The committee thus decided on a five-year program that would be divided into three separate projects: a study of supply and demand for nursing service, a job analysis of what nurses did and how they should be prepared to function, and the actual grading of nursing schools based on the facts of the other two projects. A questionnaire was used to collect information relevant to this first project, and conclusions were based on replies from hospitals, patients, nurses, physicians, and public health directors.

The report covered a wide-ranging and interesting group of problems and vividly demonstrated the economic conflict between nurses and their employers and between student service and school of nursing objectives. Specific findings included the following: educational requirements for entrance into nursing schools were minimal, most nursing schools were of poor educational quality, nursing schools existed merely to provide service to hospitals, a serious overproduction of graduate nurses had led to chronic unemployment, and salaries and working conditions were extremely poor. These findings were a serious indictment of nursing education and showed its failure to meet existing social needs for nursing service. After the findings were published, the American Medical Association withdrew from the committee without expressing a clear reason for its action.

In general, the conclusions of this committee agreed with those of the Committee on Nursing and Nursing Education in the United States and with the comments and criticisms of nursing leaders. One immediate measure recommended was the replacement of student nurses in hospitals by graduate nurses. In addition, two important resolutions were unanimously adopted by the committee:

1. No hospital should be expected to bear the cost of nursing education out of funds collected for the care of the sick. The education of nurses is as much a public responsibility as is the education of physicians, public school teachers, librarians, ministers, lawyers, and other students planning to engage in professional public service, and the cost of such education should come, not out of a hospital budget, but from private or public funds.
2. The fact that a hospital is faced with serious financial difficulties should have no bearing upon whether or not it will conduct a school of nursing. The need of a hospital for cheap labor should not be considered a legitimate argument for maintaining such a school. The decision as to whether or not a school of nursing should be conducted in cooperation with a given hospital should be based solely upon the kinds and amounts of educational experience which that hospital is prepared to offer.

— *Committee on the Grading of Nursing Schools, 1928, pp. 447–448*

Nursing Schools Today and Tomorrow (1934). In the final publication of the committee, *Nursing Schools Today and Tomorrow,* the essentials for a professional program of education were outlined. The publication contained the facts necessary for reform in schools of nursing and became a vehicle to influence public opinion in favor of nursing. Conditions that would not be tolerated in any nursing school were also specified. The weaknesses in nursing education were thus clearly described. The following recommendations on professional standards were emphasized and stressed:

a collegiate level of education; an enriched curriculum, with more and better theory and less and better practice; a better-prepared student body and faculty comparable with those in other professional schools; an organization better fitted to safeguard the professional status and freedom of the school, 'dominated by neither hospital nor treasury, nor nursing traditions'; and funds adequate to provide for such a school.

— *Stewart, 1943, pp. 214–215*

The recurring theme of adequate financial support was once again identified as the greatest problem in positioning nursing education at a higher level. Compared with other forms of professional education, the nurse stood alone with training dependent on service in the hospital. In addition, faculty were grossly unqualified; the majority of teachers in schools of nursing had not completed a high school education.

An Activity Analysis of Nursing (1934). It is possible that this study is not recognized as part of the five-year program adopted by the Committee on the Grading of Nursing Schools. As activities developed, it became evident that this part of the program dealing with the teaching of nursing and an analytical study of nursing procedures, a job analysis, could not be completed by the office staff. At the Committee's request it was turned over to Ethel Johns, a nurse editor and consultant, and Blanche Pfefferkorn, a nurse and director of studies at the National League of Nursing Education. The two were assisted by a special subcommittee that included Professor W. W. Charters, Professor Elizabeth C. Burgess, Miss Katharine Tucker, and Dr. William Darrach. As a consequence, it is more commonly known as the "Johns and Pfefferkorn Activity Analysis."

Essentially two questions were addressed: What is good nursing? and How can it be taught? An attempt was made to document the exact functions of nurses in different occupational categories: hospital bedside nursing, private duty nursing in the home, and nursing in the public health field. In addition, a list of personal activities that should be practiced by the professional nurse were described. Johns and Pfefferkorn contended that these activities ". . . have to do with matters of personal efficiency and the maintenance of good professional standards and relationships" (p. 102). These activities are particularly interesting and in many instances still very relevant to the mission of nursing.

Personal Standards

1. Providing for own economic security (savings bank, insurance, etc.)
2. Transacting own financial affairs in businesslike manner
3. Enriching own living through cultivation of artistic, intellectual, and social interests
4. Observing good standards of own environment
5. Developing pleasing qualities of speech (modulated voice, pronunciation, and adjustment to sick room)
6. Observing health standards as to mental hygiene (working relationships, social relationships, recreation, etc.)
7. Observing health standards as to personal hygiene (diet, elimination, fresh air, body mechanics, exercise, bathing, teeth, shoes, clothing, etc.)
8. Making provision for own periodic health examination and follow-up as indicated
9. Taking precautions to avoid infection or injury (use of such accepted scientific measures as vaccination, inoculation, etc., when indicated)
10. Observing special care as to personal appearance (choice of clothing, uniforms, accessories, shoes; care of hair, nails; use of cosmetics, perfume; etc.)
11. Exemplifying good health through personal habits and standards of living
12. Applying for position in businesslike way
13. Resigning position in businesslike way

Professional Standards

14. Securing adequate preparation for the practice of nursing and continuing the educational process by means of professional literature, conferences, institutes, etc.
15. Cooperating as a member of the organized profession in trying to secure an equitable distribution of nursing care for the entire population
16. Directing only well-qualified young women into nursing and assisting them in getting the best possible nursing education
17. Helping to uphold high standards and ideals in nursing
18. Contributing to the development of nursing according to one's special abilities through articles, text books, talks, etc.
19. Keeping informed on trends in nursing and allied professional fields
20. Observing courtesies which grow out of inter-professional relationships
21. Sharing in the activities of professional organizations for a sound system of nursing education

22. Sharing in the activities of professional organizations for the increased development of good nursing service
23. Studying the opportunities and needs in the nursing field and selecting that field for which the individual is best qualified
24. Participating in staff activities
25. Participating in civic activities and extending interest to national and international affairs
26. Responding when possible in times of special emergency (war, flood, drought, famine, etc.)
27. Helping to support scientific medicine and to protect the public against charlatanry and all other non-scientific medical exploitation
28. Cooperating with health specialists in their own particular fields
29. Recognizing the special responsibilities involved in professional nursing service to the community in the care of the sick, the prevention of disease, and the promotion of health (pp. 212–213)

Finally, the report included a clear and concise description of what the patient, the physician, the hospital, and the general public expected of nursing. As one scrutinizes this 1934 study, it is difficult not to draw distinct similarities between this classification and the current work on the Nursing Interventions Classification (NIC) led by Drs. Joanne McCloskey and Gloria Bulechek at The University of Iowa College of Nursing.

At the completion of the studies, it was once again clear that reform in nursing education was necessary. The findings of the grading committee provided the specific data that could be used to reinforce the debate for reform. Four basic goals were generated:

> *To reduce and improve the supply.* To make a decisive and immediate reduction in the numbers of students admitted to schools of nursing in the United States, and to raise entrance requirements high enough so that only properly qualified women would be admitted to the profession.
> *To replace students with graduates.* To put the major part of hospital bedside nursing in the hands of the graduate nurses and take it out of the hands of student nurses.
> *To help hospitals meet costs of graduate services.* To assist hospitals in securing funds for the employment of graduate nurses and to improve the quality of graduate nursing so that hospitals would desire to have it.
> *To get public support for nursing education.* To place schools of nursing under the direction of nurse educators instead of hospital administrators and to awaken the public to the fact that if society wants good nursing it must pay the cost of educating nurses. Nursing education is a public and not a private responsibility.
>
> — *Burgess, 1928, pp. 237–256*

Finally, the grading committee strongly recommended that the National League of Nursing Education undertake the accreditation of nursing schools.

Curriculum Studies and Reports

From 1914 to 1919 Isabel M. Stewart served as secretary of the Curriculum Committee of the League (originally called the Education Committee), and she was its chair from 1920 to 1937. Three important studies emerged from this committee. The first was the *Standard Curriculum for Schools of Nursing*, published in 1917. "The purpose of this study was to bring about greater uniformity in the programs of nursing schools and to help in improving the content and quality of the teaching as well as other conditions affecting the education of nurses" (Stewart, 1943, p. 211). The body of this study contained a systematic plan for the education of nurses and outlined specific courses along with their objectives, content, and methods; lists of bibliographies, equipment, and schedules completed the scheme.

Within a few years the second study was begun, and it resulted in the publication of *Curriculum for Schools of Nursing* in 1927. The word *standard* was dropped to avoid the notion that it was a requirement to be adopted by schools of nursing. This study was essentially a revision and expansion of the first. A job analysis technique was used to outline the functions and qualifications of the nurse, which constituted the practical objectives of the nursing school curriculum. Nutting and Stewart did most of the writing for these volumes, although the actual studies were conducted by the entire committee.

In 1935 Isabel Stewart urged that another revision be done to meet the current trends in nursing education necessary to comply with community needs.

> She called for a cooperative research project that would encourage participation by many people. She hoped that, through widespread involvement, schools that had been too dependent on the League's curriculum outlines might learn to build their own curriculums by taking materials from the common stock and adapting them to their different situations and stages of development. She desired a serious analysis of the philosophy of nursing education, goals to be aimed for and values to be conserved, the kind of services nurses should be prepared to give to society, the kind of individuals nursing schools should select for preparation, and the kind of preparation needed to fit them for living and serving.
>
> — *Christy, 1969c, p. 47*

The project proved to be one of the most far-reaching and ambitious efforts undertaken in this area. It included the participation of representatives of all the professional organizations, allied professions, and the community. The project called for a review and reevaluation, not only of existing curricula but of the traditional philosophies underlying them. Under the direction of Stewart, curriculum committees were organized in all of the state leagues of nursing education, with state subcommittees and local committees under these. Stewart prepared all the materials relevant to the various phases of the work for presentation to her central committee. These in turn were sent back to the state leagues, state subcommittees, and local committees. The project was a process of sharing in which participating individuals and groups were educated through their involvement. R. Louise McManus, Stewart's successor at Teachers College, emphasized the project's significance:

> I have always thought of it as one of the first major, mass studies in nursing. But more than that, it was mass education, because many people who didn't know what a curriculum was before that, had an opportunity to participate in the construction of the curriculum—and learn what it was.
>
> It was "operation bootstrap" for the profession and Miss Stewart did a masterly job. Through the materials that she prepared for the various committees she really educated the mass of nursing educators across the country.
>
> — *McManus, cited in Christy, 1969c, p. 47*

The report published by the League in 1937, *A Curriculum Guide for Schools of Nursing,* was the product of the scholarly mind and wise leadership of Isabel Stewart.

Isabel Maitland Stewart (1878–1963) was American nursing's most influential spokeswoman in the area of education for forty-five years. It was Stewart who developed the first course dealing specifically with the teaching of nursing at Teachers College. Eventually this course was expanded and developed into an entire program for the preparation of teachers of nursing. Isabel Stewart's reputation as a curriculum expert became so well established that in later years she was known as "Miss Curriculum" (Stewart, 1961, p. 184).

Stewart was born in Fletcher, Ontario, a village near the city of Chatham. Her Canadian background is particularly significant in that she became part of a nucleus of three Canadian nurses who helped to shape the destiny of nursing education:

Isabel Maitland Stewart. (Author's Collection.)

Many American nurses do not realize the debt we owe to our Canadian sisters. Three of our greatest leaders were born in Canada but spent most of their most productive years contributing to nursing and nursing education in the United States. The first, M. Adelaide Nutting, . . . was born in Waterloo, Quebec; Isabel Hampton Robb . . . came from Welland, Ontario. The third, Isabel M. Stewart, was born in Ontario also, and one might speculate on what differences there might have been in the developments in both American and Canadian nursing had these three not migrated to the United States. . . . Isabel Stewart, particularly, following in the footsteps of her mentor, M. Adelaide Nutting, had great impact on American nursing education.

— *Christy, 1969c, p. 44*

Isabel Stewart was one of nine children, all of whom were encouraged to engage in educational pursuits. Beginning her career as a schoolteacher in Canada, she soon turned to nursing and graduated from Winnipeg General Hospital in 1903. Her pursuit of further education led her to Teachers College, where she earned several degrees. Stewart became an assistant to Professor M. Adelaide Nutting and eventually succeeded her as director of the college's Division of Nursing Education, a position she held for twenty-two years. Although best known for her accomplishments as chair of the Curriculum Committee of the League, Isabel Stewart was also an active research investigator who planned and implemented studies that led to a wealth of useful information for nursing education and practice. Until her death in 1963, she remained an active participant in nursing activities. Throughout her life she filled the roles of scholar, author, educator, researcher, administrator, and leader with distinction.

Isabel Stewart's interests were wide and varied. She was deeply interested in education in all aspects, particularly the education of women. Her study of history strengthened her belief that women could not rise to the full demands of any vocation or profession without education and knowledge of the social conditions and needs of their day. Thus the fullest development of nursing was not possible without emancipation from the conditions of subjection under which women and nurses had suffered for so many years.

Early in her professional career Stewart began her contributions to nursing organizations, which provided her with an essential vehicle for improvement of professional training and curriculum in schools of nursing throughout the country. She belonged to many nursing organizations, both national and international, in which she became a prominent figure. In these organizations she worked on a multitude of committees. A prolific writer, she published numerous works through which she interpreted modern trends in both general and nursing education. Two of these publications stand out as particularly important and were directly linked to her intense love of history: *A Short History of Nursing,* first published in 1920 and written with Lavinia L. Dock, and *The Education of Nurses* (1943). An examination of the latter work can lead to an important conclusion. It was written by an individual who had the outstanding ability to select significant facts and who had the rare vision, insight, and imagination to demonstrate relationships and interpret them to professional workers. *The Education of Nurses* was the closest thing to a philosophy of nursing education ever written.

As the years went by, Stewart feared for the loss of the humanitarian aspects that had long been a vital force in nursing. Recognizing that a definite decline in the study of this area was occurring, she commented:

> I feel very strongly these days that we are failing to develop the social and humanistic side of nursing—the spirit of nursing as we used to call it—and all that goes to the *balancing* of the scientific and technical aspects—it would mean a restudy of that whole area dealing with the philosophy and history of nursing and the social sciences, and the strengthening of our cultural roots, both in nursing schools (basic) and in the preparation of graduate nurses for developing this phase of nursing.
>
> I am distressed to realize that we are doing less in this field today than we did a few years ago and there seems to be very little interest in it. Miss [Maude] Muse spoke of it the other day and she feels much as I do. It is a part of the sickness of our civilization that we have *overstressed* the scientific and technical side and have neglected the other aspects of our work and education.
>
> — *Letter from Isabel M. Stewart*
> *to Lillian A. Hudson, c. 1940–1947*

Nursing for the Future (1948)

The study called *Nursing for the Future* was initiated in connection with the postwar planning of the National Nursing Council. A grant of $28,000 was given to the council by the Carnegie Corporation in 1947 for the investigation of nursing practice and the preparation required for it. Esther Lucile Brown, a social anthropologist and director of the Department of Studies in the Professions at the Russell Sage Foundation, was authorized to conduct this study to determine the "needs of society" for nursing. Her data were obtained firsthand as she personally visited fifty geographically representative schools in the country, held three regional workshop conferences with nursing directors (representing 1250 schools), and met with individual nurses, physicians, hospital administrators, and others involved with nursing. A large number of far-reaching recommendations were published in this report, which is also known as *The Brown Report*. One of the strongest proposals was

> that effort be directed to building basic schools of nursing in universities and colleges, comparable in number to existing medical schools, that are sound in organizational and financial structure, adequate in facilities and faculty, and well-distributed to serve the needs of the entire country.
>
> — *Brown, 1948, p. 178*

The report was endorsed in principle by the boards of directors of the six national nursing organizations in existence. However, many physicians and hospital administrators were openly hostile to the following recommendations:

> That nursing make one of its first matters of important business the long overdue official examination of every school.
>
> That lists of accredited schools be published and distributed, with a statement to the effect that any school not named had failed to meet minimum requirements for accreditation or had refused to permit examination.
>
> That a nationwide educational campaign be conducted for the purpose of rallying broad public support for accredited schools and for subjecting slow-moving state boards and nonaccredited schools to strong social pressure.
>
> That provision be made for periodic re-examination of all schools listed or others requesting it, as well as for the first examination of new schools, and for publication and distribution of the revised list.
>
> That, if organized nursing committed itself to this undertaking of major social significance, the public assume responsibility for a substantial part of the financial burden.
>
> — *Brown, 1948, pp. 132–170*

Nursing Schools at the Mid-Century (1950)

A Joint Committee on Implementing the Brown Report was established by the NLNE in 1948 (it was renamed the National Committee for the Improvement of Nursing Services in 1949). Early work of this committee consisted of the collection of factual information about nursing school programs and the interim classification of schools. This was to precede the development of a more comprehensive accreditation system and program. A questionnaire was used, and the hope was to obtain information from *all* schools of nursing (ninety-six percent return rate) in the United States. Each of the participating schools was evaluated according to criteria long accepted by the profession. The schools were classified according to a total score obtained by the weighting of the various criteria of administrative policies, financial organization, faculty, curriculum, clinical field, library, student selection and provisions for student welfare, and student performance on state board examinations. This classification of nursing schools was published in the *American Journal of Nursing* in November 1949 as "Interim Classification of Schools of Nursing Offering Basic Programs." The publication of this data drew much criticism from among the ranks of nurses. In 1950 the findings were published in *Nursing Schools at the Mid-Century* and provided a method for schools of nursing to evaluate their programs.

Canadian Studies

Through the initiative of the Canadian Nurses Association, a joint committee of this association and the Canadian Medical Association was established in 1929 to undertake a nationwide study of nursing education in Canada. The

Facing page, Frans Hals, *Nurse and Child,* c. 1620. *(Gemäldegalerie-Staatliche Museen Preussischer Kulturbesitz, Berlin, 1988.)*

study was conducted by Dr. George M. Weir, a well-known educator and sociologist in the Department of Education of the University of British Columbia. The *Survey of Nursing Education in Canada* (1932), also known as *The Weir Report,* pointed out serious weaknesses that existed in the hospital schools. Important reforms were recommended: a higher educational standard, increased affiliations between schools, increased employment of graduate nurses, student tuition, and qualified instructors. The survey also recommended that "no hospital having fewer than 75 beds, exclusive of cots and bassinets, and a daily average of at least 50 patients, be recognized as competent to conduct an approved Training School" (Gibbon and Mathewson, 1947, p. 375).

Following the release of this report, the Canadian Nurses Association organized a National Curriculum Committee, which published *The Proposed Curriculum for Schools of Nursing in Canada* in 1936. This project was conducted by a special committee and chaired by Marion Lindeberg, director of the Department of Nursing Education at McGill University. The findings were similar to those in the United States and led to the closing of a number of smaller training schools. The study and the later *Supplement* became valuable guides to assist with the establishment of a more sound educational foundation for nursing in Canada.

U N I T   8

Nurses in Action

Wars of the Twentieth Century

Man's role in the grim business of war has been fully portrayed in art and literature. The exhausting strain, the danger, the suffering and the brutal death which are his portion, have all been given eloquent expression . . . But the heroic part taken by women, in the terrible ordeal of war, is only faintly heard and little noted. The mute anguish transcending tears, the infinite sacrifice and the high courage which are theirs, are voiceless amid the full throated cannon's roar, nor do they inscribe a record by fire and sword. . .

To only a few, among all the world's many gallant women, is reserved the solemn privilege of being a part of the great forces locked in battle, and of being numbered among those elect of earth who, as participants, directly govern the course of history. The nurse, because of her special training and the high calling to which her life is dedicated, brings to the battlefield indispensable attributes which she alone possesses. Voluntarily she comes in response to the utmost need of the men with shattered bodies whose cry is for the compassionate touch of a woman's hand. . . She endures all of the ordeal borne by womanhood and in addition she shares with man his bitter lot upon the field of battle.

— JULIA O. FLIKKE

Glenna Goodacre, *Vietnam Women's Memorial*, 1993. Bronze cast. 7 ft. 8 in. *(Copyright 1993 Vietnam Women's Memorial Project, Inc. Gregory Staley photograph.)*

The Vietnam Women's Memorial was dedicated on the National Mall, just yards from "The Wall" on November 11, 1993, in Washington, D.C. Glenna Goodacre modeled not only the four bronze figures but also the rawness of their emotions—their compassion, anxiety, fatigue, and dedication. It is the apparent depth of those feelings that makes the monument more than simply bronzed forms. The four figures are beautifully and poignantly portrayed: a nurse tending to the chest wound of a soldier lying across her lap; a woman scanning the sky for a helicopter or assistance, and a kneeling woman staring at an empty helmet, bowing her head in grief and despair. The memorial is a permanent tribute to women who served during the Vietnam era.

Nurses in Action

	1900	1915	1930

Daily Life

1913 Income tax becomes U.S. law

1913 Foxtrot comes into fashion

1914–1918 World War I

1917 America enters World War I

1920 League of Nations formed

1920 Nineteenth Amendment grants vote to women in U.S.

1928 Women participate in Olympic games for the first time

1929 Stock market crashes

1930 United Airlines begins hiring nurses as flight attendants

1933 Hitler becomes Chancellor of Germany

1937 Hindenburg explodes

1939 Commercial television introduced

Science and Technology

1907 Ross Harrison develops tissue culture techniques

1911 Roald Amundsen reaches South Pole

1915 Henry Ford develops farm tractor

1929 James Doolittle pilots airplanes with instruments

1930 Pluto discovered

1935 U235 identified

1936 Dr. Alexis Carrel develops artificial heart

1938 Nuclear fission discovered

The Visual Arts

1908 First glass and steel building erected

1912 Peter Pan statue erected in Kensington Gardens

1913 First Charlie Chaplin films shown

1919 Bauhaus revolutionizes teaching of painting, sculpture, architecture, and industrial arts, Germany

1928 Mary Cassatt dies (born 1845)

1931 Empire State Building completed

Medicine and Health Care

1906 Term "allergy" introduced to medicine

1922 Insulin first administered to a diabetic patient

1930 National Institutes of Health (NIH) founded

Nursing

1901 Permanent Nurse Corps established as part of the U.S. Army Medical Department

1908 U.S. Navy Nurse Corps founded as part of the Navy

1910 Florence Nightingale dies

1910 Isabel Hampton Robb dies

1915 Edith Cavell shot before a German firing squad

1918 Vassar Training Camp established, U.S.

1918 Army School of Nursing founded, U.S.

1920 Members of U.S. Army Nurse Corps granted relative rank

1923 Goldmark report issued, U.S.

1932 Wier Report issued, Canada

1945	1960	1975	1990

1939–1945 World War II
1941 Japan bombs Pearl Harbor
1950–1953 Korean War
1951 Transcontinental dial
telephone service begins
1952 TV dinners introduced

1961 Berlin Wall erected
1965–1975 Vietnam conflict
1969 Trousers become acceptable
attire for women

1989 Berlin Wall
dismantled
1991 Persian
Gulf War

1941 "Manhattan Project" of intensive
atomic research begins
1953 DNA discovered
1960 First weather lab launched into space
1962 Boeing 727 makes first flight

1950 Matisse begins work on Vence Chapel
1965 "Op" art becomes the rage

1993
Vietnam
Women's
Memorial
dedicated

1941 Penicillin first used
1941 PAP smear developed
1942 Streptomycin isolated
1949 Philip Hench discovers cortisone
1953 Lung cancer linked with
cigarette smoking
1958 Thalidomide linked with birth defects
1960 Artificial kidney introduced

1940 Nursing Council for National Defense instituted, U.S.
1942 Mobile Army Surgical Hospital (MASH) units appear
1943 United States Cadet Nurse Corps created
1945 U.S. Army and Navy nurses released from
Santo Tomas civilian prison camp
1947 Full commission rank established for nurses in
U.S. military service
1949 U.S. Air Force Nurse Corps established
1954 Annie Goodrich, internationally known nurse, dies
1955 First men commissioned as nurses, U.S.
1965 ANA position paper on nursing education issued
1966 Appointment of male nurses to regular Army, Navy,
and Air Force Nurse Corps, U.S.

It has often been said that nursing has made its greatest advances and notable achievements in connection with wars. In general, this statement is probably true, particularly when viewed from a historical perspective. One might wonder, however, why this has been the case, since injury and illness have always existed side by side with humanity. It seems that the truth of the statement lies in the fact that nations tend to recognize, respect, and value nurses when faced with the human tragedies of war. The unique circumstances of the war and the need for care of the wounded dramatically emphasize the value of nurses. Nurses are thus raised to a position of national stature.

Federal support of nursing and nursing education in the United States has been observed with each of the major wars, particularly World War II. This support has been demonstrated financially as well as through other means. In addition, the military has had a profound influence on nursing, the effects of which are still evident. Nursing, in turn, has affected the military. Its military members have shared a tradition of service; they have played an important role in the care of military personnel and their families both in times of peace and in times of war. Frequently they have assisted with the development of new techniques and innovations that have benefited medical and nursing care for both soldiers and civilians. (For example, it was Air Force nurses who solved the problem of placement of food trays for litter patients.)

War brought a sharpened awareness of the nation's dependence on nurses and the urgent need to prepare them to meet the emergency. The speeding up of military and industrial defenses mandated adjustments in the number of nurses in schools of nursing, and in nursing services. New programs were needed to expedite nursing preparedness, funds were needed for educational expansion, and intensified programs of publicity were necessary to increase the supply of applicants for nursing schools and to recruit nurses for

The Red Cross Society of Costa Rica was honored on its sixtieth anniversary in 1945 with a stamp portraying two of history's most famous nurses: Florence Nightingale, the angel of mercy, and Edith Cavell, the English nurse who was matron at Berkendael Medical Institute in Brussels. Cavell was arrested by German authorities in World War I for admittedly aiding Allied prisoners and assisting them to escape across the Dutch frontier. Despite efforts by the U.S. minister to Belgium to secure a reprieve, Edith Cavell was shot by the Germans on October 12, 1915, at the age of fifty. *(Courtesy of Howard B. Hurley.)*

Fletcher Martin, *G.I. Angel. (U.S. Army Center of Military History, Washington, D.C.)*

military and other defense services. War placed heavy demands on nurses and nursing to meet the overall crises at home and abroad. Faced with an almost insurmountable task in time of war, nurses have always risen valiantly to the occasion. Particularly remarkable was the fact that in World War II a higher percentage of nurses volunteered for military service than did any other skilled or professional group, with the possible exception of physicians. Of 274,405 active graduate registered nurses, 75,000 applied for service (Editorial, *The Saturday Evening Post*, 1945). This was one of the outstanding voluntary achievements of this war, and it spoke well for the "spirit of nursing." That nurses voluntarily went overseas was acknowledged by hundreds of soldiers:

> To all Army nurses overseas: We men were not given the choice of working in the battlefield or the home front. We cannot take any credit for being here. We are here because we have to be. You are here because you felt you were needed. So, when an injured man opens his eyes to see one of you . . . concerned with his welfare, he can't but be overcome by the very thought that you are doing it because you want to . . . you endure whatever hardships you must to be where you can do us the most good . . .
>
> — *Quoted in Shields, editor, 1981, p. 27*

Howard Chandler Christy, *The Spirit of America*, 1919. Red Cross poster. *(Courtesy of the Library of Congress, Washington, D.C.)*

Patriotism becomes prominent during times of war; feelings of allegiance and loyalty to one's country escalate. Recruitment efforts generally capitalize on this phenomenon.

WORLD WAR I

James Montgomery Flagg, *Illustration for the American Red Cross.* World War I. Watercolor. *(Courtesy of the Library of Congress, Washington, D.C.)*

The American Red Cross has actively participated in all wars that have occurred since its institution. The American Red Cross Nursing Service became the reserve of the Army and the Navy when America finally entered World War I.

A shot fired on June 28, 1914, in Sarajevo, Serbia, killed the archduke of Austria and his wife. This assassination was the precipitating factor of a series of events that ultimately forced the entrance of almost all of Europe and the world into a long and terrible war. One month later Austria declared war against Serbia, and a type of chain reaction followed: on August 1 Germany declared war on Russia and then on France, England declared war against Germany, and declarations of war from nations all over the world were rapidly issued and continued through June 1918. In 1914 no one believed that the war would last longer than a few months, nor was anyone prepared for the cost in human lives or the vast expenditure in resources.

World War I created a large demand for nurses and taxed the medical and nursing resources of the entire world. The warring countries rapidly faced extreme shortages of physicians, nurses, medical supplies, and other resources necessary for adequate health care. At the outbreak of the war the American Red Cross sent units of physicians and nurses to assist in France, England, Germany, Austria, Serbia, and Russia. However, when America finally entered the war in April 1917, the American Red Cross Nursing Service became the reserve of the Army and the Navy. Under the able direction of

David Evans, *Let Us Now Remember Many Honorable Women.* Liverpool Cathedral, England.

This memorial was dedicated to the nurses who died between 1914 and 1919 during World War I.

Jane Delano, it served as a procurement and recruitment agency and equipped nurses assigned to overseas duty. Through this agency, approximately twenty thousand nurses were assigned to military service. Many of these Red Cross nurses remained in Europe and Asia after the war to assist with the relief programs of the stricken nations.

After a long struggle to maintain neutrality the United States declared war on Germany on April 6, 1917, and many agencies were caught unprepared. Confusion and conflict arose, particularly in regard to the use of nurses' aides for service abroad. This issue was resolved by government authorities, who mandated that only trained nurses be sent to France with the Army (Stewart and Austin, 1963). As the war progressed, it became apparent that the supply of nurses was insufficient to meet both civilian and military needs. Therefore it was strongly recommended by prominent medical, hospital, and lay spokespersons that the admission and graduation requirements of schools of nursing be drastically cut and that legal requirements be waived. To counteract these proposals and other problems that might ensue, M. Adelaide Nutting, Annie Goodrich, and Lillian Wald met on June 24, 1917, and formed the National Emergency Committee on Nursing. Jane Delano, chairman of the American Red Cross Nursing Service; Lillian Clayton, president of the National League of Nursing Education; Dora Thompson, superintendent of the Army Nurse Corps; and Dr. Winford H. Smith, president of the American Hospital Association were among the other members of the committee. The stated purpose of this committee was to develop "the wisest methods of meeting the present problems connected with the care of the sick and injured in hospitals and homes; the educational problems of nursing; and the extraordinary emergencies as they arise" (U.S. Council of National Defense, 1917, pp. 1–5).

In less than two months the National Emergency Committee on Nursing was officially appointed by the federal government and became known as the Committee on Nursing of the General Medical Board of the Council of

Committee On Nursing, General Medical Board, Council Of National Defense, World War I. August 18, 1918. (Special Collections, Milbank Memorial Library, Teachers College, Columbia University, New York.)

Represented in this photograph are some of the most prominent figures in the history of nursing: S. Lillian Clayton, President, National League of Nursing Education; Anna W. Goodrich, Dean, Army School of Nursing; M. Adelaide Nutting, Chairman, Committee on Nursing, Council of National Defense; Mrs. Lena S. Higbee, Supt., Navy Nurse Corps; Dora Thompson, Supt., Army Nurse Corps.

James Montgomery Flagg, *Stage Women's War Relief*, 1918. Poster. *(Courtesy of the Library of Congress, Washington, D.C.)*

Nurses will always need to be organized and ready for service in times of disaster and national defense. They have demonstrated their skill, ability, and determination in the face of danger, war, and disaster.

National Defense. Although office space and secretarial services were provided by the government, funding was obtained through private contributions. One of the most formidable tasks facing the Committee was the need to increase the existent supply of student nurses. A recruiting campaign was thus initiated in which a variety of techniques were used. Publicity in the form of pamphlets, posters, and even motion pictures was created and dispersed. Speeches were given and newspaper and magazine articles were written and published, all with the intent of enticing young women into service by entering schools of nursing. Typical of such activity was a *Ladies' Home Journal* editorial:

> Have you felt that you could best answer the war's appeal to you by entering the nursing service? Then this is the day of your opportunity, provided you are in earnest and wish to set your patriotic impulses free in the place where they will do the most good.
>
> That place is in a regular nurses' training school, such as is conducted in nearly every hospital in America. Many women, untrained in nursing, have been disappointed to learn that their services were not wanted on the field of battle, nor even in a base hospital.

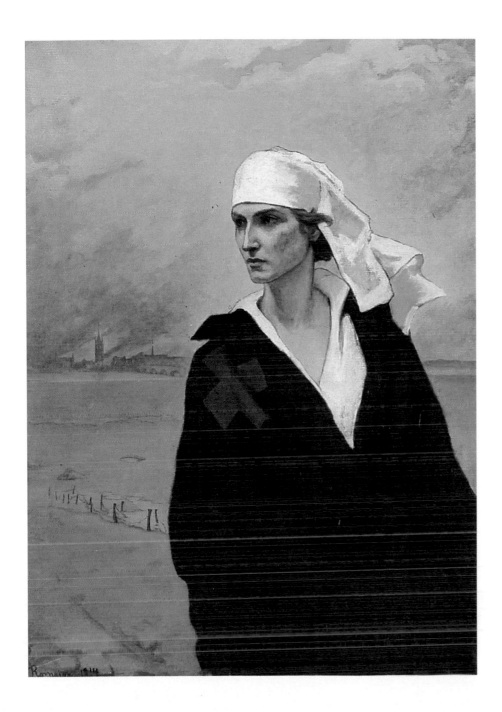

Romaine Brooks, *La France Croiseé (The Cross of France)*, 1914. Canvas, approx. 118.1 × 86.4 cm. (*National Museum of American Art, Washington DC/Art Resource, New York.*)

357

It is the professional nurse only who has been called and accepted, and more than a thousand of her are now in active service. More thousands will follow soon. They are the finest of their profession, and they go gladly; but do you realize that each one is leaving behind her important work in civil life, which must now be done by someone else?

We have no right to expect—though we may hope for—a short war. We must put away makeshift methods and think of a year from now, two years, perhaps even three years. The woman who enters training today is the woman who a little later will be prepared to take the place at home of the nurse who has gone, or even to follow her to the Front.

The Red Cross earnestly hopes that many young women, particularly those with the advantages of a good education, will let their desire to be of service take a most practical form and prepare to enter a profession which has been called upon to do so noble a work.

— *Taft, 1917, pg. 5*

The Committee also asked existing nursing schools to do their part. They requested that schools enlarge their facilities, including dormitories and clinical facilities. More instructors were to be acquired to handle increasing student numbers; working hours were to be shortened to attract greater numbers. These methods proved to be successful as the numbers of students entering nursing schools increased dramatically.

Vassar Training Camp

The Committee on Nursing was also interested in attracting women with better educations into nursing. A plan thus evolved for a three-month intensive theoretical training program for college graduates who wished to enter nursing schools. The original concept was proposed by Mrs. Minnie Comnock Blodgett, a trustee of Vassar, who partially financed the project. This program, known as the Vassar Training Camp of 1918, was soon under way at Vassar College under the chairmanship of Isabel M. Stewart. It was in actuality a three-month preparatory course for college graduates seeking admission to schools of nursing. More than four hundred college graduates participated in the program. At the completion of the intensive course the college graduates entered some thirty-three affiliated schools of nursing for a period of two years and three months. The nursing schools had committed themselves to accepting a specified number of these students. Since the students wore the uniforms of the affiliated schools, they became known as "Vassar's Rainbow Division." Five other universities (Western Reserve University in Cleveland, University of Cincinnati, University of Iowa, University of Colorado, and University of California) offered similar programs. This cooperative effort between universities and schools of nursing provided a higher standard of teaching and the advantages of an institution of higher learning. The far-reaching contributions of the camp were reiterated by Katherine Densford Dreves, a member of this program who became an influential leader in nursing:

First, the camp brought college recognition to nursing . . . the fact that prestigious Vassar College chose the camp for its major war effort helped (1) to bring nursing out of its hospital cloister into higher education and (2) to challenge colleges increasingly to accept responsibility for nurse preparation.

Then, the camp helped immeasurably to interest college women in nursing. The camp brought into nursing the first very large group of well-educated, versatile women, almost half of whom went on to complete the entire nursing course. Also, the camp enlisted national recognition of nursing by the public and of the need for public and private support of nursing.

— *Dreves, 1975, p. 2002*

Cecile R. Johnson, *Pediatric Unit at a U.S. Naval Hospital. (National Archives and Records Administration, Washington, D.C.)*

Portrait of *Anna W. Goodrich*, Dean of the Army School of Nursing. *(National Library of Medicine, Bethesda, Maryland.)*

The unfavorable report on nursing conditions in the army given by Annie Goodrich was accompanied by a proposal for an Army School of Nursing. After much controversy, the school was finally approved with Goodrich as its first dean. She was the driving force behind many significant events in nursing.

Army School of Nursing

In May 1918 the secretary of war authorized the establishment of the Army School of Nursing (also known as the Army Training School) at Walter Reed Hospital, Washington, D.C., with branches in other military hospitals across the country. The proponents of this school had presented the plan, prepared largely by the school's first dean, Annie W. Goodrich, before the twenty-fourth annual convention of the National League of Nursing Education (NLNE). Goodrich had been appointed chief inspecting nurse of the Army hospitals at home and abroad and was charged with the evaluation of the quality of nursing services in military hospitals. Her unfavorable report was accompanied by the proposal for an Army School of Nursing. Viable arguments for the establishment of the school were presented:

> It would attract a high type of young women who would appreciate the opportunity to acquire a professional education while giving patriotic service; since the service of student nurses was an acceptable method of providing civilian hospitals with nursing service it could be assumed that such service could provide equally satisfactory care for military patients; because affiliations would be required for experience not available in military installations some civilian hospitals could anticipate sharing the service of the Army school students; the graduates of the school, whether they remained in the ANC or not would constitute an important addition to the nursing resources of the nation.
>
> — *Roberts, 1954, pp. 138–139*

The convention voted its support, and a budget was approved in June 1918. The chief distinction of the Army School of Nursing was that it was a separate educational unit with an independent federal fund budget that was specifically for educational purposes (Stewart, 1943). The course, based on the new *Standard Curriculum for Schools of Nursing* (1917), covered three years and gave nine months' credit to college graduates. No tuition was required; board, lodging, laundry, and required textbooks were provided. The majority of clinical experiences were provided in military hospitals; clinical experiences in pediatrics, obstetrics, gynecology, and public health were obtained through affiliations. Applications were received from thousands of enthusiastic women. The first graduating class (1921) numbered five hundred students, probably the largest class of nurses ever graduated at one time. A total of 937 women completed the course before the school officially closed its doors in January 1933.

Annie Warburton Goodrich (1866–1954) was the driving force behind many significant events in nursing. She was described as a crusader, statesman, dean of American nurses, most beloved of American nurses, and militant angel (Christy, 1970). Goodrich was known nationally and internationally for her leadership ability, which facilitated the promotion of nursing toward a professional status. She received many honors and served as president of the International Council of Nurses (ICN) (1912–1915), the American Nurses Association (ANA) (1916–1918), and the Association of Collegiate Schools of Nursing (ACSN) (1934–1936). A quote by Lillian Wald describes the strength of this almost legendary figure:

> Whether on platform or in committee or in conference, she inevitably suggests a torch, a spirit afire, and an apparently frail physique emphasizes this flaming attribute as the symbol of her genius. Though she seems to burn steadily she appears never to be consumed.
>
> — *Quoted in Robinson, 1946, p. 349*

Annie Goodrich was designated as the third member of a group referred to as "the triumvirate" by Mary M. Roberts. M. Adelaide Nutting was the leader and occupied the tip of the pyramid; she was the educator who originated most ideas concerning developments in nursing schools; Lillian D. Wald, who occupied the second point in the triangle, was the practitioner and accepted founder of modern public health nursing; Annie W. Goodrich was the last of the trio, the skillful implementer who combined the ideas and desires of the other two (Christy, 1970). Goodrich worked closely with Wald while the latter was director of the Henry Street Settlement House in New York and Goodrich simultaneously held the position of professor at Teachers College under Nutting.

Goodrich believed in collegiate nursing education and actively campaigned for that goal to be realized. Her positions as first dean of nursing at Yale University and at the Army School of Nursing epitomized this educational philosophy.

> It is desirable that nursing education should find its place in the university, which is another way of saying that it belongs where all educational expressions have been increasingly placed, and for the reason that universal knowledge is here assembled and distributed in accordance with the needs of the students as future builders of the community.
>
> — *Goodrich, 1932, p. 173*

Her philosophy encompassed university preparation not only for teachers and administrators of nursing but also for the practicing nurse. Throughout her life Annie Goodrich fought the battle of educational standards for nursing along with other nursing leaders. Undoubtedly, her success at Yale University was the crowning achievement of her life. Her dream of university preparation for *all* nurses, however, has still not been realized. In her eyes, therefore, nursing is not functioning to its fullest capacity: "Our place has been found in the institutions of the sick, but we shall never render our full service to the community until our place is also found in the University" (Proceedings of the Eighteenth Annual Convention of the American Society of Superintendents of Training Schools, 1912, p. 43).

Nursing at the Front

Conditions of warfare had changed a great deal since the time of the Spanish-American War. Military nursing needed to be revised and modernized to account for such things as submarine warfare, air attacks, shrapnel lacerations and wounds, poison gas, and trench warfare. The nurse's powers of observation and technical skills were challenged by shock, hemorrhage, communicable diseases, infected wounds, and the inhalation of poison gas. World War I was also the first war in which nurses were exposed to the perils of actual battles. Nurses and the troops were constantly threatened by frequent shelling, faced with the deaths of colleagues, forced to tolerate sordid living conditions, and exposed to communicable diseases. "Confronted with overwhelming suffering and awesome responsibility, nurses abandoned their customary obedience to authority and assumed independence in judgment" (Beeber, 1990, p. 39). Perhaps the most crucial aspect of this war was the idea that nurses were faced with the dilemma of caring for soldiers who would return to battle if they were able. How could they justify healing for destructive purposes? Reverence for all life against the violent destructiveness of war was indeed a contradiction. The effect of war upon these nurses' lives transformed their image of themselves in radical and irreversible ways (Donahue, 1995). Films about the war generally depicted nurses as melodramatic, sentimental, and romanti-

James Montgomery Flagg, *Not One Shall Be Left Behind*, 1918. Poster. *(Courtesy of the Library of Congress, Washington, D.C.)*

Nurses, as well as other groups, answered the call for patriotic service during World War I.

USS *Higbee* in Boston Harbor, May 1945.
(National Archives and Records Administration, Washington, D.C.)

The USS *Higbee* was the first fighting ship named after a woman in the service, Lenah S. Higbee, the second superintendent of the Navy Nurse Corps.

The First Commissioned Hospital Ship, Red Rover. *(National Archives and Records Administration, Washington, D.C.)*

accordance with the requirements of naval service, the Navy Nurse Corps was reduced after the war. By 1935, with the Government Economy Act, the number in the corps had dropped to 332.

American nurses on active duty faced not only the horrors and dangers of war but other types of conflicts and frustrations as well. These arose primarily because the nurses had no military rank. Army and Navy nurses had not been designated by Congress as either officers or enlisted personnel, although they had military status and were subject to military discipline. Consequently the nurses could not assume the responsibilities for teaching and directing orderlies and corpsmen and for handling administrative problems as heads of wards and nursing services. Following the war, with the help of legal and other advisers and the support of the Votes for Women Amendment (passed in 1920), nurses appealed to Congress. After a long, slow, and difficult battle, relative rank was granted to members of the Army Nurse Corps by amendment of the National Defense Act of June 4, 1920. At that time nurses were given officer status ranging from second lieutenant through major, but pay and allowances were not the same as for men. (In 1942 Navy nurses were accorded relative rank.) In 1944 nurses in both the Army and the Navy were given full military rank for the duration of World War II and six months longer. Finally, in 1947, full commissioned rank for nurses in the military services was permanently established. Florence A. Blanchfield became the first woman to be given the permanent commission of colonel in the regular Army. The Army-Navy Nurse Act of 1947 also provided for an Army Nurse Corps section in the Officers' Reserve Corps.

The first men were not commissioned as nurses until 1955—through the Bolton Amendment to the Army-Navy Nurse Act. Since that time, other legislative acts have improved the conditions of military nurses, including Public Law No. 90130, which removed most promotional restrictions on the careers of nurse officers in the Army, Navy, and Air Force. Numerous rank and privilege "firsts" have occurred in military nursing and will continue at a steady pace.

George W. Bellows, *Edith Cavell Directing The Escape Of Soldiers From Prison Camp,* 1918. Signed lower left by Mrs. George Bellows. Oil on canvas, 114.3 × 160.0 cm. *(Museum of Fine Arts, Springfield, Massachusetts, The James Philip Gray Collection.)*

Edith Cavell, an English nurse, had organized the first school for nurses in Brussels, Belgium. There she cared for soldiers of all armies and directed the escape of Allied soldiers from prison camps during World War I. She was arrested by the Germans and executed on October 12, 1915.

The story of World War I cannot be left without at least mentioning one famous nurse heroine, Edith Cavell (1865–1915). She was an English nurse who founded a school of nursing in Brussels, Belgium, in 1909 and was its superintendent. Cavell remained at the school when the war started and helped to organize an underground escape route for Allied soldiers. She also faithfully cared for sick Germans. Although she could have escaped and saved herself, she chose to remain at her post. Despite diplomatic efforts to obtain

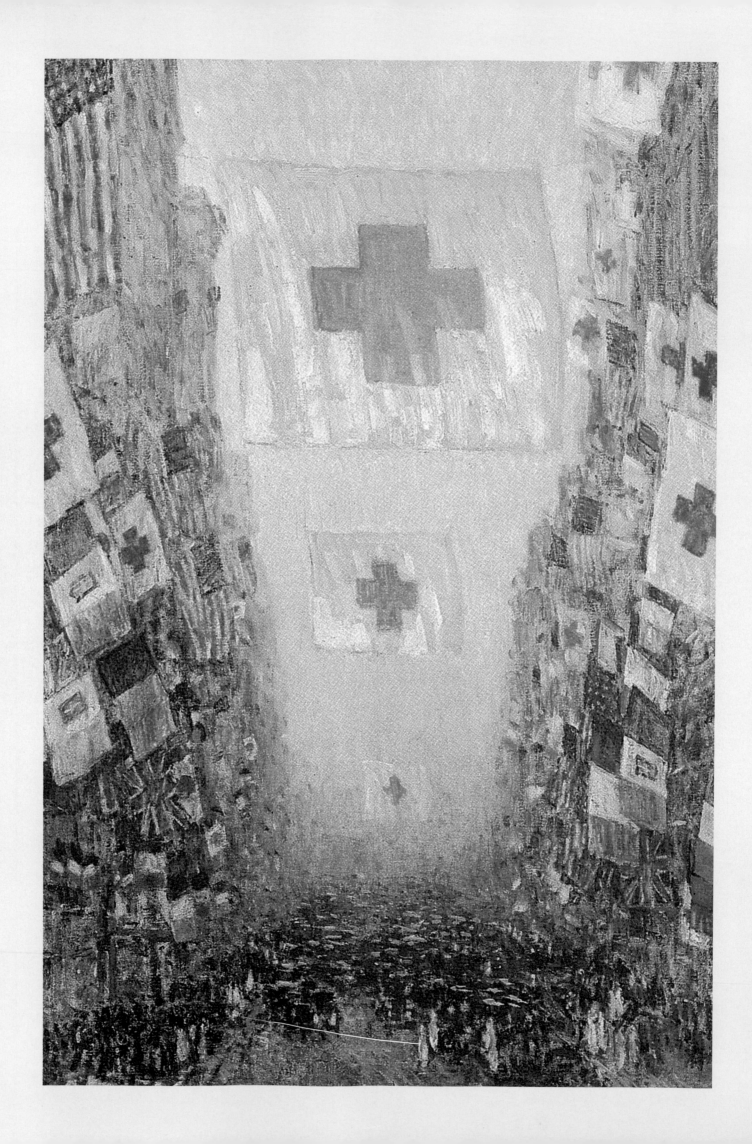

a reprieve for her, Edith Cavell was executed before a German firing squad on October 12, 1915. The charge was harboring British and French soldiers and assisting them with escape from Belgium. Cavell did not deny the charges and faced her death with tremendous courage. It is reported that the following were her last words:

> I have no fear or shrinking; I have seen death so often that it is not strange or fearful to me. I thank God for this ten weeks' quiet before the end. Life has always been hurried and full of difficulty. This time of rest has been a great mercy. They have all been very kind to me here. But this I would say, standing as I do in view of God and eternity: I realize that patriotism is not enough. I must have no hatred or bitterness towards anyone.
>
> — *Quoted in Judson, 1941, p. 281*

WORLD WAR II

> It took the second World War to bring the American nurse to her national stature. Serving in embattled lands whose names the public had never heard before, in hospital ships on all the seas, and in air ambulances evacuating the wounded by plane, the nurse came into her own as comforter and healer. Feminity in foxholes, with mud-caked khaki coveralls over pink panties, captured the imagination of the public and the fighting men of America.
>
> — *Robinson, 1946, p. 358*

The period between World War I and World War II was a time of great unrest because the defeated nations were dissatisfied with their lot. Depression on a worldwide scale led people to accept any type of leadership so long as it might restore them to prosperity. Bolshevism conquered Russia; Benito Mussolini and Fascism assumed control of Italy; Hitler and the National Socialist German Workers' Party (Nazis) steadily became more powerful in Germany; Spain underwent civil revolution; England and France were engaged in internal disagreements. It is no wonder that an era of dictatorship emerged and began to flourish in a number of nations. Major shifts in alignment also were observed as Italy and Japan, formerly in the Allied camp, joined with Germany in the so-called Axis, which opposed the United Nations.

The League of Nations had been established after World War I in an effort to preserve international peace. This organization was to act as a body of arbitration between nations. Members of the league would be committed to arbitration on all matters of dispute; hostilities would be postponed for three months after a decision was reached. The United States did not join this organization because of a traditional policy of remaining free from foreign entanglements. The league proved its value for a time but then began to weaken because it had no adequate means of enforcing its decisions.

During the late 1930s, as international relations slowly deteriorated, war broke out once again in Europe. From the time of the Treaty of Versailles, which had ended World War I, Germany had been denouncing the Polish Corridor. This strip of land had been awarded to the newly formed state of Poland, and the German city of Danzig had been placed under the League of Nations. In 1939 Hitler demanded that Danzig be returned to the Reich and that Germany be allowed to build a road across the Polish Corridor. A series of events occurred that terminated in the invasion of Poland by Germany without a formal declaration of war. Two days later Great Britain and France declared war on Germany. The United States had no desire to become involved in war. However, in 1940, anticipating the possibility that such a step might be unavoidable, it repealed the Neutrality Act of 1935. At this point the United States began to gear up for war. On December 7, 1941, the Japanese bombed Pearl Harbor, Hawaii, in a surprise air raid that ultimately

Facing page, Childe Hassam, *Celebration Day,* 1918. Oil on canvas, 90.2 × 59.7 cm. *(Eleanor and C. Thomas May Trust for Christopher, Sterling, Meredith, and Laura May.)*

In *Celebration Day,* also known as *Red Cross Day,* the red and white banners of the Red Cross form a majestic processional as they recede up Fifth Avenue in New York City.

Norman Rockwell, *Rosie to the Rescue,* cover of the *Saturday Evening Post,* September 4, 1943. *(Copyright 1943 the Norman Rockwell Family Trust. Printed by permission of the Norman Rockwell Family Trust, Poughkeepsie, New York.)*

Women became a powerful force in the workplace during World War II. By the time Pearl Harbor was bombed, twelve million women were working outside the home, many of them in factories.

369

This stamp is one of a set of four, each in a different color, that was issued by Australia in 1940 to commemorate her participation in World War II and particularly honoring her servicemen, represented by the sailor, soldier, and aviator. Her nurses have a prominent place of honor in this interesting design. *(Courtesy of Howard B. Hurley.)*

changed the course of world events. On December 8, 1941, the United States declared war on Japan; two days later Germany and Italy retaliated and declared war against the United States. The world was immediately plunged into a terrifying conflict known as the "total war." Nursing and health care services were once again radically affected as every man, woman, and child of belligerent countries became involved.

When war had been again threatening the country in 1940, Isabel Stewart wanted nursing to be prepared, to avoid mistakes, and to profit from the achievements of World War I. That summer, according to Stella Goostray, she wrote to the president of the National League of Nursing Education and emphasized

> the need of some official nursing committee or commission to think through the position that nursing should take with respect to national defense and the many adjustments that may be called for within the next few months . . . I believe we should have such a commission or board that is representative of the nursing profession as a *whole* and that it should be at work *now,* and not wait until Miss Beard calls on us to do something in connection with the American Red Cross. . . . I do not want us to be stampeded into doing things we will be sorry for.
>
> — *Goostray, 1954, p. 304*

In July 1940 the Nursing Council for National Defense was instituted at Goostray's suggestion. The council included the six national nursing organizations (ANA, NLNE, National Organization of Public Health Nursing [NOPHN], ACSN, National Association of Colored Graduate Nurses [NACGN], and American Association of Industrial Nurses [AAIN]), the federal nursing services, and representatives from such organizations as the American Hospital Association. Major Julia Stimson of the Army Nurse Corps was chairman of the council. With the declaration of war in 1942, the organization's name was changed to the National Nursing Council for War Service and Stella Goostray became its head. Plans were formulated to promote a national inventory of registered nurses, determine the role of nurses and nursing in the defense program, expand facilities of existing accredited schools of nursing, and supply supplementary nursing services to hospitals and public health agencies.

As more and more graduate nurses withdrew from civilian agencies to enlist in the Army and Navy Nurse Corps, the council tackled the problem of recruitment of students for schools of nursing. This work was assigned to the Committee on Education Policies and Resources. Isabel Stewart was appointed chairwoman of this committee, the first one constructed under the aegis of the council. The preliminary investigations of the committee indicated that financial aid to assist schools, to improve the preparation of faculty members, and to assist candidates who could not otherwise afford to enter nursing was a matter of primary importance.

The United States Cadet Nurse Corps

Convinced of the possibility of getting a federal appropriation for nursing education for defense needs, Isabel Stewart began to pursue avenues through which such a goal might be achieved. Commissioner Studebaker of the United States Office of Education was sympathetic to the cause and invited her to Washington to prepare a plan for a request of funds. This she did with the assistance of nine other committee members. "The Proposal," as it came to be known, investigated the country's need for professional nursing services in both military and civilian situations, plans needed to meet that need, and the cost of such a program. It rapidly became apparent that nursing schools could not be expected to increase their enrollments and to increase instructional or housing facilities without financial assistance. The government needed to be

Cecile R. Johnson, *Night Duty. (National Archives and Records Administration, Washington, D.C.)*

persuaded that federal aid for nursing education was a legitimate and imperative defense measure. The committee soon made these findings:

> Uncle Sam was spending large sums in training his sons for national defense, but he had provided little or nothing for the preparation of his daughters who were to serve in the national forces. Apart from the experiment with the Army School of Nursing during the first World War, and the stipends to nurses given through the Social Security Act, practically no federal funds had been appropriated for nursing education up to this time. . . . A plan was prepared and, after many vicissitudes, submitted in a lull to Congress. Finally, in June, 1941, with the assistance of friends of nursing education in Congress, a law was passed authorizing the expenditure of $1,200,000 for the current fiscal year to assist in the training of nurses for national defense. The administration of this fund was entrusted to the United States Public Health Service.
>
> — *Stewart, 1943, p. 283*

The first support for nursing education from federal funds specifically appropriated for that purpose thus occurred. The Appropriations Act for 1942 (effective July 1, 1941) was passed with inclusion of funds for nursing education through the efforts of Frances Payne Bolton, a Congresswoman from Ohio and a friend of nursing. In July 1942 this federal appropriation was increased to three and a half million dollars. This major feat resulted largely from the leadership of Stewart, who served on the advisory committee for the initial project. The sum that was to be applied to "refresher," postgraduate, and basic programs was inadequate for existing needs, but it paved the way for future financial assistance to nursing schools.

Subsequently a Nurse Training Act (Public Law No. 74, Seventy-Eighth Congress) was introduced into Congress in 1943 by Frances Payne Bolton. An appropriation of sixty million dollars was voted at this time to cover the cost of an accelerated and expanded program of education for students entering approved schools of nursing, and later the amount was increased. The bill, commonly known as the Bolton Act, created the United States Cadet Nurse Corps. It provided for a thirty-month basic program, free tuition and fees, free uniforms, monthly stipends for students in approved basic schools of nursing, and grants for postgraduate work.

The program of the Cadet Nurse Corps was administered by the United States Public Health Service, Division of Nursing Education, which was headed by Lucile Petry. (Petry was appointed assistant surgeon general of the United States Public Health Service in 1949. She was the first woman to hold this position.) This program proved to be a major incentive for the improvement of standards in nursing education because schools had to meet requirements developed by the NLNE to obtain the federal monies. Nursing schools were also required to admit all qualified applicants, regardless of race or religion. An intensive publicity and recruiting campaign was launched. The desirability of a student reserve with benefits of an "attractive uniform," liberal scholarships, and subsistence grants was given wide press. Students who entered pledged themselves to serve where needed (military or civilian agencies) for the duration of the war and six months thereafter. The potential overcrowding of available space from the enormous influx of nursing students into this program was assisted by the passage of the Lanham Act (1941), which provided funds for dormitories, libraries, classrooms, and other physical facilities that were needed.

Quotas based on national nursing needs were established for the Cadet Nurse Corps: 125,000 for the first two years, with 65,000 recruited during the first twelve months and 60,000 the following year. Both yearly quotas were exceeded, and the total number who joined the corps was 179,000. The program was a unique experiment that achieved remarkable success. In addition, from the start the National Nursing Council had ensured the removal of

Honorable Frances Payne Bolton. (National Archives and Record Administration, Washington, D.C.)

Frances Payne Bolton was a congresswoman from Ohio who became a friend of nursing. She strongly supported the development of the Army School of Nursing and introduced the bill into the House of Representatives that created the U.S. Cadet Nurse Corps.

Cadet Nurse, The Girl With a Future, 1944. Poster. (National Archives and Records Administration, Washington, D.C.)

A recruitment poster emphasizing the wartime need and educational opportunities for those interested in nursing. This massive campaign to recruit people into nursing programs offered a free education. The only payback was a pledge to serve where needed for the duration of the war and six months after. President Roosevelt had signed the bill that created the Cadet Nurse Corps on June 15, 1943.

all barriers resulting from various forms of discrimination. Some important racial barriers were therefore removed. The way was paved for the acceptance of black students into a greater number of nursing schools and for the enlistment of black nurses into the Army and Navy. A committee of the council, the Coordinating Committee on Negro Nursing, was set up to assist with the recruitment of well-qualified black students and the provision of better educational opportunities for these students. In 1944 the council also openly campaigned for racial equality in the military nursing services.

First Anniversary of the U.S. Cadet Nurse Corps, July 1944. (National Archives and Records Administration, Washington, D.C.)

Dr. Thomas Parran, Surgeon General of the U.S. Public Health Service *(left)* and Miss Lucile Petry, Director of the U.S. Cadet Nurse Corps *(right)*, hold the new official flag of the corps at ceremonies in Washington, D.C., marking the first anniversary of the group. Comprising nearly one hundred thousand student nurses, the corps made it possible for hospitals to release graduate nurses for specialized positions on the home front and behind fighting lines. The fiftieth anniversary of the Cadet Nurse Corps was held in 1993.

Nursing at the Front

The role of the nurse in war had been almost revolutionized since the time of Florence Nightingale in the Crimean War. By World War II, nurses constituted an integral part of the military structure. Their contributions could no longer be ignored. Wherever American troops were stationed around the world, nurses could be found. They were accustomed to organization, had a working knowledge of war that had been gained through personal experiences, and were prepared to meet the demands of modern warfare. By the end of this war, the romance between the nurse and the American GI would be real, built on mutual admiration and respect. The bravery of the nurses under the most rigorous and demanding situations was witnessed by many soldiers, who wrote of these experiences:

> They were 24 hours with plenty of things dropping all around—planes being shot down. Let me tell you they quickly learned to dig fox holes. I have seen them digging them with a spoon—two things they soon learn to do—wear helmets and dig foxholes. . . . They were pretty hard put for food. They had no water except in their canteens when unloaded. [When I arrived with the equipment] . . . they welcomed the "old man" with food and equipment. They had no tents. Each nurse was given one blanket in half shelter tent, their "B" and "C" ration and a musette bag. They were wearing fatigues and steel helmets. They used the ground for their bed—but they were there ready to go and waiting for us . . .

> — *Quoted in Aynes, 1973, p. 245*

Franklin Boggs, *Night Duty*, 1945. *(U.S. Army Center of Military History, Washington, D.C.)*

More than fifty thousand Army nurses served at the battlefront during World War II. Here an Army nurse checks on a coughing patient during her vigil of night duty. The artist, Franklin Boggs, slept in this ward in the South Pacific. He was impressed with the effect of the flashlight's beam on the green mosquito nets. He reported: "The night sounds of the jungle cannot be painted, but are quite unforgettable."

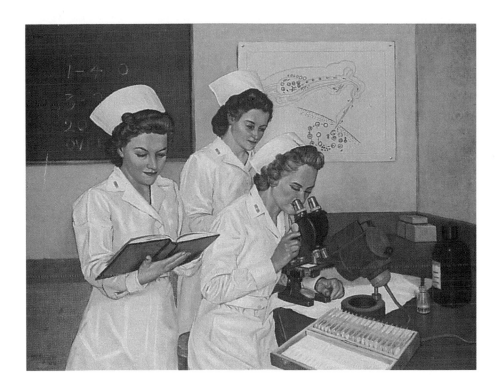

Manuel Tolegian, *Laboratory Warfare*, 1945. *(U.S. Army Center of Military History, Washington, D.C.)*

The Army Medical Department's war on disease is constant. Its laboratories are battlefields staffed by doctors and nurses. This painting illustrates a former training center for members of the Army Nurse Corps at Camp White, Oregon.

The global scope of World War II presented a sharp challenge to military nurses. By the end of the war, nurses had been stationed on the soil of approximately fifty nations scattered over the face of the globe. They worked and lived in the installations of the Army and the Navy, in hotels and other adapted structures, in cantonment barracks, in tent hospitals, and in Quonset and other prefabricated huts. Speed in rendering care was probably the biggest factor that kept the death rate below that of World War I.

> The sulfonamides, the advent of penicillin, DDT, new developments in antimalarial therapy, and the ready availability of blood and blood derivatives, plus the heroism and ingenuity of the medical corpsmen, were among the factors which contributed to that favorable result.
>
> — *Roberts, 1954, p. 344*

Nursing care also contributed to the statistics and made a great difference in the recovery of sick and wounded soldiers.

The peak strength of the Army and Navy Nurse Corps was nearly sixty-nine thousand during World War II. These nurses gave care in front-line situations, field hospitals, evacuation hospitals, base hospitals, hospital ships and trains and in the air. Army nurses served at nine stations and fifty-two areas. Navy nurses served on a dozen hospital ships and in more than three hundred naval stations. Both served wherever the American soldier could be found. More than sixteen hundred nurses were decorated for meritorious service and bravery under fire. They received honors that included the Distinguished Service Medal, Silver Star, Distinguished Flying Cross, Soldier's Medal, Bronze Star Medal, Air Medal, Legion of Merit, Army Commendation Medal, Purple Heart, and Gold Star. A total of 201 nurses died; 16 of these deaths were the result of enemy action. Throughout the war, nurses in both the Army and the Navy were held as prisoners by the Japanese in the Philippines at Santo Tomas civilian prison camp near Manila. They continued to give nursing care under terrific hardships until their release in 1945. Eleven Navy nurses were interned for a period of thirty-seven months.

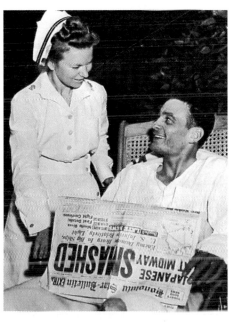

Battle of Midway, June 1942. (National Archives and Records Administration, Washington, D.C.)

Liberated Prisoner of War Nurses, March 1945. (Bureau of Medicine and Surgery Archives, U.S. Navy. Courtesy of Laurie K. Glass.)

Flight nurse talking with patients aboard a C-54 air evacuation plane before takeoff from Andrews Air Force Base. *(U.S. Air Force Photo.)*

A new field of military nursing opened up in World War II—flight nursing. Both the Army and the Navy instituted flight nurse programs for assistance with the extended use of air transport for the evacuation of wounded soldiers. Established through the Air Surgeon's Office in September 1942, this program prepared qualified nurses to rapidly convert transport planes (C-45 Commandos, C-47 Skytrains, and C-54 Skymasters) into flying ambulances. These transports had dual functions; they were used to transport cargo and troops to battle and then became ambulances for the return trip. They were not protected from enemy fighters, since they were not marked with the Geneva Red Cross as noncombatant (Kalisch and Scobey, 1983). Flight nurses performed under great pressures and were instrumental in providing effective nursing care in frequently dangerous circumstances. The nurses were specially trained to give nursing care to the wounded on stretchers piled three tiers deep on either side of a cargo plane that had been converted into a rough ambulance. They were also taught to perform duties related to ground medical installations.

Admittance to the program began with application for commission in the Army Nurse Corps; this was followed by a minimum of six months in the Army Air Force unit hospital. Application could then be made for admittance to the flight nursing school. After completion of these requirements, an automatic designation of "flight nurse" was still not granted. The nurse was required to submit a request to the commanding general of the Army Air Forces for the designation. The first class of Army Nurse Corps flight nurses was graduated from the School of Air Evacuation at Bowman Field, Kentucky, on February 18, 1943. Many nurses desired entrance to the program because flight nurses represented the elite of the corps.

Music had frequently been used in the military to relieve tension and boost morale. The "Song of the Army Nurse Corps" was officially adopted by January 1944. "The marching music was composed by Lou Singer and the lyrics written by Hy Zaret, a professional doing his bit as a private in the Special Services in New York. . . . Army bands at home and overseas played it. . . ." (Aynes, 1973, p. 243):

> We march along with faith undaunted beside our gallant fighting men;
> Whenever they are sick or wounded, we nurse them back to health again;
> As long as healing hands are wanted, you'll find the nurses of the Corps,
> On ship, or plane, on transport train, at home or on a far off shore;
> With loyal heart we do our part, for the Army and the Army Nurse Corps.

This achievement occurred through the effort of Edith A. Aynes and was supported by Colonel Blanchfield, who wrote the foreword:

> There is no burden so heavy, no night so long that it cannot be eased by music. The members of the Army Nurse Corps should be encouraged to sing, for in song there is a contentment that means happier times, good fellowship, better care for their patients and a more optimistic outlook for the entire Corps.
>
> — *Aynes, 1973, p. 243*

A final newcomer in the federal nursing services was the Air Force Nurse Corps, established within the Air Force Medical Service in July 1949. An Army Air Force regulation was published on June 8, 1949, that provided for the separation of certain Air Force activities that were formerly the responsibility of the Army Medical Department (Vreeland, 1950). The purpose of this enforcement was twofold: the complete separation of Army and Air Force

The Song of the Army Nurse Corps, by Hy Zaret and Lou Singer. (Copyright 1944 by MCA Music, A Division of MCA Inc., New York. All Rights Reserved.)

Franklin Boggs, *Air Evacuation*, 1945. *(U.S. Army Center of Military History, Washington, D.C.)*

A flight nurse administers oxygen to a wounded soldier. This plane was bound for Australia, one stop on the long journey to the United States and a hospital near home.

medical activities and the establishment of the Air Force Nurse Corps. Procedures were developed whereby nurses in the Army who were on duty with the Air Force and nurses who were stationed at Army installations could request to be transferred to the Air Force Nurse Corps. Of Army nurses on active duty, 1,199 transferred from the Army to the Air Force, becoming the nucleus for the Air Force Nurse Corps. One year later the corps prepared to assist with the air evacuation of battle casualties from the Korean area. This was to become a vital key to the survival of the soldier wounded in the Korean War.

The Nurse Draft Bill

The large number of graduate nurses engaged in military service was still not enough; voluntary enlistments were not meeting anticipated needs. During what were to become the closing months of the war, steps began to be taken to draft nurses into military service. An article by the well-known columnist Walter Lippmann, which appeared on December 19, 1944, included a charge of gross neglect against the Army. Lippmann contended that the Army had not provided adequate numbers of nurses to care for wounded soldiers:

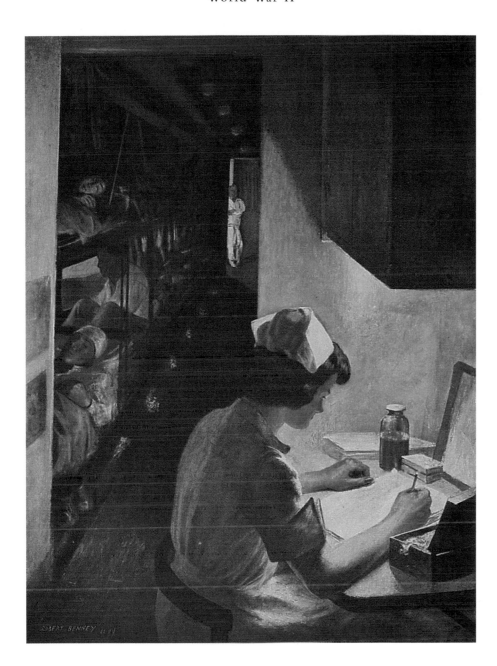

Robert Benney, *Night Vigil,* 1945. *(U.S. Army Center of Military History, Washington, D.C.)*

The Army Nurse checks the patients' charts while aboard a hospital train in World War II. Some of the wounded men sleep soundly, others fitfully.

The last thing our people will put up with is that sick and wounded American soldiers should suffer because the Army cannot find enough women to nurse them. Yet, I am reporting only the stark truth, which is well known to the Army and to the leaders of the medical profession, when I say that in military hospitals at home and abroad our men are not receiving the nursing care they must have, and that with casualties increasing in number and in seriousness, this will mean for many of the men brought in from the battlefields that their recovery is delayed, and even jeopardized.

— *Lippmann, 1944*

It was not long before President Roosevelt, in his State of the Union message on January 6, 1945, came forth with an unprecedented request for a draft of women nurses. The ANA went on record as approving such a move provided that the Selective Service legislation include *all women.* The Nurse Draft Bill quickly passed the House of Representatives but became bogged down in the Senate. The threat of the draft initiated an overwhelming mass of applications from nurses for war service, and the result was an excess of nurses in the military. The conclusion of the war on the European front made the draft bill virtually unnecessary, and it was quietly withdrawn in May 1945.

James Montgomery Flagg, *Your Red Cross Needs You,* 1942. Poster. *(Courtesy of the Library of Congress, Washington, D.C.)*

The Red Cross Nursing Service was planned on a large scale by the voluntary affiliation of the American Nurses Association with the Red Cross officials.

THE KOREAN WAR

The Korean War broke out on June 25, 1950, and thrust nurses once again into service in combat areas. The nurses of the armed forces—Army, Navy, and Air Force Nurse Corps—were called upon as a result of the invasion of South Korea. Although this action was not officially designated as a "war," the realities of casualties were nonetheless harsh. The United States was essentially forced to play a role in a situation created by the conflicting ideologies of the freedom-loving Western world and communism. Fears of an acute nurs-

John Groth, *A Nurse at Work,* Korean War. Watercolor. *(U.S. Army Center of Military History, Washington, D.C.)*

ing shortage prompted the Joint Committee on Nursing in National Security, along with representatives of the six national nursing organizations, to recommend the following:

> That all possible means be developed for recruiting more students for schools of nursing.
>
> That as many practical nurses be trained and employed to help professional nurses as hospitals and other community agencies could utilize to good advantage.
>
> That nurses be withdrawn systematically from the civilian services for military duty according to a plan that ensured their employment at the highest level of skill for which they were prepared.
>
> That state and local advisory boards of nurses be organized and be given the authority by the government to review assignment of nurses to the armed forces and to civilian agencies.
>
> That, if there was total mobilization, nurses be redistributed within the fields of nursing and within community agencies so that the most essential civilian needs would be taken care of first.
>
> That major effort be directed to improving sound basic nursing education and to increase enrollment in schools of nursing that offered effective programs.
>
> That selected nurses be encouraged to prepare for responsibilities as teachers, supervisors, and administrators, as well as for the special fields, in order to safeguard essential nursing service. That administration of nursing services be improved so that nursing skills would be used to the best advantage and their full value would reach more people.
>
> That nursing service be stabilized as much as possible and turnover of staff held to a minimum through the adoption and application of sound personnel policies for nurses and allied workers.
>
> — *Joint Committee on Nursing in National Security, 1951, pp. 78–79*

During World War II the Army had experimented with and demonstrated the need for a new type of hospital that would be located as close to the front as was relatively safe, about eight to twenty miles. This new unit first appeared in late November 1942 and was tried out under actual combat conditions in Korea. The Mobile Army Surgical Hospital (MASH) could be moved at a moment's notice. It was basically a sixty-bed unit with the flexibility to expand five or six times beyond its standard bed capacity. Within a few hours several hundred patients could be admitted and treated. The hospital was usually staffed by ten physicians, twelve nurses (two were anesthetists), and ninety corpsmen. It could be set up in any type of location that was available—a barn, church, or schoolhouse or in the tents that were carried with it (*American Journal of Nursing,* 1951, p. 387). An Army helicopter detachment was attached to each MASH unit to provide care as close to the front as possible and to provide for immediate evacuation for the critically ill.

The MASH unit became the first hospital to which the wounded were sent and was a great factor in maintaining morale.

> The proximity of the unit to the front, its trained personnel, its adequate supply of whole blood, and its rapid helicopter and ambulance evacuation services all contributed greatly to the reduction of mortality rates in Korea as compared with those during World War II: the mortality rate among wounded soldiers who reached hospitals in Korea was half the corresponding rate during World War II.
>
> — *Kalisch and Kalisch, 1978, p. 543*

John Groth, *Receiving Tent*, Korean War. Watercolor. *(U.S. Army Center of Military History, Washington, D.C.)*

John Groth, *Recovery Tent*, Korean War.
Watercolor. *(U.S. Army Center of Military
History, Washington, D.C.)*

John Groth, *Field Hospital Ward*, Korean
War. Watercolor. *(U.S. Army Center of Military History, Washington, D.C.)*

John Groth, *Nurses in the Operating Tent,*
Korean War. Watercolor. *(U.S. Army Cen-*
ter of Military History, Washington, D.C.)

Cecile R. Johnson, *Evening Rounds.*
(National Archives and Records Administra-
tion, Washington, D.C.)

Russell Connor, *Korean Mother and Child.*
(National Archives and Records Administration, Washington, D.C.)

A pattern of action was followed as patients were admitted: pulse rates and blood pressures were taken and recorded on tags attached to each litter; infusion of whole blood was started; penicillin was given to everyone with an open wound; clothing was cut away and wounds exposed; critical cases were identified; and patients were sorted on the basis of treatment. Those designated as seriously wounded were transported either to southern Korea or to medical centers in Japan. The majority of cases comprised chest, abdominal, or extremity injuries.

The fledging Air Force Nurse Corps faced its first major test during this war. The members' primary responsibility was the care of patients airlifted during the Korean conflict. The volume of patients was staggering. As many as 3,925 patients were aeromedically evacuated on one day, December 5, 1950 (Chow and others, 1978). The corps had mobilized its resources and accelerated training programs. By the end of the war, more than 350,000 patients had been evacuated by propeller-driven cargo aircraft. Rapid air evacuation in the Korean War served to virtually eliminate the hospital ship as the means for transporting the wounded. Although three hospital ships—*Consolation, Repose,* and *Haven*—were present in Korean waters during the conflict, they were used as floating hospitals; they transported patients only when en route to Japan for renovation. It had been proven that air transportation was the cheapest and most efficient method for transport of the wounded.

John Groth, *Nurses Tent,* Korean War. Watercolor. *(U.S. Army Center of Military History, Washington, D.C.)*

Throughout the ground fighting and during the prolonged peace negotiations that lasted for two years, until July 27, 1953, nurses served throughout the Korean peninsula. Fewer nurses served in Korea than in previous wars, but they had once again made a tremendous contribution to advances in the delivery of care to the wounded.

THE VIETNAM WAR

The Vietnam War became the longest conflict in which American troops were committed in the history of the United States. It was a war like no other that evoked conflict and controversy initially at home. It was an extremely unpopular war; thousands of people marched in protest and hundreds were arrested trying to storm the Pentagon. Student unrest erupted on campuses across the country as the war dragged on and American casualties escalated. The futility of American intervention was felt, and this resulted in problems never before experienced by veterans of other wars. "There was widespread resistance to fighting, extensive drug usage, and racial conflict among American troops. Profound guilt, feelings of stasis, impotence, psychic numbness, and a deeply embedded antiestablishment anger were common" (Kalisch and Kalisch, 1978, pp. 634–635). Deep, lasting wounds occurred that were not always caused by enemy action. An appropriate name for this conflict could well be the "forgotten war" because there is a silence, and at times a mystique, that still pervades discussions of this war. This is consistent with published accounts in the nursing literature, which are on the increase but yet fewer in number than those of either World War I or World War II.

Certainly the Vietnam War was a different war for a variety of reasons. Television portrayed the war in homes throughout the United States and the world, but reality was difficult to ascertain. Conscientious objectors fled to Canada, went underground, or were jailed. Minorities were drafted in disproportionate numbers. And even though it was not labeled as such, *it was a war* in which over fifty-eight thousand Americans were killed, including eight female and two male nurses who died of illness or injury sustained in Vietnam (Fischer, 1990; Freedman and Rhoads, 1987; Lippard, 1990; Spelts, 1986; Walsh and Aulich, 1989). The Vietnam War was also a war of contrast.

America's interest in Southeast Asia began in 1950. At that time President Truman sent a thirty-five-man military advisory team to assist the French with their fight against the North Vietnamese. In 1954 the French garrison at Dien Bien Phu fell to communist forces; this was followed by a subsequent agreement between France and North Vietnam to partition Vietnam. The agreement was, however, contingent on free reunification elections. South Vietnam believed that free elections were impossible in North Vietnam and refused to prepare for them. Other events occurred, including President Eisenhower's offer of economic aid and training for the South Vietnamese army. By 1960 North Vietnam had formed the National Liberation Front (Viet Cong) of South Vietnam. The number of American "military advisers" steadily grew in proportion to increased terrorism in South Vietnam. The involvement of American military nurses did not begin until March 1962.

The first contingent to arrive in the Republic of Vietnam were thirteen Army nurses assigned to the Eighth Field Hospital, Nha Trang. Navy Nurse Corps officers were assigned to the Station Hospital, Headquarters Support Activity, in Saigon. By February 1966, three hundred military nurses of the Army, Navy, and Air Force were serving. More than two hundred were members of the Army; thirty-seven (not including flight nurses assigned aboard medical air evacuation aircraft) were Air Force; and thirty-nine were Navy, including the twenty-nine serving aboard the hospital ship *Repose*. This ship

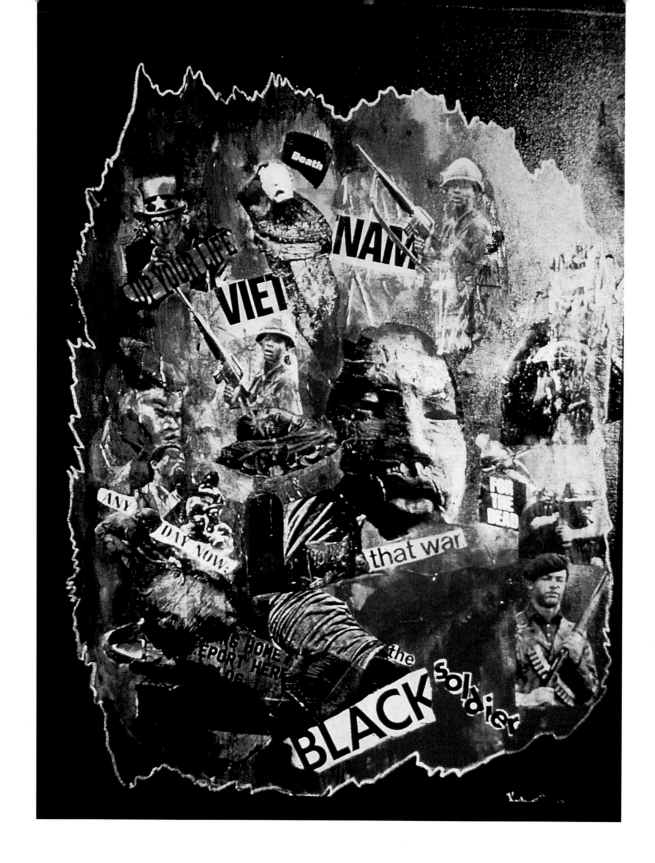

Kay B. Brown, *The Black Soldier,* 1969, Collage.
(Courtesy of Kay B. Brown, Washington, D.C.)

The Vietnam War was a "different war" in many
respects. It was different for people of color who
enlisted and were drafted in disproportionate numbers. Many of their white middle- and upper-class
counterparts, on the other hand, received either
college or medical deferments or left the country in
protest. Military minorities also bore the brunt of
combat as they served primarily in the infantry
with reported race and class oppression in concert
with the horrors of battle.

was later joined by the *Sanctuary*. Both were equipped to give optimal medical and nursing care to the wounded. Between March 1962 and March 1973 more than five thousand nurses served in Vietnam (Shields, 1981). As with the Civil War, there are discrepancies with numbers of women and nurses who served in Vietnam. There does not seem to be an accurate count. For example, the Department of Defense stipulates that about seventy-five hundred American women served on active military duty in Vietnam; the Veterans' Administration indicates more than eleven thousand (Hardaway, 1988; Norman, 1990; VVA, 1985).

The Vietnam nurses were not, however, prepared for the kinds of injuries they saw. The American napalm, white phosphorus, and antipersonnel bombs and small arms used by both sides inflicted massive, multiple injuries. Traumatic amputations, enormous blast wounds, and flesh burned down to the bone were frequent occurrences. The war was also a dirty war in which traumatic injuries were penetrated with dirt and debris. "Wounded men in an alien world thousands of miles from home were astonished and reassured at the sight of an American woman so close to the battlefield sharing this

Naval Hospital, Da Nang, Vietnam, 1965. *(National Archives and Records Administration, Washington, D.C.)*

View of the main street of the hospital compound after the 1965 attack by the Viet Cong. Surgery was once performed on the left, and the labs were originally located on the right.

R.D. Moser, Navy Nurse Tends a Patient in the Intensive Care Ward of the Hospital Ship USS Repose, 1967. *(National Archives and Records Administration, Washington, D.C.)*

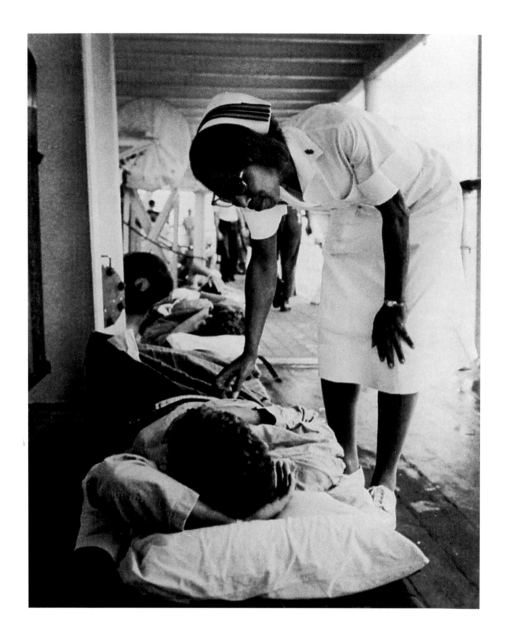

grotesque experience. The men seemed to gain a sense of security and comfort from the women's presence, a sense of a more normal way of life, a reminder of home" (Holm and Wells, 1993, p. 46). As in other wars, the presence of female nurses lent reassurance, comfort, and emotional support to a devastating experience.

Nurse casualties also occurred in Vietnam. The only nurse and only woman, however, to die as a result of hostile fire was First Lieutenant Sharon A. Lane of Canton, Ohio. Lieutenant Lane died of shrapnel wounds she received during an enemy rocket attack on June 8, 1969, while on duty at the 312th Evacuation Hospital, Chu Lai. Her memory and spirit will live along with those of the thousands of men killed in action in Vietnam and elsewhere. The essence of her being is poignantly described by Colonel Maude M. Smith, ANC (ret.), in an imaginary monologue:

Message from Sharon
A Reading

I am Lieutenant Lane. Do you remember me?
I was taken from your midst beyond the China Sea
Yes! I am Sharon Lane and I am here with them
The very many thousand valiant young men
Yes! I am with them now where it's evermore serene
Indeed! I am treated regally—as if I were a queen
We were sad to leave you though little was our choice
But lasting peace is ours now we say with one voice
We rest in summer meadows that are always green
The beauty that surrounds us is bright fresh and clean
Friendly birds sing songs amid heavenly flowers
And time is not measured in mere moments or in hours
Butterflies flit gently over clover that is sweet
And joy and love abound on the paths where we all meet
We do not dwell in sorrow on the days missed of our youth
In the cause of freedom—in man's epic search for truth
We only plead that you will think it carefully through
Before another brutal war claims other young folk too
I was caring for a soldier
Leaning over his bed
A bit of shrapnel pierced my neck
In seconds I was dead
I didn't even have a chance
To breathe a quick good-bye
To gesture—to scream
Or to say a prayer or cry
It happened very suddenly
A long time ago
And I am not regretful
I do want you to know
That all of us up here have received the answers now
To our souls' burning questions that suffice somehow
Enjoy earth's awesome wonder the while that you are there
But accept in your hearts that here too it is fair
The ones who are so dear to you abiding here with me
We know you're only human and can't see as we now see
We have learned these lessons well so early in life's game
That death is not the end of thought and all men are the same
We are part of a unity in which mortal beings share
A mystical oneness of which we're quite aware
We also know our sacrifice shall not have been in vain
If it has meant that nevermore shall war destroy again
Please keep the sacred trust of peace that we all place in you
The sort of trust you put in us—the faith that we kept too
Yes! I am Sharon Lane. Love binds me to you yet
As it does the gallant men. Lest you forget!

— Smith, 1984, p. 3

An Air Force nurse checks the identification of an injured man during the Strike Command exercise, Goldfire I, designed to test newly developed Air Force tactical support techniques against current conventional Army-Air Force techniques in 1964. (U.S. Air Force Photo.)

Paul Ortlip, *Mother and Child—Widow Village*, Vietnam, 1967. (*National Archives and Records Administration, Washington, D.C.*)

The appointment of male nurses to the regular forces of the Army, Navy, and Air Force Nurse Corps was made possible by a congressional bill in 1966. Frances P. Bolton, representative from Ohio, had initially introduced the bill in 1961 and resubmitted it in 1963. She again introduced legislation in January 1965, which was followed by an identical bill by Samuel S. Stratton, representative from New York, in May 1965. As a result, the number of male nurses in the services steadily rose. At one point all-male nursing units were established. These were dissolved as the presence of the female nurse was again recognized as an important morale booster.

No front lines in the traditional sense existed in Vietnam; nor were there secure road networks in combat areas. Therefore the hospitals could not follow and support tactical operations, and ground evacuation was next to impossible. All hospitals became fixed installations, and helicopters became the primary means of evacuation. Inflatable rubber shelters known as Medical Unit, Self-contained, Transportable (MUST) hospitals became operational in Vietnam. They, too, were fixed but could have been moved under proper conditions. These semipermanent structures were equipped with integral electrical power, air conditioning, heating, hot and cold water, and waste disposal. Sophisticated medical equipment and facilities combined with quality nursing resulted in the best care ever available to those in combat.

A massive exodus of Vietnamese refugees took place at the end of the Vietnam War in April 1975. Military nurses worked diligently to provide nursing care to these homeless people in refugee camps and during air evacuation to the United States. They also contributed to the teaching of Vietnamese nurses and physicians while aiding in the health care of Vietnamese villagers.

Sgt. Ronald A. Wilson, *Anatomy of a Dustoff*, Vietnam, 1967. (*U.S. Army Center of Military History, Washington, D.C.*)

The term "dustoff" was derived from the speed of landing, unloading the wounded, and the quick takeoff causing a lot of dust. A medical corpsman accompanied the patients.

AT WAR IN THE PERSIAN GULF

The most recent war, commonly referred to as the Gulf War, is in actuality the Second Gulf War. The original or First Gulf War was the conflict between Iran and Iraq that took place between September 1980 and August 1988. The Second Gulf War occurred between Iraq and the U.S.-led coalition and was precipitated by Iraq's invasion and occupation of Kuwait (Hiro, 1992). The genesis of this war can be traced to the history of the Middle East, but the more immediate basis can be traced to Iraq's need to increase the price of oil on the world market to meet its foreign debt. Saddam Hussein was deeply in debt as a result of his drive to create the most powerful armed forces in the Middle East and his eight-year war with Iran. According to his point of view, the Organization of Petroleum Exporting Countries (OPEC) was bowing to Western pressures to keep oil prices low. Since oil sales were almost Iraq's entire source of funds, Hussein had to do something to increase prices. He was also convinced that Kuwait was illegally pumping more than its share of oil from the Rumalia oil field, which stretches across the Iraq-Kuwait border, thereby keeping some of Iraq's income. In addition, Hussein did not accept the existing boundary between Iraq and Kuwait as binding, since it had been imposed by old colonial powers. "In sum, seizing Kuwait would restore to Iraq what was rightfully its own—including whatever assets Kuwait possessed, such as the gold in its banks—and simultaneously enable Iraq to eliminate a $4 billion debt owed to Kuwait" (Blair, 1992, p. 11).

On August 2, 1990, Iraqi troops crossed the border into Kuwait. The main column led by Soviet-designed T-72 tanks and supported by fighter aircraft and helicopter gunships overwhelmed the Kuwaiti border guards and marched toward Kuwait City. The Iraqis were in control of the country by the end of the day. The United States immediately froze Kuwaiti and Iraqi assets and imposed a trade embargo on Iraq. Other countries such as Britain and France followed suit. At the initiation of President George Bush, the United Nations Security Council passed Resolution No. 660, which condemned the invasion and called upon Iraq to withdraw all troops from Kuwait. Further resolutions followed. Ultimately, Operation "Desert Shield" became a reality with the Washington ordering of military intervention (Hiro, 1992). Operation "Desert Shield" became "Desert Storm" (code name for the air campaign of the U.S.-led coalition) on January 16 and 17, 1991. After 209 days of the Gulf crisis and warfare, a temporary ceasefire began on February 28, 1991 as the coalition forces suspended combat operations. "The armed force of the Coalition that defeated Iraq totaled 737,000 men and women in ground units, aboard 190 vessels, and flying or maintaining 1,800 aircraft. While the United States provided the bulk of the Coalition forces—with 532,000 troops, 120 ships, and more than 1,700 aircraft—thirty-four other nations provided personnel and equipment in action or in support of Desert Storm" (Blair, 1992, p. 125).

One potential legacy of this conflict is that the Persian Gulf War and its popular support forced Americans to reexamine the Southeast Asian conflict and the way in which the country had treated its veterans. The Gulf War entered the daily lives of the citizens of the world through the media and exposed them to the everyday happenings of those fighting for peace. Although Vietnam was the first television war, there was no aspect of the Gulf War that was not directly affected by the mass communications media. The media helped to confirm not only the superiority of Western technology but also the courage of both allied servicemen and servicewomen and their willingness to participate no matter what the risks. Perhaps more far-reaching is the fact that this war may well become a historic turning point. A whole new level of international cooperation may have been achieved that may continue to progress.

Facing page, above, Black Hawk Helicopter, 1991. (Official U.S. Navy Photo by JO2 Pete Hatzakos.)

An Army UH-60A Black Hawk helicopter lifts off from the helicopter pad at the Navy Fleet Hospital 5, located in Saudi Arabia after delivering a Marine wounded in action supporting Operation Desert Storm.

Facing page, below, Medical Personnel, 1991. (Official U.S. Navy Photo by JO1 Joe Gawlowicz.)

Medical personnel tend to a simulated casualty during a drill aboard the hospital ship USNS *Comfort* (T-AH-20). The vessel was deployed to the Persian Gulf during Operation Desert Storm.

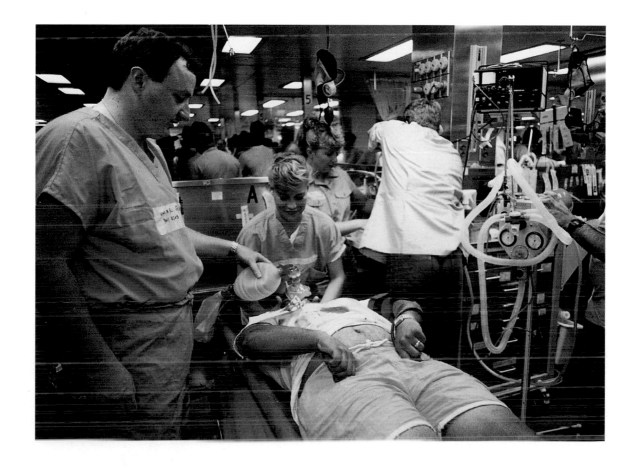

Several thousand nurses from the United States were deployed with Operation Desert Storm to provide nursing care for the five hundred thousand troops sent to Saudi Arabia and the Persian Gulf. They were sent to desert sites where troops were stationed. Nursing was also represented by other countries, as in the case of Great Britain. Nearly six thousand British medical personnel, including nurses, were part of the operations. Within a week of Iraq's invasion of Kuwait, nurses both on active duty and in the reserves were in action in the Middle East. Both women and nurses were involved in the military conflict in crucial ways. About thirty-two thousand women went to this war; women made up more than ten percent of the U.S. military and staffed almost forty percent of military medical units (David, 1991). There was a certain irony here, since Saudi Arabian women were not permitted to drive cars or even show their faces. Because of Saudia Arabian customs, American military women were not permitted to wear shorts, jog, or go shopping unless accompanied by a man. Yet, they shared all duties except those on the front lines.

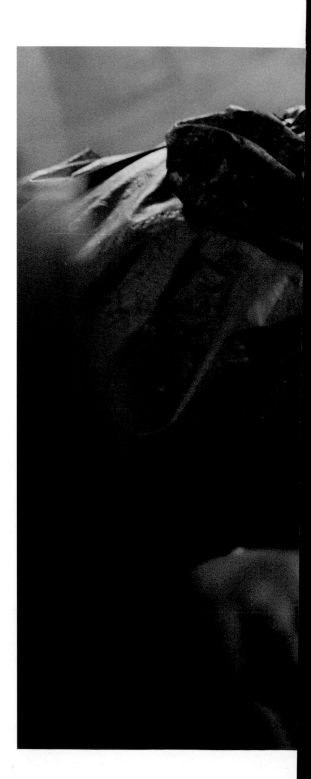

David C. Turnley, *Lt. Linda McClory,* 1991. *(Permission of David C. Turnley/Detroit Free Press.)*

Lieutenant Linda McClory of the 5th MASH Unit cares for a soldier wounded by a grenade during Operation Desert Storm. Almost forty percent of the military medical units are staffed by women, the largest number in any specialty.

This war confirmed again the courage of military nurses and affirmed their willingness to care for the sick and the wounded. All branches of the military were represented. Although much has been written about the history, military aspects, and chronology of the Gulf War, information about the role of nurses is sparse. The reality is, however, that nurses, too, were faced with the threat of biological and chemical warfare and SCUD attacks and tolerated the brown, desolate, dry Gulf landscape.

They put together 'hospitals' from tents to serve as super first-aid stations. In battle, crews of RNs and techs would work close to the scene of action, keeping men from bleeding to death and pushing oxygen and IV fluids. Once stabilized, the wounded would be transported to field hospitals, tended in flight by aerovac crews trained to deal with the impact of altitude on trauma patients.

— *American Journal of Nursing, 1990, p. 7*

David C. Turnley, *Amy Stuart,* 1991. *(Permission of David C. Turnley/Detroit Free Press.)*

During Operation Desert Storm, Amy Stuart, a nurse in the 5th Mobile Army Surgical Hospital, snoozes in her tent with a comforting friend. This was one means to escape the bloodshed of war, if only temporarily.

USNS Comfort, 1987. *(Official U.S. Navy Photo by National Steel and Shipbuilding Co.)*

A starboard bow view of the hospital ship USNS *Comfort* (T-AH-20) underway during sea trials in the Pacific Ocean.

USNS Mercy. *(Official U.S. Navy Photo by National Steel and Shipbuilding Co.)*

A port quarter view of the hospital ship USNS *Mercy* (T-AH-19) underway during sea trials in the Gulf of Mexico.

Field hospitals were typically assembled from eight or nine tents tunneled together; wounded were received as air evacuation teams delivered them. Navy nurses also functioned on the thousand-bed hospital ships, the USNS Comfort and the USNS Mercy, which were deployed to the Gulf. These ships were considered the world's largest trauma centers. Overall, nurses were equipped to handle at least fifteen thousand casualties daily (Kalisch and Kalisch, 1994).

As with previous wars, progress in health care occurred. Frozen blood was prepared for the first time for transfusion. Monoclonal antibody treatments were available for large wounds and multiple-system trauma; improved anti-chemical treatments were in place. The aftermath of this war on nurses remains to be seen, but it is possible that they will also suffer from the unknown and elusive disease (Persian Gulf syndrome) taking its toll on military personnel who served. Posttraumatic stress disorder may also be experienced.

IN HONOR OF . . .

"Mother" Mary Ann Bickerdyke Memorial, located on the lawn of the Knox County Courthouse, Galesburg, Illinois. *(By permission of the Galesburg Public Library, Galesburg, Illinois.)*

A considerable number of memorials have been dedicated to nurses and nursing. The majority can be categorized as ecclesiastical, military, or educational. Those related to military nursing bear testimony to the strong relationship between war and nursing. They represent a variety of methods for bestowing honor, such as through statues, cornerstones, scholarships and loan funds, buildings, chapels, hospital ships, and stained glass windows. One of the most impressive is the Nurses' Monument in Arlington National Cemetery. This monument, which symbolizes the "Spirit of Nursing," was dedicated to Army and Navy nurses. Carved by Frances Luther Rich, the daughter of actress Irene Rich, the monument is made of Tennessee marble. At the unveiling ceremonies on November 8, 1938, Julia C. Stimson, superintendent of the Army Nurse Corps (ret.) and current president of the ANA, made the dedication to "their tenderness and compassion, their competence, courage and human qualities . . . the spirit of nursing of the past, of today, and of the years to come" (*American Journal of Nursing,* 1939, p. 90). The Nurses' Monument, which overlooks the graves from the top of a "hilly slope," was rededicated on March 11, 1971, by the chiefs of the Army, Navy, and Air Force.

A second imposing monument was erected to the memory of a single individual, Mary Ann Bickerdyke from Galesburg, Illinois. Affectionately known as "Mother Bickerdyke" by the sick, wounded, and dying soldiers, she served as a nurse under fire in nineteen battles during the Civil War. This monument was erected on the Public Square in Galesburg in 1903, an event made possible by an appropriation of five thousand dollars by the state of Illinois. On the 125th anniversary (1962) of Knox College in Galesburg, Mary Ann Bickerdyke was remembered with a commemorative cover that was franked with the 1950 U.S. four-cent stamp honoring nursing.

Perhaps the erection of the most recent memorial, the Vietnam Women's Memorial, will finally call attention to the great advances and notable achievements made by nurses during wartime. The service of these "forgotten veterans" is not well known and has received relatively little attention. However, on Veterans' Day, 1993, in Washington, D.C. a dramatic event was witnessed by thirty-five thousand people. On this day the Vietnam Women's Memorial was dedicated to honor the strength, compassion, and service demonstrated by more than 250,000 women during the Vietnam War. Approximately eight thousand nurses served in Vietnam. The dedication was a result of a decade-long struggle spearheaded by Diane Carlson Evans, a former Army nurse and Vietnam veteran. She had been a head nurse at a frontline Army unit in Pleiku, a village near the Cambodian border. This memorial project was not without controversy and rejection. However, with incredible tenacity, perseverance, and teamwork, obstacles were overcome and the project became a reality.

Judy Waid, *Nursing: A Tradition of Caring,* 1991. *(Copyright Judy Waid and District Three, Ohio Nurses Association, Youngstown, Ohio.)*

This second edition medallion is dedicated to all registered nurses of the past and present who have unselfishly served our country in peace and in war, and to those of the future who will do so. It has been those unrecognized heroes and heroines who have cared for American soldiers and dramatically reduced the casualty statistics of all conflicts.

401

Frances Luther Rich, *Spirit of Nursing,*
1938. Tennessee marble. Arlington
National Cemetery, Arlington, Virginia.
(Photograph courtesy of Morton Broffman.)

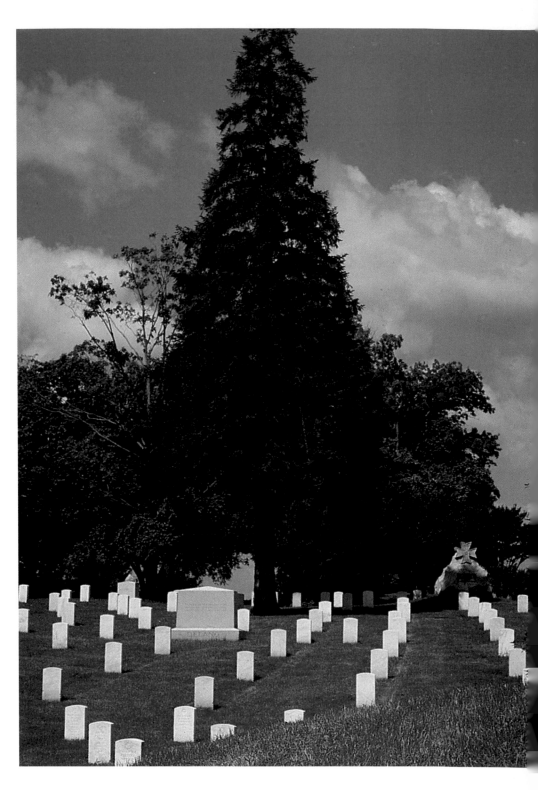

The memorial, a seven-foot bronze sculpture by artist Glenna Goodacre,
beautifully and poignantly portrays four figures: a nurse tending to the chest
wound of a soldier lying across her lap; a woman scanning the sky for a helicopter or assistance; and a kneeling woman staring at an empty helmet, bowing her head in grief and despair. The memorial is a symbol of healing that is
set in a grove of trees three hundred feet from the low, black wall that is the
Vietnam Veterans Memorial. At last—but only after exhausting years of convincing people of the need to honor female veterans, rallying financial support, lobbying Congress, and obtaining government support and permission—there is a visible symbol in the nation's capital that honors women's
patriotic service.

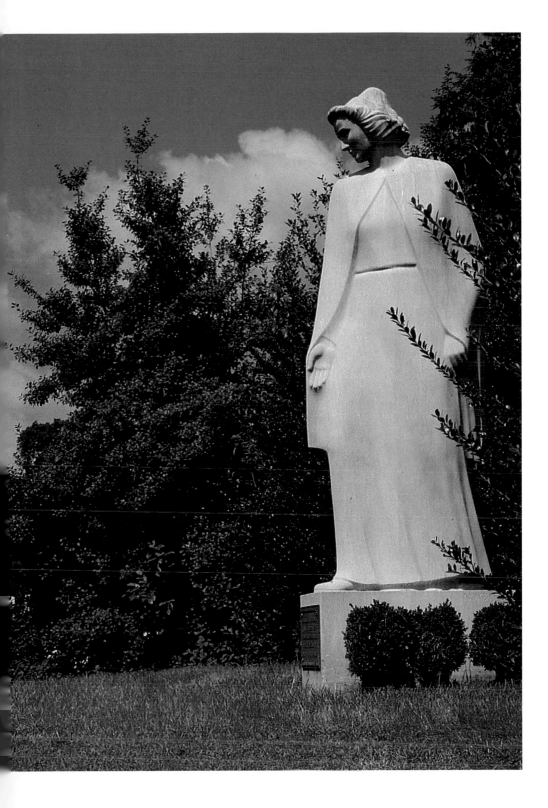

The Spirit of Nursing monument, which looks over the graves at Arlington National Cemetery, stands as a constant reminder of the compassion and bravery of the nation's military nurses. *(Photograph courtesy of Morton Broffman.)*

In 1968, Americans did not want to hear about the suffering of soldiers in an unpopular war, did not want to hear from nurses who served in Vietnam. Yet, nurses have given undeniable, beneficial service under extreme circumstances during every war in which they have served. Their legacy is profound, as is their legacy to society of the whole of nursing. Public recognition of their services, however, has been slow to evolve. Nurses have invested in the future of this country as they have diligently worked with tenderness, compassion, and expertise to comfort the suffering and save lives. It is time that they become *loudly heard and greatly noted* (Donahue, 1995).

✿ IMAGINE A WAR, ANY WAR, WITHOUT NURSES ✿

U N I T   9

The Age of Expansion

A Biblical Fable on Our Origins

In the beginning, God created nursing.
He (or She) said, I will take a solid, simple,
significant system of *education* and an adequate,
applicable base of clinical *research*, and
On these rocks, will I build My greatest gift
to Mankind—nursing practice.
On the seventh day, He—threw up His hands.

And has left it up to us.

— MARGRETTA M. STYLES

Winona Chenevert, *Nursing: Courage, Heart, Brains*, 1991. Oil on canvas, 83.82 × 91.44 cm.
(By permission of Pro-Nurse, Gaithersburg, Maryland.)

This was the second painting designed and commissioned by Melodie Chenevert, RN, and executed by her sister-in-law, Winona Chenevert. Nursing is often pictured as the heart of health care. But being a nurse requires much more. It requires courage and brains as well. These qualities often go unrecognized in nurses just as they did in the characters of *The Wizard of Oz*. The original painting hangs in the Pro-Nurse headquarters from which posters are available.

405

The Age of Expansion

	1920	1930	1940	1950

DAILY LIFE

1941 U.S. Savings Bonds and Stamps go on sale

1945 "Bebop" comes into fashion

1945 Atomic bombs dropped on Hiroshima and Nagasaki

1948 Gandhi assassinated

1953 Queen Elizabeth II crowned

SCIENCE AND TECHNOLOGY

1941 Donald Bailey invents portable military bridge

1942 Enrico Fermi splits the atom

1942 Bell Aircraft tests first U.S. jet plane

1948 Long-playing record invented

THE VISUAL ARTS

1940 Lascaux caves discovered with prehistoric wall paintings, France

1945 Trial of Hans van Meegeren, Dutch painter who forged great paintings

1946 British Arts Council inaugurated

1951 Cinerama invented by Fred Waller

MEDICINE AND HEALTH CARE

1944 Quinine synthesized

1945 Vitamin A synthesized

1950 Antihistamines become popular

NURSING

1920s First doctoral program in nursing education (EdD) at Teachers College

1934 New York University begins PhD and EdD programs in nursing

1950s "Progressive patient care" set into motion

1950s–1970s Emergence of nursing theoretical and conceptual frameworks

1952 Dr. Hildegard Peplau publishes *Interpersonal Relations in Nursing*

1953 Team nursing introduced

1954 Eurovision network founded

1956 Andrea Doria sinks

1957 Words "beat" and "beatnik" come into vogue

1961 Dag Hammarskjöld killed in air accident

1962 *The Sunday Times* issues first color supplement

1964 300 spectators killed in soccer match riots in Lima, Peru

1968 Mickey Mouse celebrates fortieth birthday

1971 Cigarette ads banned from U.S. television

1972 Death of eleven Israeli athletes at Olympics in Munich

1977 Passenger service of Concorde supersonic transport begins

---

1957 U.S.S.R. launches first earth satellites

1959 De Beers manufactures synthetic diamond

1965 First flight around the world over both poles

1978 First ascent of Mt. Everest without artificial oxygen supply

1980 "Baby Fae" receives baboon heart transplant

1959 Joan Miró creates murals for UNESCO building in Paris

1968 Sotheby's of London sells four hundred impressionist and modern paintings in three days

1975 Life-sized pottery figures (six thousand) from third century BC found in northwest China

1982 Vietnam Veterans War Memorial dedicated in Washington, D.C.

1956 Albert Sabin develops oral polio vaccine

1966 Michael De Bakey implants plastic arteries leading to external artificial heart, providing bypass during valve replacement surgery

1976 Discovery of viral cause of multiple sclerosis

1981 Acquired Immune Deficiency Syndrome (AIDS) identified

1981 Valve inserted into skull of human fetus to prevent hydrocephalus

---

1955 American Nurses' Foundation established for research grants to graduate nurses

1960s Growth of specialization in nursing

1963 Loeb Center for Nursing and Rehabilitation established at Montefiore Hospital

1965 The "nurse practitioner" introduced at the University of Colorado

1965 American Nurses Association position paper on nursing education released

1969 American Association of Colleges of Nursing established

1970s Advent of primary nursing

1971 National Black Nurses Association established

1971 M. Lucille Kinlein establishes herself as independent practitioner

1973 American Academy of Nursing established

1978 International History of Nursing Society formed

As the end of the twentieth century is approaching, nursing stands poised between the past and the future. The question of what lies ahead is open to speculation, since the state of nursing's art is ever changing and responsive to societal needs. The twentieth century has been marked by many changes in the healing arts; some are in striking contrast to earlier epochs in history.

Maurice Cliot, *Aspirine—Usine de Rohne,* early twentieth century. Poster. *(Philadelphia Museum of Art. Gift of William H. Helfand.)*

The emerging recognition of the professional role of the nurse led to the use of nurses in advertising. It is possible that this is one of the first advertising posters in which a nurse is used to promote a product.

Yet many of the extraordinary innovations that have occurred are continuations of contributions from the past. These changes have resulted from an interplay of numerous factors that have arisen in an increasingly technological age.

There is little doubt that nursing practice has been forced to make severe accommodations within this larger societal context as knowledge has continued to increase and attitudes and values have shifted. Nursing practice has expanded and extended in both horizontal and vertical directions. Some believe that this expansion has been too great and that professional growth comes by limiting functions rather than by extending them; they believe that the focus of concentration should be on the functions that are of a professional nature and integral to nursing. They argue that nursing has gone too far and that it has begun to encroach on the medical domain. Others believe that the expanded roles in nursing fulfill a vital need and provide health care services where either none exist or services are limited. In addition, the assumption of additional functions by nurses is viewed as necessary so that the best possible care be rendered. Whatever the case, the changing environment has called for an education to keep pace with the modern world. Yet the struggle for the

Vignettes of the New York Ambulance Service. Engraving. *Harper's Weekly,* May 24, 1884. *(National Library of Medicine, Bethesda, Maryland.)*

inclusion of educational programs for nursing in institutions of higher learning still continues at a time when education is needed more than ever to develop individuals who can deal with the problems of adjustment in modern life. Alfred North Whitehead, a scientist and philosopher, issued a warning in 1929 that is relevant to nursing's current educational situation:

> In the conditions of modern life, the rule is absolute, the race which does not value trained intelligence is doomed. Not all your heroism, not all your social charm, not all your wit, not all your victories on land or at sea can move back the finger of fate. Today we maintain ourselves. Tomorrow science will have moved forward yet one more step, and there will be no appeal from the judgment which will then be pronounced on the uneducated.
>
> — *Whitehead, 1929, p. 22*

The education of nurses for the future must provide for the society of the future. At the same time, the full potentialities of individual nurses and nursing at large must not be sacrificed.

The scientific, technological, and societal movements of the twentieth century have had a significant effect on the development of health care and on the direction of nursing services. A wide spectrum of change has occurred and catapulted society from the horse-and-buggy era to the space age. Diseases such as smallpox, diphtheria, and cholera, which virtually devastated populations in the past, are now rare or nonexistent. Scientific advances have made it possible for humans to prolong life: sophisticated diagnostic methods permit visualization of the most minute internal structures of the human body; anesthetic agents and improved asepsis enhance surgical practice; grafts and transplants of healthy structures or even mechanical devices are used to replace diseased organs; miracle drugs wipe out formerly hopeless infections and bacterial diseases; the inner workings of the cell are open to scrutiny through physical and chemical means; and the hospital has moved from pesthouse to comprehensive health care center.

Artist's depiction of the complex of The University of Iowa Hospitals and Clinics, 1995. *(Courtesy of The University of Iowa Hospitals and Clinics, Iowa City, Iowa/Warren Paris.)*

Visiting nurse wrapping the leg of an elderly woman, c. 1920s. A bird cage and crutches are in the background. *(Courtesy of the Visiting Nurse Association of Maryland.)*

Visiting nurse wrapping the leg and brace of a child while mother, father, and siblings watch, c. 1920s. *(Courtesy of the Visiting Nurse Association of Maryland.)*

Other current events and social issues were also influencing, either directly or indirectly, the health care delivery system and the roles and functions of its providers. During the first fifty years of the twentieth century many factors gave impetus to the progress of nursing: two world wars, self-organization of nurses, government and nursing legislation, problems of social welfare, support of health care fields by national foundations, and the complexities of medicine. In the latter part of the century other social movements profoundly influenced health care and nursing; these included the rise of consumerism (the increased awareness and expectations of the patient for quality in health care delivery), changes in work and leisure patterns, the fight for civil rights, progress in public health, the development of voluntary and governmental health care organizations, and the struggle for equal rights for women. All these factors—combined with the internal forces in nursing of consciousness raising, role innovation, and the drive for professionalization—shaped the role of the nurse and nursing (Reeder, 1978).

As the twentieth century witnessed improvements in the general standard of living; significant progress in transportation, communications, and other areas; and the lengthening of the life span, industrialization transformed rural America into an urban society. The social scene was marked by increasing change and complexity in nearly every field of endeavor. Urban centers rapidly became overcrowded because of an unprecedented population expansion and the unrestricted immigration of millions of poor Europeans. Health problems were aggravated, and problems in the provision of adequate health care

C.J. Taylor, *Remember Hospital Sunday.* Cover of *Puck,* December 22, 1886. *(Courtesy of the Library of Congress, Washington, D.C.)*

This cover appeared as a plea for public support of volunteer hospitals. The woman helping the injured man is wearing a hair band with the word "charity" written across it.

were intensified. Hospital services were broadened to provide for middle-class patients as well as the indigent and homeless. Consequently the whole concept of nursing had to be reevaluated and changed to fit the needs of this age of reform.

THE CHANGING SCENE IN NURSING

Numerous changes have occurred in nursing throughout the course of the twentieth century. The advent of new drugs, new techniques, and new technologies has placed new responsibilities on nurses and has mandated radical changes in nursing care. The patient care of today is of necessity different from that given at the time of Florence Nightingale, since nurses are expected to perform many tasks formerly performed by physicians. Before the 1930s few graduate nurses were employed by hospitals because most nursing care was given by nursing students. At that time "nursing" included a variety of non-nursing tasks such as scrubbing floors, carrying trays, and cleaning equipment, in addition to the so-called routine care of patients. The students were left with relatively little time to give adequate nursing care—let alone incorporate a holistic approach to that care.

By the 1940s many more tasks and procedures were being performed by nurses as a result of the introduction of new innovations in health care. Nurses' functions then included blood pressure measurement, suctioning in a variety of conditions, transfusion assistance, oxygen administration, medication injection, and other more sophisticated techniques. Nurses were also assisting in operating rooms, delivery rooms, and outpatient facilities. More and more individuals were being admitted to hospitals to have greater numbers of procedures performed as these institutions became safer and more efficient. This phenomenon was significantly enhanced by the advent of hospitalization insurance and prepayment plans for hospital care. In *Nursing for the Future*, Esther Lucile Brown reported that in one large teaching hospital more than a hundred procedures (exclusive of operating, obstetrical, and outpatient services) were being performed by nurses. This finding is substantiated by Dennison:

> [Nurses] managed the apparatus for Wangensteen suction, tidal irrigation, and bladder decompression. They irrigated eyes, cecostomies, colostomies, and draining wounds. They did artificial respiration, applied sterile compresses, and painted lesions . . . They did catheterizations, sitz baths, and turpentine stupes. They gave insulin and taught the patient or his relatives to give the drug and examine urine. They administered approximately 1500 medications daily, by mouth or hypodermic. They assisted with lumbar punctures, thoracenteses . . . and phlebotomies.
>
> — *Dennison, 1942, p. 777*

Nursing shortages occurred periodically throughout the twentieth century. Even the belief that there would be an oversupply of nurses for civilian work after World War II was dashed. Many nurses stopped practicing to devote time to their family responsibilities. Many nurses did not return to practice, their answer to an authoritarian and paternalistic system in which they had no participation in planning or decision making. Many refused to be involved in a work structure that offered few rewards, long hours, hard physical labor, and very low salaries.

Compounding this situation were other significant events that led to the gradual development of a new organizational pattern for hospital care. The demonstrated success of resuscitation stations on the front lines in World War II led to the emergence of special units for patient care. Postanesthesia and recovery rooms were established to prevent postoperative complications. Eventually this change was to transfer to a broader concept, the intensive care

unit, after the use of Mobile Army Surgical Hospital (MASH) units in the Korean conflict. Progression from the intensive care unit to the intermediate care, self-care, long-term care, and home care units was thus possible. This concept of "progressive patient care" was set into motion and was in operation by the middle 1950s (Haldeman and Abdellah, 1959). This development of specific types of units, although advantageous in many respects, created the need for specialized nursing skills and varying nurse–patient ratios in some areas, which contributed further to the nursing shortage.

As the ranks of nurses continued to diminish and new nursing demands increased, "team nursing" was introduced. This new, different method of assignment used fewer well-prepared personnel. It was designed to fit particular assignments to the background and expertise of the provider of service. In philosophic terms team nursing was a system whereby different types of hospital nursing personnel could be placed into teams to provide quality nursing care for groups of patients. The professional nurse would directly supervise all patients and team members. In addition, team conferences would be held for planning and evaluation, nursing care plans would ensure continuity of care, and in-service education and on-the-job training would be provided as necessary (Lambertsen, 1953). However, the quality of nursing care and patient satisfaction diminished as fewer registered professional nurses were giving direct care to patients. The work was indeed coordinated, but the nursing care was fragmented. This was particularly disastrous as major advances in diagnostic and treatment procedures and the development of sophisticated technology continued. The 1950s and 1960s were a revolutionary time for health care:

> A sampling of major advances during the two decades includes the development of the heart-lung machine, open heart surgery, high-frequency implements for blood coagulation, and new vaccines, pharmaceuticals, and monitoring devices. The expanding field of medical science had made nursing care increasingly more complex and had made demands of increasing gravity on nurses as well. To effectively give care, nurses needed to be able to identify very subtle changes in patients' status, learn new sophisticated treatment techniques, increase their ability to interpret laboratory data, recognize delicate physiological interrelationships, and closely monitor the efficacy of potent and sometimes experimental forms of drug therapy.
>
> — *Fitzpatrick, 1983, pp. 34–35*

It became clear that a different approach to nursing care was needed, one that would provide both quality and holistic framework. A movement was begun in the 1960s to close the gap between the professional nurse and the patient. It was initiated as an important innovation in 1963 through the efforts of Lydia Hall, who was the inspiration behind the philosophy and work of the Loeb Center for Nursing and Rehabilitation at Montefiore Hospital in New York. The overall purpose of this center is to provide continuous, high-quality nursing care that emphasizes the facilitation of healing, prevention of complications, promotion of health, and prevention of recurrences and new illnesses. Nursing care is given solely by professional nurses in a setting that enhances the movement of the patient from the general hospital to home. The nurse is the *primary factor* in patient care and coordinates the combined efforts of the patient, the family, and the nurse in the solving of problems that might hinder ultimate recovery. Medicine and allied fields are viewed as ancillary treatment. In this structure the assumption is made that less medical care is needed; more professional nursing care and teaching are needed (Hall, 1963). Slowly, other such attempts were made by acute care hospitals under the guise of "comprehensive" or "total" nursing care. However, nurses were frustrated in their efforts by inadequate staffing, emphasis on efficiency, and lack of regard for patient orientation.

416

It was not until the 1970s that the combined goal of nursing care by professional nurses and total patient care (holistic approach) began to be realized with the advent of primary nursing. The primary nurse is responsible for the patient's total care for the entire hospitalization period, twenty-four hours a day, seven days a week. High-quality nursing care is promoted through this modality because the primary nurse assumes responsibility for the entire spectrum of functions, including teaching, consultation, comprehensive care with continuity, planning and evaluation of care, documentation of progress, discharge planning, and referrals to ancillary services or agencies (Marram, Barrett, and Bevis, 1979). When the primary nurse is not physically present, an associate nurse follows the plan of care. In this system nurses truly can be patients' advocates, they can be accountable for their own practice, and they can make decisions based on available data.

Although primary nursing has grown in popularity since its inception, its success has depended on adequate staffing, administrative support, and technically and educationally prepared nurses. It has been received favorably by patients, and it has been hoped that it will gain total recognition and acceptance by health care delivery systems. The best argument for the implementation of primary nursing is that it has the greatest potential for placing the patient in an environment conducive to the attainment of wellness.

Some primary nurses now engage in private practice or share a private practice with a physician. One such "independent practitioner," M. Lucille Kinlein, hung out her shingle in May 1971. Others engage in various alternative methods of care. For example, Dr. Delores Krieger, a professor of nursing at New York University, has repopularized the theory of therapeutic touch. She has achieved national recognition for her expertise in this area and has taught many nurses and other individuals to use this therapy.

Although great strides have been made in nursing, problems continue. Working conditions and environments are still sources of conflict. Nurses continue to voice their concerns regarding inadequate staffing, low wages, long hours, unsafe practices, nurses' inability to use their own knowledge, judgment, and decision-making abilities, and other circumstances that prohibit the rendering of high-quality nursing care. When all attempts at communication have failed, nurses have turned to organization through local units of the state professional organization or other types of bargaining units.

The nurses of today are expected to be many things to many people and to function in a variety of settings. They are to be excellent caregivers, adequate researchers, seekers of knowledge, and thinkers grounded in scientific and logical thought. Nurses are involved with scientific and technical advances and with all types of new roles that have broadened their opportunities but increased their scope of responsibilities. They are slowly but steadily moving toward a goal of holistic treatment for all individuals in a structure that is not always supportive. Nurses will continue to meet the challenges of the future identified by Florence Nightingale:

> No system can endure that does not march. Are we walking to the future or to the past? Are we progressing or are we stereotyping? We remember that we have scarcely crossed the threshold of uncivilized civilization in nursing; there is still so much to do. Don't let us stereotype mediocrity. We are still on the threshold of nursing.
>
> In the future, which I shall not see, for I am old, may a better way be opened! May the methods by which every infant, every human being will have the best chance of health, the methods by which every sick person will have the best chance of recovery, be learned and practiced! Hospitals are only an intermediate state of civilization never intended, at all events, to take in the whole sick population.
>
> — *Nightingale, 1860*

Facing page, Winslow Homer, *The Nurse,* 1867. Oil on wood. *(Collection of Mrs. Norman B. Woolworth, New York.)*

The connotations of the word "nurse" have changed throughout history. A woman who cares for and tends young children became synonymous with a nurse. Homer's painting originally included a baby looking over the woman's shoulder. The baby's shawl is still visible.

A.E. Foringer, *The Greatest Mother In The World*, World War I poster. Lithograph. *(National Archives and Records Administration, Washington, D.C.)*

Nursing Research

Nursing research is new, yet old. Florence Nightingale is generally regarded as the first "nurse researcher," since her nursing reforms were based on careful investigation. Undoubtedly the first research report ever written by a nurse was "Notes on Matters Affecting the Health, Efficiency and Hospital Administration of the British Army" by Nightingale. It was hurriedly prepared within a year of her return from the Crimea in 1856 and printed privately by her for distribution among influential government officials and friends. This report combined the techniques of both qualitative and quantitative research. In one thousand pages she reported detailed observations of medicine and nursing in the Crimea and documented facts and figures with vital statistics.

In recognition of her great contribution to the field of social statistics, Nightingale was made a fellow in the Royal Statistical Society in 1858 and was granted an honorary membership in the American Statistical Society in 1874. Sir Francis Galton acknowledged her preeminence in statistics. Queen Victoria regretted that she could not have Nightingale, with her exceptional abilities, in the War Office. One author's comments illustrate her deep commitment to this field of endeavor:

> Miss Nightingale's attitude towards the application of statistics in the field of social dynamics was very similar to that of Thomas Buckle; they both deplored the fact that a wealth of data was available, but unapplied. Her typically practical philosophy demanded that if statistics were to be useful, they must be used. They must aid in the establishment of preventive measures. . . .
>
> Florence Nightingale was determined to make statistics an active reality which would influence the general welfare as well as the health of man. . . .
>
> — *Newton, 1949, p. 33*

Florence Nightingale's "coxcomb" diagram showing the extent of needless deaths from April 1854 to March 1855 in British military hospitals during the Crimean War. Each colored wedge is proportional to the number of casualties being represented. From her book *Notes of Matters Affecting the Health, Efficiency and Hospital Administration of the British Army*, 1858. *(By permission of the Houghton Library, Harvard University, Cambridge, Massachusetts.)*

Florence Nightingale recognized the value of medical statistics as a method for improving medical care in both military and civilian hospitals. She developed graphical representations of statistics, which she called "coxcombs." These were polar-area charts; those statistics being represented were proportional to the area of a wedge in a circular diagram.

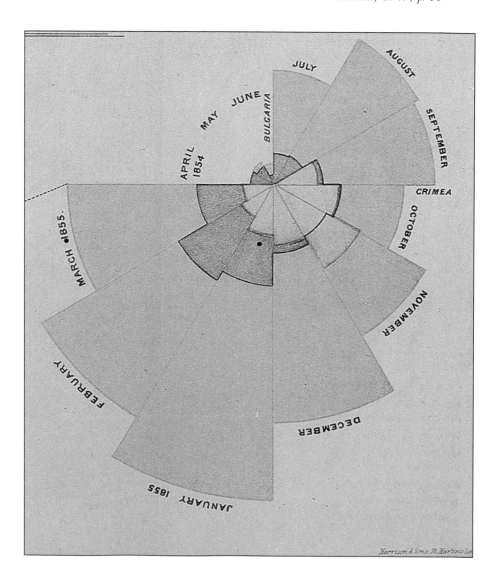

Although the Nightingale tradition of education was transmitted to the United States, the approach to and use of research was not. In addition, the "training schools" in the United States were not conducive to the development of critical thinking or problem solving. Inquiring minds were not fostered through the prevailing atmosphere of rigid discipline and unquestioning obedience. These elements, which were strong influences within nursing schools, reduced individualism, creativity, critical thinking, and assertiveness. They served to place students and graduate nurses in a subservient role, a position where they remained for many years. In some instances, even currently employed nurses believe that nursing is still held to a subservient role and that gains made to improve the situation are being consistently eroded.

The environment in which nursing operated was not conducive to nursing research; nor were nurses prepared with the skills to pursue it. Relatively few research studies in nursing were conducted in the United States before 1930. In this era nursing was helplessly swept along with rapid hospital expansion and the proliferation of training schools for nurses. These insistent demands shoved the need for studies into the background. It was also during this time that professional nursing organizations had their beginnings. It is no wonder that the early leaders were thus diverted from independent research and writing to the improvement in training of nurses and organizational activities.

The need for nursing research was recognized by the early leaders, who were committed to the scientific method of collecting and interpreting data to generate new knowledge for the improvement of nursing care. Probably the earliest American research report, written by M. Adelaide Nutting, was *The Educational Status of Nursing* (1912). A comprehensive analysis of nursing during this period, the report revealed the appalling practices and conditions under which student nurses functioned. Other reports followed during the first half of the twentieth century, as did studies of nursing practice, nursing services, nursing education, nursing service administration, and virtually every field related to nursing. The majority of these were done by individuals who were not nurses.

Leadership ability in the area of nursing research was demonstrated early by Isabel M. Stewart. Although her activities and interests in this area were not widely known, they were nonetheless significant. Intrigued by the time and motion studies for improvement of efficiency in industry and home economics, Stewart began to investigate the potential of this technique for nursing. She visited Dr. and Mrs. Frank Gilbreth, who set up beds in the living room of their home in Providence, Rhode Island, for use as a laboratory. This was the beginning of Isabel Stewart's attempt at an activity analysis of nursing to differentiate between nursing and nonnursing functions. This minimal study still provides standards of nursing care that are useful in current nursing practice. From this meager beginning Stewart continued her pursuits and conducted research in nursing and nursing education. She studied philosophical, educational, and historical research methods and incorporated these into her books and other writings. Eventually she published the *Teachers College Nursing Education Bulletin,* possibly the first research journal in nursing. This was done in the face of opposition from other nurses, whose concept of research was limited to test-tube methods. In an editorial in 1929 Isabel Stewart explained her position:

> If nursing is ever to justify its name as an applied science, if it is ever to free itself from these old superficial, haphazard methods, some way must be found to submit all our practices as rapidly as possible to the most searching tests which modern science can devise. Not only bacteriological and physiological and chemical tests are needed, but economic and psychological and sociological measurements also, if they are appropriate and workable. There is not much use waiting for someone outside our own body to recognize our critical situation and to offer to do the work for us. Some help may be secured from physicians and from

experts in other fields, but most of the experimentation that is done will have to be carried on in all probability by our own members. Nurses may not be prepared to make the more difficult studies at once, but if a few will prepare themselves to start in a small way and to show what can be done, others will undoubtedly become interested, and in time, resources will be found, if the results warrant them.

— *Stewart, 1929, p. 3*

Stewart firmly believed that students should receive a research orientation, and she involved them in studies and projects that were needed or were under investigation. Thus she incorporated research training into the program of graduate study in nursing education. She recognized, however, that not all individuals were "fitted" for investigation, so she proposed that a few minds could take a lead in such activities. With that goal in mind, Stewart consistently urged that graduate students have more advanced preparation in research. Student reaction was positive, as described by McManus:

> Inspired, prodded and encouraged by Miss Stewart, an increasing number of students did undertake doctoral study. Without her interest, support, and patient understanding, I know I could and would not have persevered toward that goal; I am sure this is true of many others of her students. . . .
>
> Miss Stewart laid the firm foundation for nursing research and research preparation in the Division of Nursing Education at Teachers College.

— *McManus, 1962, p. 6*

As a lasting tribute to Stewart's impact on nursing research, Teachers College in 1961 opened a fund with a goal of four hundred thousand dollars to establish the *Isabel Maitland Stewart Research Professorship in Nursing and Nursing Education*.

A series of events eventually transpired that led to a decided commitment to the incorporation of nursing research in the overall structure of nursing. Sigma Theta Tau initiated a research fund in the 1930s to develop an awareness of the need for research. The Association of Collegiate Schools of Nursing (ACSN) sponsored a special forum on nursing research in 1941. The House of Delegates of the American Nurses Association (ANA) approved a research program in 1950. This program was designed as a long-term research project to study (1) nursing functions in a variety of settings and geographical locations and (2) nurses' relationships with their co-workers and associates. Membership fees were used to fund these studies, which included interviews, activity classifications, and observational studies of nurses on the job. Teachers College established the Institute of Research and Service in Nursing Education during the early 1950s to provide a full-time mechanism for studying and developing nursing education through research. Launching of the journal *Nursing Research* in 1952 was evidence of nursing's promotion and communication of research and scholarly productivity. The first issue was sent to approximately eight thousand subscribers across the United States and to twenty-two other countries. Increasing numbers of nursing researchers quickly adopted this journal as necessary and basic reading. In 1955 the American Nurses Foundation was organized as a membership corporation of the ANA. The purposes of this foundation were to provide research grants to graduate nurses for scientific and educational projects; to conduct studies, surveys, and research; to provide grants to public and private nonprofit educational institutions; and to publish scientific, educational, and literary work. The ANA Board of Directors had donated one hundred thousand dollars to the Foundation specifically for use during 1955 for studies of nursing functions. This donation was followed by the establishment of a Commission on Nursing Research (1970) and a Council of Nurse Researchers (1972) in the ANA.

Government funds for nursing research began to be allocated at the end of World War II. Between 1940 and 1956, small grants were awarded to numerous individuals and institutions for various research projects through the

Nursing Research, cover of the first issue, 1952. *(By permission of the American Journal of Nursing Company, New York.)*

Department of Health, Education and Welfare. An extramural grant program in nursing research was originated in the United States Public Health Service's Division of Nursing Resources in the fiscal year 1956. Monies were awarded to qualified researchers for projects in nursing. This was the first time grants from federal sources were made available for nursing research. Federal support of research training for nurses was also provided in a twofold approach: through special predoctoral fellowships established by the Division of Nursing Resources in 1954 and in 1962 through nurse-scientist graduate training grants to both assist institutions with development of nursing research competence and provide stipends for graduate nursing students preparing for research. Finally, the integration of research in nursing into all nursing collegiate educational programs was accomplished in the 1970s.

The value of nursing research, which has already been demonstrated, will become even more important as nursing continues its march toward professional status and excellence in performance. Research has proven to be a mechanism of generating new knowledge for nursing that will ultimately ensure quality of nursing care. A growing acceptance of nursing research has occurred as this area has become recognized as an effective method for cost containment. The most efficient and effective modes of nursing can be identified through nursing research.

Nursing Theory

Nursing has been one of several "semiprofessions" involved in an extensive campaign to achieve full professional status. One characteristic associated with established professions is the acquisition of a unique body of scientific knowledge through vigorous training. Discussions regarding the development of nursing theories to assist with this generation of knowledge and to assist with the definition and identification of the unique role and functions of nursing have taken place since the middle 1960s and early 1970s. The origins of nursing theories, however, go back much farther. Some individuals in nursing identify Florence Nightingale as the first nursing theorist. She, indeed, followed principles related to cleanliness, fresh air, good food, rest, sleep, and exercise. She was the first individual to define and describe nursing in her *Notes on Nursing: What It Is and What It Is Not.* She did have significant thoughts, ideas, and principles, although at times they were disjointed. Yet one must systematically analyze these according to defined criteria to establish whether they constituted a theory.

The struggle to clearly identify a unique knowledge base for nursing (nursing science) has been continuous, particularly in relation to defining and describing the functions of nursing. Definitions of these functions were published by the ANA in 1932, 1937, and 1955. However, they lacked specificity and prompted individual nurses to write their own. Two of the pioneers in this area were Virginia Henderson and Hildegard Peplau. Henderson's definition of nursing was first published in 1955, and it was revised in 1966.

> The unique function of the nurse is to assist the individual (sick or well), in the performance of those activities contributing to health or its recovery (or to peaceful death) that he would perform unaided if he had the necessary strength, will, or knowledge. And to do this in such a way as to help him gain independence as rapidly as possible.
>
> — *Henderson, 1966, p. 15*

In 1952 Peplau published *Interpersonal Relations in Nursing,* which described four phases of the nurse-client relationship and led to numerous studies in the communication area. She brought interpersonal theories from psychiatry into nursing as a basis for the analysis of these interactions in terms of therapeutic quality. It is possible that this work was one of the first proposed theoretical frameworks for nursing. Ida J. Orlando (1961) offered communications theory for the description of what she labeled "a deliberate nursing approach." Imogene M. King (1971) later began to explain the intricate transactional process between nurse and patient.

A significant catalyst in the movement for the development of nursing theory was Martha E. Rogers, whose work was a vivid testimony for nursing to be recognized as a science:

> The science of nursing is an emergent—a new product. The inevitability of its development is written in nursing's long commitment to human health and welfare. With today's rapid and unprecedented changes, new urgency has been added to the critical need for a body of scientific knowledge specific to nursing. Only as the science of nursing takes on form and substance can the art of nursing achieve new dimensions of artistry.
>
> The science of nursing aims to provide a body of abstract knowledge growing out of scientific research and logical analysis and capable of being translated into nursing practice.
>
> — *Rogers, 1970, pp. 83, 86*

The need for and development of nursing theories were prominent issues in the 1970s. Several "theories" and "conceptual frameworks" emerged through the diligence of such individuals as Sister Callista Roy, Martha E. Rogers, Imogene M. King, Dorothea Orem, and Margaret A. Newman. A question still posed by some in nursing, however, is whether any of these are

Virginia Henderson

Hildegard E. Peplau

Ida J. Orlando

Imogene M. King

indeed *theories* or whether they are all *conceptual frameworks.* Indeed, many of the nurses who fall into the category of theorist do not consider themselves theorists, nor did they intend to develop a theory. Marriner-Tomey (1994) clustered the theorists into the following categories, which are particularly useful for the analysis and synthesis of their work:

Philosophies (analysis, reasoning, and logical argument used to identify nursing phenomena)
    Florence Nightingale: Modern Nursing
    Ernestine Wiedenbach: Helping Art of Clinical Nursing
    Virginia Henderson: Definition of Nursing
    Faye Glenn Abdellah: Twenty-one Nursing Problems
    Lydia E. Hall: Core, Care, and Cure Model
    Jean Watson: Philosophy and Science of Caring
    Patricia Benner: From Novice to Expert—Excellence and Power in
        Clinical Nursing Practice

Conceptual models or grand theories (broad in scope and usually require further specificity and distribution of theoretical statements for empirical testing and verification)
    Dorothea E. Orem: Self-Care Deficit Theory of Nursing
    Myra Estrin Levine: Four Conservation Principles
    Martha E. Rogers: Unitary Human Beings
    Dorothy E. Johnson: Behavioral System Model
    Sister Callista Roy: Adaptation Model
    Josephine G. Paterson and Loretta T. Zderad: Humanistic Nursing
    Betty Neuman: Systems Model
    Imogene M. King: Theory of Goal Attainment

Nursing theories in middle range (more precise than grand theories that focus on developing theoretical statements to answer questions about nursing)
    Hildegard E. Peplau: Psychodynamic Nursing
    Ida Jean Orlando: Nursing Process Theory
    Joyce Travelbee: Human-to Human Relationship Model
    Joan Riehl-Sisca: Symbolic Interactionism
    Helen C. Erickson and Evelyn M. Tomlin: Modeling and
        Role Modeling
    Ramona T. Mercer: Maternal Role Attainment
    Kathryn E. Barnard: Parent-Child Interaction Model
    Madeleine Leininger: Cultural Care Theory
    Rosemarie Rizzo Parse: Man-Living-Health
    Joyce J. Fitzpatrick: Life Perspective Rhythm Model
    Margaret A. Newman: Model of Health
    Evelyn Adam: Conceptual Model of Nursing
    Nola J. Pender: The Health Promotion Model

Martha E. Rogers

Margaret A. Newman

Dorothea E. Orem

Sister Callista Roy

Charles Emile Callandre de Champmartin, *After Death, Study of a Severed Head,* 1818-1819. Oil on canvas, 45.6 × 55.6 cm. *(A.A. Munger Collection. Photograph copyright 1994, The Art Institute of Chicago. All rights reserved.)*

The emphasis on dying in early nursing educational programs was on the care of the patient after death, which entailed postmortem care and getting the body ready for the morgue. Since the 1960s, nursing has steadily incorporated all aspects of the dying process — physical, psychological, and spiritual—into holistic nursing practice.

Nursing is beginning to be recognized as a legitimate science, but a continuing momentum is necessary to achieve this goal. The united efforts of nurse scholars and practitioners of nursing are needed to assist with the identification of a knowledge base for nursing and to formulate a theory or theories to validate professional practice. There is no doubt that differing conceptualizations of nursing will contribute to its ongoing evolution and will enrich the discipline's knowledge of the environment, health, human beings, and nursing.

Educational Advancement

The history of education in nursing at the master's level is rather vague because information about these programs was not available until midcentury. What is known about the earlier programs is that they differed in organization and structure, varied in requirements, admitted students at differing times throughout the year, and used a variety of labels. Even more significant, initially all the postdiploma programs were considered "postgraduate education" and were identified as such. Therefore it was difficult to differentiate between some baccalaureate and master's level programs.

The growth of university nurse educational programs sparked graduate study in nursing. The lack of prepared nurses for teaching and administrative positions was apparent, and the need to rectify this weakness was pressing. Master's degree programs were thus initiated and soon became viewed as the level for specialization in teaching and administration. Fitzpatrick (1983) described the following phases in this development that incorporate primary influences and changes.

Origins: 1939–1952. The phase of origins relates to the difficulty in tracing the development of nurse education programs. However, several important events were occurring. Baccalaureate programs of varying types were increasing in number. *Nursing for the Future* (1948) was published, and an accreditation system was established in 1949—both promoted the elucidation of the nature of collegiate education. An informal group of representatives from five New York schools was convened by R. Louise McManus. This group proposed baccalaureate education as a beginning level and the master's as the specialized degree.

Transitional Stage: 1953–1964. It was during the eleven years of the transitional stage that master's level was recognized as the advanced level of nursing education. A conference on graduate education was sponsored by the National League for Nursing (NLN) in 1954 and 1955. Guidelines were formulated for organization, administration, curriculum, and testing, and a Subcommittee on Graduate Education in Nursing (of the NLN) was created. The emphasis in content at the master's level vacillated and moved from both clinical and functional role preparation in all programs for teachers, administrators, and clinical specialists to the elimination of double preparation in the late 1960s, as clinical specialization became extremely popular. A shift occurred once again in the 1980s, as the position in favor of double preparation gained momentum.

Regionalization. Regional planning in graduate education was begun in the 1950s with the development of two organizations: the Southern Regional Educational Board (SREB) and the Western Interstate Commission on Higher Education (WICHE). Both were committed to better nursing through strong master's degree programs to prepare faculty. The Western Interstate Commission for Higher Education in Nursing (WICHEN), was begun in the western area of the country in 1955 to promote graduate and professional education in the health fields. These programs contributed greatly to graduate education that was research based.

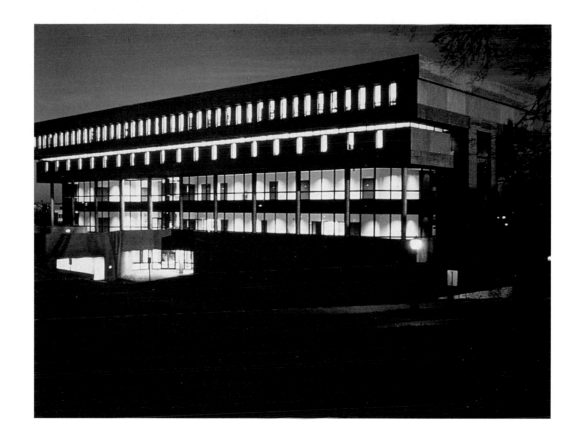

Maturing of Education at the Master's Level: 1964–1975. Master's level education in nursing matured and became an important credential for nurses in leadership positions during these years. Increased interest in research and an expanding number of graduate programs in clinical specialties occurred. The Nurse Training Act of 1964 (Title VIII of the Public Health Service Act, H.R. 10042) provided a comprehensive financial package for nursing school construction, faculty development, special projects grants, student loans, and merit scholarships. Between 1964 and 1971, more than $334 million was appropriated by Congress for nursing education.

Master's level graduate study has become firmly entrenched in the structure of nursing education. There are continuing discussions regarding both the purpose and the product of such an education. Consequently the emphasis in content periodically shifts in relation to prevailing philosophies, nursing care needs, social forces, and health care reform. However, educational upgrading is apparent: the number of nurses attaining master's degrees is rapidly increasing.

Social forces that have affected the development of nursing have also influenced the development of doctoral education in nursing. Although the first graduate courses and graduate programs of study originated in 1899 at Teachers College, many years passed before a bona fide doctoral program came into being. The first doctoral program in nursing was initiated at Teachers College, Columbia University, about 1920 and led to a doctorate in nursing education (Ed.D.). The evolution of additional programs was a slow process directly related to nursing's continuing struggle for respect, credibility, recognition, and power. One author has summarized the difficulty of this growth in the following way.

> The evolution of the nursing profession has occurred within a political context that has placed many constraints upon the developmental process. Conflicts within administrative hierarchy, the effects of sexism, and circumscribed roles for

The University of Iowa College of Nursing, Iowa City, Iowa. (Photo: Larry Perkins, The University of Iowa, Medical Photography.)

women are but a few of the constraints. In this context, doctoral education for nurses and in nursing is but another step in the overall struggle for independence and recognition of worth.

— *Grace, 1978, p. 114*

Other factors inhibited a rapid growth in doctoral preparation for nurses, including the following: nursing was perceived solely as a practice discipline; there was a fear that nurses might become too knowledgeable and pose a threat to the medical hierarchy; a retarded growth in master's degree programs resulted in an inadequate pool of doctoral candidates until the 1960s; the nature, orientation, and direction of the nursing doctorate was not clearly defined; and a body of scientific knowledge was lacking.

In 1934 New York University followed Teachers College with doctorates in philosophy (Ph. D.) and education (Ed. D.) in nursing. In 1954 the University of Pittsburgh established a doctoral program in maternal-child nursing. The first doctorate in nursing science (D.N.S.) in psychiatric nursing was initiated at Boston University in 1960. Since there were so few doctoral programs in nursing before 1960, most nurses who sought doctoral preparation were forced to pursue degrees in other fields. Education was the most popular field; the natural, behavioral, and biological sciences were the other chosen areas of study. In 1964 the University of California–San Francisco established the doctorate in nursing science in several nursing specialties.

According to Styles (1977), the history of doctoral education divided itself into two logical components: the early years, which were dominated by doctoral education *for* nurses, and the current years, with their emphasis on doctoral education *in* nursing. This is consistent with Grace's discussion

Nurse With a Newborn Baby. (Courtesy of The University of Iowa Hospitals and Clinics, Department of Nursing, Iowa City, Iowa.)

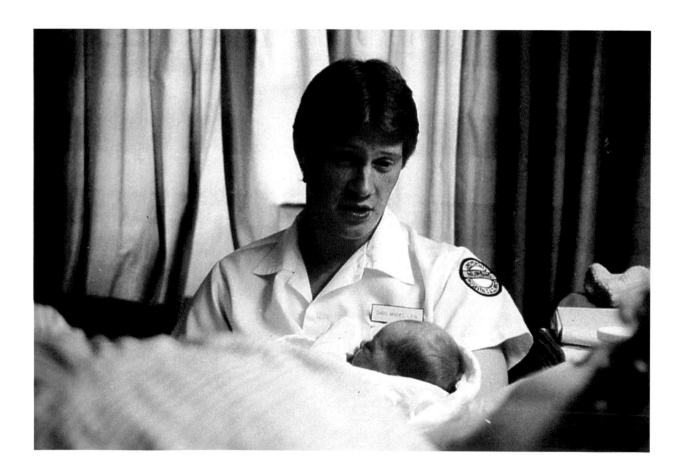

(1978) of the evolution of specific forms of doctoral programs in nursing. The first form was that of the functional specialty, with an emphasis on the methodologies and knowledge base necessary for teaching and administration. The second form involved preparation in basic scientific disciplines upon which the science and art of nursing rest. This movement was greatly enhanced by the nurse-scientist program of the federal government, in which grants were awarded to finance the education of nurses in closely related disciplines. The intent was for these graduates to return to faculty positions and provide input into basic science and research content in nursing. The third, current form is doctoral programs *in* nursing.

Two doctoral degree programs in nursing are now offered: the Ph. D., or academic doctorate with emphasis on nursing research, and the D.N.S., or professional doctorate with emphasis on nursing practice. There is disagreement as to which type will best prepare a nurse to assume power and position and to exert influence in the health care system. Which will better prepare the nurse for the generation and application of new knowledge? Which will better enable the nurse to conduct and use nursing research? "Inasmuch as the problem also has plagued every other scholarly discipline and profession, the question of which is the appropriate doctoral degree for a nurse has never found and continues to find little consensus" (Metarazzo and Abdellah, 1971, p. 404).

The Age of Specialization

The concept of nursing specialties was literally unheard of before the influence of Florence Nightingale and the advent of modern nursing. Each nurse was expected to provide for patients no matter what illness caused the need for nursing care. In hospitals patients were not segregated according to diseases until the early decades of the twentieth century. This change may have been the initiating factor in the movement toward specialization, since patients were placed in specific areas according to medical diagnoses. Yet, until World War II most nurses worked as general staff nurses in hospitals, as public health nurses, and as private duty nurses. The scientific and medical advances made during and after this war resulted in a vast body of knowledge that gave impetus to medical specialties. These were deemed necessary so that expansion and use of the knowledge could occur.

Eventually the trend toward specialized care units gained momentum, and various nursing roles evolved. These roles became known as *expanded* roles and *extended* roles. Although the terms are frequently used interchangeably, there is a difference between the two. The *extended role* refers to a physician extender with a cure orientation; the physician retains authority and decision-making power. The *expanded role* is an expansion or broadening of care-oriented nursing in which the nurse collaborates with the physician when such collaboration is indicated in specific situations.

The first nursing specialists have existed since the late nineteenth and early twentieth centuries: the nurse-midwife and the nurse-anesthetist. The training of nurse-midwives was a direct response to the need for improvement in maternal-child care, the unregulated practice of untrained midwives, and the unavailability of obstetricians in poor rural areas. The role of nurse-anesthetist developed as part of the increasing sophistication in surgery in the early 1900s, when it was recognized that trained assistants were needed to administer anesthetics. No longer was it safe or satisfactory to have untrained medical students or attendants providing anesthesia. These early specialists were recruited from the available pool of trained nurses to meet very specific societal demands and needs. Opposition from particular specialty groups in medicine and legal barriers to practice were among their greatest struggles. The same struggles continue to occur with current nursing specialization.

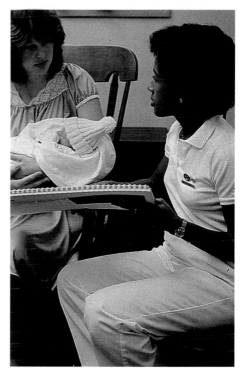

Nurse Talking With a Patient. (Courtesy of The University of Iowa Hospitals and Clinics, Department of Nursing, Iowa City, Iowa.)

P. Buckley Moss, *Medical Team*, 1993, off-set lithograph from watercolor, image size: 20.16 × 22.22 cm; paper size: 27.45 × 27.13 cm. *(The Moss Portfolio, Mathews, Virginia, Copyright P. Buckley Moss.)*

"Collaboration" is the buzzword of the nineties. With continued movement toward primary care services, collaboration between nurses and physicians and among other health care professionals will become even more important. Such an approach will do much to help ensure continuity of care.

Although nurse anesthetists and nurse midwives were initially trained and supervised by physicians, the development of autonomous clinical specialization in nursing has not been well received by medical groups. Opposition to the training and clinical practice of nurse midwives and nurse anesthetists continues to be an issue . . . the nurse midwifery and nurse anesthetist conflicts have resulted in underutilization and inappropriate use of these highly skilled nurse specialists. Debate and ambivalence regarding their role continues to confuse the American public. The resolution of territorial disputes between nursing and medicine is long overdue. However, it can be anticipated that debate and conflict will continue as long as highly skilled nurse specialists are perceived as a "threat to the other groups' social and/or financial status or its power or base of control."

— *Krampitz, 1981, p. 62*

The need for legal restrictions on nursing practice or the placement of nursing practice under the direct supervision of medicine is a concern heard consistently in discussions of specialization in nursing. This is not surprising, since it has been documented historically that physicians have often tried to keep nursing under restraint. Now, as before, nurses need to define and control their nursing practice and heed the words of Lavinia Dock:

Nothing, I think dear Editor, is more trying to one's toleration than to see men—most of whom never did and never can comprehend what a woman's work really is, what its details are, or how it ought to be done—undertaking to instruct and train women in something so unquestionably her own special field as nursing. I do not limit this statement to men only, but will say that physicians, be they men or women, cannot teach nursing, any more than nurses can teach medicine. Medicine and nursing are not the same; and how-ever much we may learn from the physician about disease and its treatment, the whole field of nursing—as nursing is realized by the *patient* (the centre of the question)—is unknown to him. I agree that he can criticise nursing intelligently, but he cannot show how it ought to be done or do it himself, except in rare instances.

We need, then, to recognize those qualities and characteristics in our work which are superior to what men can teach us, and to hold firmly to them, refusing to give them up, and most unremittingly should we resist all attempts to take our right of teaching our own work out of our hands, putting nurses out of their true relation to their own calling, and bringing up a set of imperfect imitators of pseudoscientific men, mere satellites of the medical profession, who will be neither doctor nor nurse.

— *Dock, editorial, 1901*

One other early nurse specialist bears mentioning—the industrial nurse. This specialty arose in response to the hazards and abnormal health conditions in shops, factories, and other fields of industrial labor. Initially, little concern was given to the care of injuries. In its early stages industrial nursing was a home visiting service; patient referrals were initiated by physicians. Ada Mayo Stewart was the first nurse in this specialty. She was hired by Fletcher D. Proctor in 1895 to act as a visiting nurse for the families of the employees of his Vermont Marble Company. The growth of industrial nursing was a slow one until the massive boom in the defense industry during World War II. Nurses were then rapidly employed in all types of manufacturing plants, a practice that in most instances was continued even after the war.

The 1960s witnessed another distinct growth period of specialization in nursing that has continued to the current time. All types of specialty areas—coronary care units, surgical intensive care units, medical intensive care units, burn units, dialysis units, oncology units—were developed in hospitals and necessitated the changing of nursing roles. In addition, gaps identified in the health care system of the United States in this era led nursing to experiment with the role of "clinical specialist" or "nurse clinician." This new concept allowed nurses to use their expertise, based on in-depth knowledge, for advanced nursing practice. Once again, nursing efforts were partially thwarted as hospital administrations frequently would not pay for such services and

Emergency Treatment in the Court of the Palais Royal. (National Library of Medicine, Bethesda, Maryland.)

During the revolution in July 1830, the court of the Palais Royal was used to treat the casualties of the revolt.

would assign responsibilities to the specialist head nurse or staff nurse. The specialist was thus prohibited or prevented from functioning in the clinician role. All obstacles to this role have not yet been overcome, but clinical specialists currently function in a variety of settings, including hospitals, outpatient facilities, in conjunction with individual or groups of physicians, and in private or joint practice with other nurse specialists or physicians, or both. In 1954 the first *graduate* level program to prepare clinical specialists was developed by Hildegard E. Peplau at Rutgers University; the specialty area of the program was psychiatric nursing.

The "nurse practitioner" was also introduced in this period as the result of a specific demonstration funded by the Commonwealth Foundation at the University of Colorado in 1965. Henry Silver, a pediatrician, and Loretta Ford, a public health nurse of the University of Colorado, collaborated in this venture. This demonstration project resulted in the establishment of the pediatric nurse practitioner (PNP) program, which was designed to prepare nurses to give comprehensive well-child care in ambulatory settings. The nurses were further taught to make judgments about acute or chronic conditions in children and to perform as primary practitioners in childhood emergencies. One effect of these innovations was the development of numerous new titles in nursing, such as *nurse clinician, clinical nurse specialist,* and *nurse practitioner.* All of these differed in meaning, requirements for preparation, and expected per-

Edvard Munch, *The Sick Child*, 1885-1886. Oil on canvas, 119.5 × 118.5 cm. *(Copyright 1995 The Munch Museum/The Munch-Ellingsen Group/ARS, New York.)*

Scenes of sickness and death became common in the late nineteenth century. This painting was inspired in part by the death of the artist's sister Sophie from consumption; the sorrowing woman was their Aunt Karen. It is clearly an indictment of a perceived social and cultural sickness as well as a tubercular epidemic, a "vivid study of the ravages of a degenerative disease." The woman kneels at the bedside of the child, who is looking toward the window. It is almost as though the child, knowing that nothing more can be done, is comforting a person who has reached the end of her endurance.

Munch provided a physical link in the painting, the joining of the hands, signifying the love that unites the two figures. The hands seem to be fused into one, making the sufferer and griever become a single unit.

> Yet on a higher psychological level the two are separated, each absorbed in her own immediate emotions. . . . Her (the sick child's) pale face and fiery red hair against the white pillow, painted with turbulent impasto, create a feverish atmosphere of sickness. The expression on her face seems to convey spiritual exaltation as she approaches death. (Loshak, 1994, p. 24).

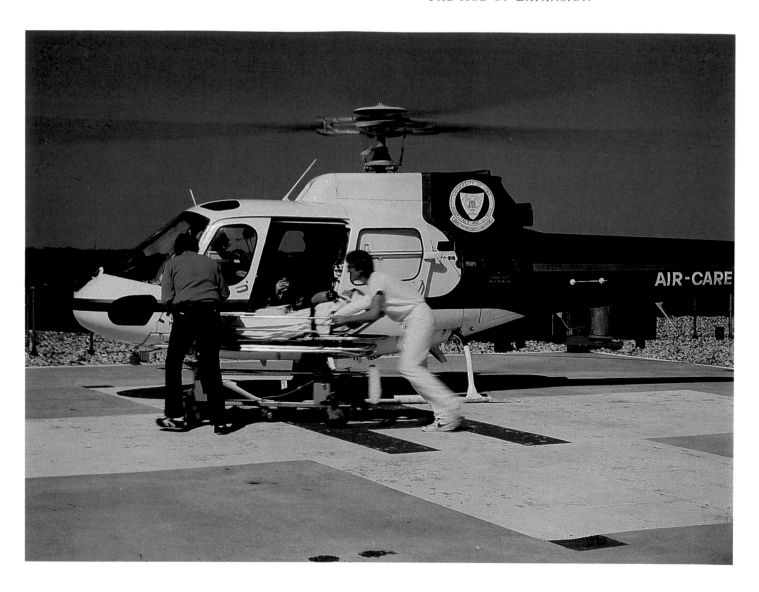

Heliport at the University of Iowa Hospitals and Clinics. (Courtesy of The University of Iowa Hospitals and Clinics, Department of Nursing, Iowa City, Iowa.)

Heliports are now a common fixture associated with large medical centers. Helicopters and other aircraft have replaced the horse and buggy. Air care has become an important part of the health care delivery system. Accident victims and patients in a variety of critical situations are quickly transported to an institution where intensive and specialized care can be provided.

formance. It is clear that standard titles are lacking, as demonstrated by a list of more than eighty different titles for nurse practitioners generated by Grippando (1977, p. 253). In addition, about twenty-seven organizations now represent various types of specialized nursing practice, and the list continues to grow. The ANA, however, defined its position on the issue through a social policy statement:

> The specialist in nursing practice is a nurse who, through study and supervised practice at the graduate level (master's or doctorate), has become expert in a defined area of knowledge and practice in a selected clinical area of nursing. Specialists in nursing practice are also generalists, in that they hold a baccalaureate in nursing, and therefore are able to provide the full range of nursing care. In addition, upon completion of a graduate degree in a university graduate program with an emphasis on clinical specialization, the specialist in nursing practice should meet the criteria for specialty certification through nursing's professional society.
>
> — *American Nurses Association, 1980*

The role of the nurse is constantly changing, and nursing practice is becoming more sophisticated. New theories, techniques, skills, and tools are being used in practice to meet the current needs of a society that is highly technological, complex, and dynamic. Specialization has led to the development of revised or new curricula in basic educational programs and the establishment of new programs in graduate education to prepare nurses to acquire the knowledge, skills, and responsibilities consistent with this role.

CONTINUED GROWTH OF ORGANIZATIONS

The American Nurses Association and the National League for Nursing have continued to represent the interests of nursing since the restructuring process in 1952. Their combined achievements and contributions are many. Each has served to promote and improve conditions in nursing service, practice, education, research, and a number of other related areas. Each has undergone some reorganization in programs in an attempt to keep pace with societal changes and demands. This period of change has resulted in advantages and disadvantages for both organizations.

The NLN adopted a new structure in 1967 to provide greater flexibility so that the national board of directors and the constituent leagues could enjoy a closer working relationship. The membership continued to include individuals and agencies, in addition to the Assembly of Constituent Leagues for Nursing with six regional assemblies for planning, coordination, and implementation of programs—the councils of Associate Degree Programs, Baccalaureate and Higher Degree Programs, Diploma Programs, Practical Nursing Programs, Hospital and Related Institutional Nursing Services, and Home Health Agencies and Community Health Services. Other changes occurred including those related to the administration of examinations for licensure. States had used the State Board Test Pool Exam (SBTPE) until 1982, when the first National Council Licensure Examination (NCLEX) was given. The National Council of State Boards of Nursing comprises members, executive secretaries, and directors of boards of nursing of the United States and territories. In 1992 the NCSBN voted to develop a Computerized Adaptive Test (CAT), which was implemented in 1994.

The various issues that arose in the organization were dealt with in the most feasible manner possible. One action that evoked a tremendous response from agency members was a historic statement entitled "Nursing Roles—Scope and Preparation," issued by the NLN in February 1982. Through this statement a baccalaureate degree was recognized and accepted as an important credential for professional nursing.

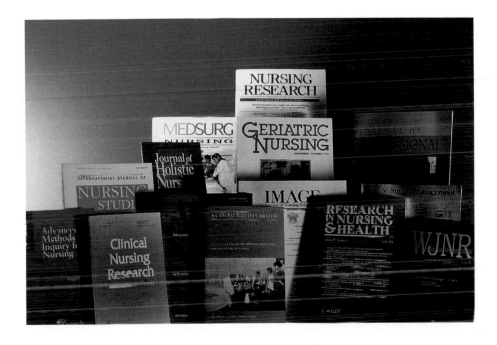

Nursing Journals, 1995. (Photo: Steven Warner, The University of Iowa College of Nursing, Iowa City.)

Nursing scholarship has progressed steadily since the first few nursing journals were initiated. Numerous journals are now available that cover a wide range of subject matter, including specialty areas, education, administration, research, organizations, and practice. The world of nursing has shrunk as international nursing journals have increased in number. Information about nursing in many countries is now available through this medium; nurses can now publish in journals worldwide.

The ANA has continued its efforts on behalf of individual nurses through its programs on economic and general welfare, its certification of practitioners, the development of standards for practice, and other significant activities in the service, practice, education, and research areas. Although the organization's classic "position paper" that was issued in 1965 did much to aid the advancement of nursing, it also intensified controversy over the future direction of the hospital diploma program. This paper, prepared by the ANA Committee on Education, was adopted as a proposal for study by the ANA House of Delegates in 1964. It was released in 1965, proposed and approved by the ANA membership in 1966, and reaffirmed in 1978, when the ANA passed the Entry Into Practice Resolution at the national convention. The statement and resolution, predicated on the need for improved nursing practice, concluded as follows:

> The education for all of those who are licensed to practice nursing should take place in institutions of higher education; minimum preparation for beginning professional nursing practice should be a baccalaureate degree; minimum preparation for beginning technical nursing practice should be an associate degree in nursing; education for assistants in the health service occupations should be short, intensive preservice programs in vocational education rather than on-the-job training.
>
> — *American Nurses Association, 1965*

At the 1982 ANA convention the House of Delegates voted for a major bylaw change that mandated the restructuring of the ANA commencing in 1984. The essence of this change was that state nurses' associations would be the units of membership in the ANA; the individual member would belong to ANA through state membership. Two objectives were to be achieved through this "federation model": the strengthening of the ANA while allowing for flexibility and the granting of autonomy of state nurses' associations.

All nursing organizations have served to effect some aspect of change and provide the necessary communication for collective action. Consolidation of the organizations was achieved in 1952 to increase efficacy and efficiency and to ensure collaboration. Since that time, additional associations have arisen, usually in response to a major issue facing either a group or the entire profession. The current proliferation of nursing organizations may serve to dilute the profession and create disunity. Therefore caution must be exercised and measures taken to prevent these possibilities from occurring. The newer organizations are added testimony to the complexities and technologies that are being experienced within the society.

National Black Nurses Association

The National Association of Colored Graduate Nurses (NACGN) existed for almost four decades, until the ANA House of Delegates in 1948 voted to rapidly remove all barriers that prevented full participation of racial minority nurses in the association. To bypass some state associations, the ANA offered individual membership to black nurses, and in 1949 approximately 634 black nurses belonged to the organization. A special committee was also set up to explore comparable functions of the NACGN and the ANA.

> Encouraged by the developments on the national level, the black nurses voted in 1949 to dissolve NACGN, and formal dissolution occurred on January 31, 1951. The struggle for professional parity, they thought, was over. The dream of recognition and equality was finally to be realized.
>
> — *Smith, 1975, p. 225.*

Logo for the National Black Nurses Association. *(Courtesy of the National Black Nurses Association, Washington, D.C.)*

This stamp was issued in 1966 by the Republic of Guinea, Africa. Depicted is the emphasis on maternal and child health, which has been a popular subject. Care and concern for the baby are exhibited on the faces of those gathered around. *(Stamp courtesy of Medical Economics Publishing, New Jersey.)*

The intent of black nurses was to become a part of the mainstream of organized nursing and of the ANA. This was apparently not the total answer for blacks and other minorities. "In many sections of the country, nurses are organizing in ethnically identifiable associations, because they have not felt they were integrated into the professional association" (Shaw, 1975, p. 8). Thus emerged the National Black Nurses Association, Inc., in 1971, a structure that would not duplicate the functions of the ANA but would complement them so as to meet the special needs of black nurses. This organization was begun through the efforts of Lauranne Sams as the vehicle to assist with voiced concerns of black nurses. Some of these concerns were the absence of black nurses in positions of leadership; limited opportunities for black nurses to share in shaping ANA policies and priorities; loss of identity of black nurses; and limited recognition of their contribution to nursing. Membership was open to all licensed nurses (R.N. and L.P.N.) and nursing students. "Its future is uncertain, as would seem to be true of other emergent nursing organizations organized around race, sex, specialization, and division of labor" (Smith, 1975, p. 226).

American Association of Colleges of Nursing

Developments among the professional nursing associations included the establishment of the American Association of Colleges of Nursing (AACN) in 1969 as the Conference of Deans of College and University Schools of Nursing. The name was changed in 1973 to indicate its separation from the NLN. The AACN, which is a national association of nursing deans from colleges and universities, was created to provide administrators of baccalaureate and graduate degree nursing programs with an outlet for review of developments in the health care field. Its numerous activities are executed to improve the practice of professional nursing by elevating the quality of degree programs. Schools of nursing are represented by their respective deans, who discuss common concerns. Through a concerted effort, the AACN has continually influenced public policy related to nursing and nursing education.

Numerous stamps illustrating the treatment of those inflicted with tuberculosis have been issued by countries throughout the world. The war against tuberculosis became a united effort. Public health campaigns led to a significant decrease in cases. Currently, tuberculosis is once again on the rise as resistance to the drugs of choice has increased. This stamp was issued by Afghanistan in 1967. (*Stamp courtesy of Medical Economics Publishing, New Jersey.*)

Logos for the American Association of Colleges of Nursing. *Left*, original logo, *right*, present logo. (*Courtesy of the American Association of Colleges of Nursing, Washington, D.C.*)

National Federation for Specialty Nursing Organizations and the American Nurses Association

As the number of nursing specialty organizations increased in the early 1970s, the numerous groups expressed the desire for unity and communication. They were dissatisfied with the ANA and believed that it was not concerned with the needs of the specialty groups. The American Association of Critical-Care Nurses called for a meeting in January 1972 to provide a forum to communicate and seek mechanisms for support and cooperation. The First National Congress in Nursing, as the meeting was called, was held at the Western White House in San Clemente, California.

At about the same time, in April 1972, the ANA Board of Directors decided to call a similar meeting "to explore how the organizations can work toward more coordination on areas of mutual interest" (National Federation for Specialty Nursing Organizations, 1984, p. 3). They invited the presidents and staff of nursing organizations, and mutual concerns were identified.

The First National Congress in Nursing was a historic event in which support and cooperation between specialty groups and the ANA were sought. It was decided that the group convened by the ANA and the National Nurses Congress would merge. A third meeting was held in Denver in June of 1972. The title of the organization was determined to be The Federation of Specialty Nursing Organizations, and the ANA and twelve specialty groups became charter members. This organization has more than doubled its charter membership since its inception in 1973. It currently represents over 360,000 nurses and approximately thirty-four specialty groups throughout the United States who have differing clinical backgrounds. The name of the organization was changed to the National Federation for Specialty Nursing Organizations (NFSNO) in 1981.

Auguste Rodin, *Young Woman and Winged Child,* c. 1885. Marble, 43.2 × 44.4 × 33.1. cm. *(Copyright 1995 Board of Trustees, National Gallery of Art, Washington, D.C. Gift of Mrs. John W. Simpson.)*

American Academy of Nursing

The American Academy of Nursing was established in 1973 under the auspices of the ANA. Membership in this academy is limited to graduate nurses who are members of the ANA. A nurse who becomes a Fellow in the American Academy of Nursing (F.A.A.N.) has provided documentation of outstanding contributions to nursing. Potential members are nominated and voted on by current members. Election to this group is considered an honor because members represent a selected group of leaders in the profession. The Academy currently comprises more than one thousand members. Meetings are held annually, primarily to enter into dialogue about nursing issues and to work on reports, studies, and position papers related to major nursing and health care issues.

Nurses Coalition for Action in Politics

Nurses for Political Action was started in 1972 as the first national organization of nurses to enter the political arena. It soon became affiliated with the ANA and has been regarded as its legislative and political action arm (Kalisch and Kalisch, 1978). The name was eventually changed to Nurses Coalition for Action in Politics (N-CAP) in 1974. Nurses Coalition for Action in Politics was organized as a nonpartisan and nonprofit association. Its expressed goal is the attainment of substantial political influence on national policy related to health care delivery. This group encourages and assists nurses to become social and political activists. It continues to strive for support for nursing from legislators and government officials.

American Association for the History of Nursing

Early American nursing leaders supported and promoted the study of nursing history and advocated its incorporation into curricula of schools of nursing. In particular, M. Adelaide Nutting, Lavinia L. Dock, and Isabel M. Stewart became known as authorities on nursing history through the publication of their classic works on the subject. Dedicated to fostering greater understanding of and respect for nursing's past, they were committed to the belief that to understand and deal with problems and trends in nursing education and nursing practice nurses needed to be familiar with their history. These leaders believed that no one can get a true picture of current situations without finding out how the issues developed and what their underlying causes were. This general philosophy was expressed by Stewart:

> History can often help individuals to deal more effectively with persistent issues and conflicts by throwing light on their origins, and by indicating long-term trends that show the general direction in which things are moving. Educators who know something of the historical foundations of a system of education are also in a better position to evaluate the materials that have gone into it, to capitalize its assets and to eliminate what is no longer useful.
>
> — Stewart, 1943, p. viii

There has been no consistent support for historical inquiry. In fact, emphasis on the historical foundations of nursing has decreased over time to the point that few nursing history courses are currently available in schools of nursing. Nor are there sufficient nursing faculty available who are prepared to teach them. In an effort to revive an interest in nursing history, a small number of interested nurses and historians began meeting as a historical methodology interest group in 1978 as part of a federally funded project for the development of nursing research in the Midwest. Originally called the

American Association for the History of Nursing logo. *(Courtesy of the American Association for the History of Nursing, Washington, D.C.)*

The origin of the concept of nurse as mother has perpetuated the notion that only women can nurse; the assumption is that the maternal instinct is necessary to provide the motivation for the care of the suffering, sick, or helpless. In years past, the saying has been, "Little girls grow up to be nurses; boys grow up to be physicians!"

International History of Nursing Society, the name of the group was changed in 1980 to the American Association for the History of Nursing. The membership comprises individuals, nurses and nonnurses, who are interested in achieving the purpose of the association—to educate the public about the history and heritage of the nursing profession by:

a. Stimulating interest and national/international collaboration in promoting the history of nursing.
b. Encouraging research in the history of nursing.
c. Promoting the development of centers for preservation and use of materials of historical importance to nursing.
d. Serving as a resource for information related to nursing history.
e. Producing and distributing to members of the public educational materials regarding the history and heritage of the nursing profession.

— *American Association for the History of Nursing, Bylaws, May 1983*

The movement, although slow, has begun to return nursing history to the curricula of schools of nursing, to foster historical research, and to collect, restore, and preserve historical materials relevant to nursing's rich heritage.

John Sloan

UNIT 10

An Era of Change and Challenge

In order to advance the discipline toward the future, the new tomorrow, nurses have to unite themselves in an effort to construct new organizational and legal structures and thus bring more clarity in their roles as professionals. They can no longer allow others to do the job for them. This has become even more important within the context of the 'Health for All' movement, that encourages nurses to redirect their attention from primarily hospital care to 'health for all,' the healthy and the sick in the community. Although this challenge has received a positive response from many nurse practitioners, the question is whether the discipline is ready to accept this challenge with competence and vision. Is nursing ready to take on a role as a pathfinder or trendsetter and engage in *anticipatory nursing* or are its members waiting for directions given by other disciplines, who are often less well equipped to act as a liaison between the policy-makers and planners of care and the public at large?

— HANNEKE M. TH. VAN MAANEN

John Sloan, *Professional Nurse*, 1893. Watercolor, 27.3 × 22.86 cm. *(The Delaware Art Museum, Wilmington, Delaware. The John Sloan Collection.)*

From its beginnings, the nursing profession has continually endeavored to excel in patient care but has also grown and developed into a discipline that studies, researches, and creates new knowledge. As the end of the twentieth century approaches, nursing stands poised between the past and the future.

Nurses of today are expected to be many things to many people and to function in a variety of settings. They are to be excellent caregivers, adequate researchers, seekers of knowledge, and thinkers grounded in scientific, humanistic, and logical thought. Nurses are involved with all types of new roles that have broadened their opportunities and increased the scope of their responsibilities. They continually strive to provide holistic and quality care for all individuals in structures that are not always supportive.

An Era of Change and Challenge

DAILY LIFE

1970 Television sets in use worldwide: 231 million

1971 Women granted vote in Switzerland

1971 Cigarette ads banned from United States television

1971 India and Pakistan go to war

1972 Tasadays, a tribe with Stone Age culture, discovered living in southern Philippine cave

1974 Smallpox epidemic kills 10,000–20,000 in India

1976 North and South Vietnam unite as one country after twenty-two years

1980 Fifty nations boycott Olympics after Soviets invade Afghanistan

SCIENCE AND TECHNOLOGY

1970 First synthesis of gene announced in Wisconsin

1971 Three Russian cosmonauts die upon reentry into Earth's atmosphere

1971 Human growth hormone synthesized in California

1972 Pocket calculator introduced

1976 Discovery of viral cause of multiple sclerosis

1978 Discovery of a moon orbiting Pluto

1981 First successful space shuttle flight occurs

1981 Scientists identify Acquired Immune Deficiency Syndrome (AIDS)

1981 IBM unveils its first personal computer

1983 Compact disc is launched

THE VISUAL ARTS

1970 Henri Matisse exhibition in Paris

1971 Kennedy Center for Performing Arts opens in Washington, D.C.

1972 Michelangelo's *Pieta* seriously damaged by hammer-wielding vandal

1973 Pablo Picasso dies (born 1881)

1978 Norman Rockwell, American illustrator and painter, dies (born 1894)

1982 Vietnam Veterans War Memorial dedicated in Washington, D.C.

MEDICINE AND HEALTH CARE

1970 Nuclear-powered heart pacemakers implanted in three patients in France and Britain

1977 Last documented case of smallpox diagnosed in southern Somalia

1977 World Health Assembly establishes goal of "Health for All by the Year 2000"

1978 World Health Organization declares primary health care the strategy for achieving health for all

1978 First "test-tube baby" born in London

1981 WHO formulates strategy for health promotion, disease prevention, and curative and rehabilitative services

1982 First artificial heart implanted

1982 Combined heart-lung and kidney-pancreas transplant done

NURSING

1973 North American Nursing Diagnosis Association (NANDA) formed

1975–1980 Community Nursing Center (CNC) movement begins

1980 Nursing Case Management Model pioneered at New England Medical Center, Boston

1984 Series of famines in Ethiopia

1985 World Bank organizes famine relief fund for Africa

1986 Chernobyl nuclear power plant accident occurs

1988 Famines in Ethiopia, Sudan, and Bangladesh

1989 Tienanmen Square Massacre in China

1989 Berlin Wall dismantled in East Germany

1989 Kenya calls for ban on ivory imports

1984 Apple introduces Macintosh microcomputer with mouse

1984 AIDS virus isolated

1984 Internet opened to public use

1986 Space shuttle *Challenger* explodes

1987 International scientists confirm ozone hole over Antarctica and postulate link with chlorofluorocarbon emissions

---

1985 Claude Monet's *Impression, Sun Rising*, the painting that gave Impressionist movement its name, is stolen in Paris

1986 Film companies begin to colorize black and white films

1984 First frozen embryo baby born

1985 Lasers used to clean out clogged arteries

1990 Contemporary managed care movement begins in United States

1990 English and French engineers meet under the sea as portions of English Channel tunnel linked together

---

1985 Nursing Minimum Data Set (NMDS) developed

1986 National Center for Nursing Research (NCNR) founded

1988 Sigma Theta Tau becomes an international organization

1989 International Classification of Nursing Practice (ICNP) project starts

1992 International Nursing Center established by American Nurses Association

1992 *Nursing Interventions Classifications* (NIC) published

1993 NCNR receives status of institute: National Institute of Nursing Research

1994 Barbara Fassbinder, RN, infected with HIV in 1986, dies

1994 *The Online Journal of Knowledge Synthesis for Nursing* created

*T*he last ten years in health care might appropriately be called the "decade of the paradoxes" in which a transformation has been taking place in the very core of society. Along with almost unimaginable technological advances have come profound questions relative to life and death, which have provoked serious doubts about the value of technology. Who will receive lifesaving organs when not all can? Will the rich, the elderly, and the poor receive quality, if not equal, care? How and by whom will decisions be made in the face of limited resources? Will health care be available to all? Other contradictions in health care such as those that concern diseases, in vitro fertilization, surrogate mothers, the elderly, access to care, financial resources, and governmental control can also be readily identified. These paradoxes are interwoven with the strands of technology, bureaucracy, and healing. Bulger (1988) comprehensively discussed these three strands in relation to the American system of health care, but his statements can easily be applied to global societies without much alteration. Although his writing is several years old, it is still applicable to the current system. He pleads for a reintegration of technology, bureaucracy, and healing into a new, more humane, and more effective approach to health care. This "postmodern paradigm" would preserve ". . . liberty, freedom, hope, and a sense of human progress which incorporates suffering and death, all united through a sense of belonging and community" (pp. 86–87).

As the twenty-first century rapidly approaches, numerous questions are being raised in an attempt to guide health care policy toward greater social harmony, to alleviate social dilemmas created by competing sets of values, and to confront the realities of current health care economics. Instability, volatility, and incredible change are forcing a reexamination of societal values along with changing consumer expectations of health care. Those values of individualism, competition, cost containment, efficiency, and technology that are currently driving health care policy and health care systems are also influencing nursing's ability to provide quality care. A look to the past demonstrates the evolution of the changing scene in nursing practice. In the 1960s and 1970s nurses were the almost exclusive providers of patient care. By the mid-1980s, diagnostic-related group (DRG) reimbursement forced nurses to understand the necessity for cost containment and reduced lengths of stay. Currently business and economics have become the buzzwords as nursing care costs are coming under even closer scrutiny (Kalisch and Kalisch, 1995). As health care increasingly runs along business lines, competition occurs through mergers, acquisitions, and the expansion into new markets. What becomes clear is that quality of care is not the major focus of the competitiveness. Reduced revenues have even led to a reduction in the registered nurse workforce as unlicensed assistive personnel are hired to reduce labor costs and act as nurse extenders. It is clear that new and creative approaches to health care and nursing care are needed.

THE HOSPITAL SCENE

Now is a time of transition for health care institutions and health care in general. The issue of allocation of scarce health-related resources has become almost paramount, leading to serious ramifications for institutions, health care personnel, and consumers around the globe. Ethical questions of the past were related to affluence; the problems of today deal with scarcity. Yet, efforts to control costs have been erratic, with various reasons given to explain high costs. Initially the problem of increasing hospital costs was attributed to poor management. Why was it that an individual could obtain better service in a hotel or in a restaurant at a cheaper cost? In the 1960s the rise of health care costs was drastically influenced by what were referred to as thousands of

Facing Page, Test-Tube Triplets, 1990. (Photo by Nick Kelsh.)

Test-tube triplets Jonathan, Nicholas, and Holly Cakebread celebrate their first birthday outside stately Bourn Hall Clinic in Cambridge, England. Bourn Hall is among the world's leading in vitro fertilization clinics. The triplets were conceived in the clinic, where their mother's eggs were fertilized with their father's sperm after the parents failed to conceive naturally. Although there are relatively low odds that pregnancy will occur with the attachment of fertilized eggs to the mother's uterine wall, childless couples still opt for the relatively expensive procedure.

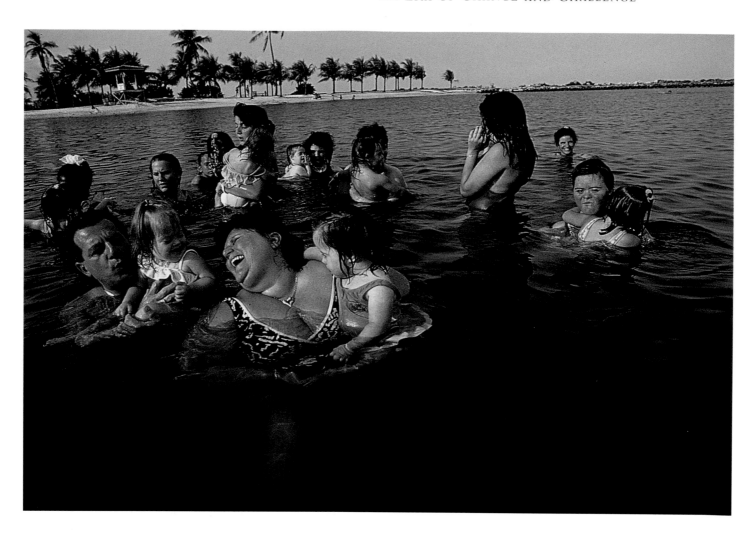

Giraldi Family. (Copyright 1994 Andy Levin. All rights reserved.)

Camille Giraldi, an RN, and her husband Michael, an MD, have made it their lifetime mission to help children with Down's Syndrome. Their "Up With Downs" foundation has provided a home for dozens of Down's children and has helped inform the public about Down's people. This picture, taken at the beach in Miami, shows Camille and Michael with some of their extended Down's family.

"small-ticket" items like new laboratory tests and radiological examinations. The emergence and dissemination of "big-ticket" items such as computerized axial tomography (CAT) scans, lasers, transplantations, and nuclear magnetic resonance imaging (MRI) devices accounted for increased costs in the 1970s and 1980s. Currently more and more health care institutions have turned to business, industry, and the marketplace for the answers to managing costs. Debates about health care reform, decreasing revenues, and strategies for change continue throughout the world. But one thing remains clear: resultant changes in health care have affected and will affect nurses financially, environmentally, and clinically and present one of the greatest challenges nurses have ever faced.

Historically and traditionally the majority of sick and injured people were cared for by families. Eventually early hospitals emerged that provided services for those who had no home or family, including orphans, soldiers, travelers, the impoverished, nuns and monks (religious orders), and in some cases the insane. These early hospitals functioned in a variety of roles as hostels, hotels, and hospitals in which care was primarily custodial and religiously motivated. Consequently the caregivers were primarily men and women with a religious calling. During the time of the Reformation, another change in the hospital structure took place. As previously discussed and using England as an example, the religious orders were suppressed and the hospital commenced as a secular institution. Other events occurred in the eighteenth century, such as the Industrial Revolution, the migration of populations to cities, and changes in the workplace environment and family structures, that necessitated the expansion of hospital systems again to care primarily for the poor, but this time, the urban poor. Even with the establishment of Nightingale's St. Thomas School of Nursing in the nineteenth century, hospitals were still sanctuaries for those devoid of family care, the mentally ill, and the poor (Bullough and Bullough, 1984). Hospitals were not numerous and were essentially insignificant, since no "respectable" person entered them for treatment. The wealthy continued to be cared for at home for a number of reasons including available financial resources. In Rosenberg's analysis (1987) of the evolution of American hospitals, his description of the internal structure of hospitals during this time is enlightening:

> It (the hospital) was in its internal structure a very different institution from that we know in the late twentieth century. It was not directed by a bureaucracy of credentialed administrators; it was certainly not dominated by the medical profession and its needs. Lay trustees still felt it their duty to oversee every aspect of hospital routine. The hospital was very much a mirror of the society that populated and supported it, a society rooted in deference and hierarchy, a society in which traditional attitudes toward the responsibility of wealth were very much alive. Medical men needed and used the hospital; they could not control it (p. 5).

With the advent of the twentieth century, major changes occurred and have continued in hospitals throughout this century. Hospitals grew in size, spread widely, became more formal and bureaucratic, and began treating not only the indigent but also the wealthy and respectable. In addition, many decisions that shaped modern hospitals were directly related to medical ideas and values. Events such as childbirth that had occurred in the home moved into the hospital; medical specialties emerged and escalated. Hospitals no longer remained charitable institutions; they often became profit-making institutions, particularly with the evolution of health insurance and government intervention. The hospital eventually became synonymous with high technology and bureaucracy; the alleviation of pain and suffering—and potentially cure—was rendered at enormous economic and emotional cost.

Currently, new organizational and administrative structures, job restructuring, decreased hospital stays, increased patient acuity, the rise of consumerism, and mergers are reshaping health care and hospitals. Hospital closures and "downsizing" (the negative connotation of the term "downsizing" is one factor that has led to the use of the term "rightsizing") are occurring in the face of cost-containment pressures and a shrinking hospital industry, even in countries that have national health care systems. There is a trend toward privatization in Norway and the United Kingdom as a result of issues of efficiency and provision of services to low-income immigrant workers from developing countries. Canada is facing a major issue of hospital restructuring and closure, in addition to the requirement to develop a more comprehensive primary health care service (Buchan, 1993). Regionalization has occurred in New South Wales; the state was divided into twelve regions. Further subdivision occurred, leading to the establishment of twenty-three area health services under the Area Health Services Act of 1986 in which ". . . hospitals and other health care agencies within a defined geographical area are to be grouped together under one management board" (Duffield, 1988, p. 127). Integrated health care systems are on the rise. A primary shift from inpatient to ambulatory care has resulted in the need to develop new strategies for the provision of adequate, high-quality patient care. With the reduction in inpatient days, home-delivered medical and nursing services are becoming vital, viable components of these systems. Correspondingly, the nursing shortages of the 1980s have given way to a situation in which experienced nurses and new graduates are having difficulty finding employment. The need for recruitment of nurses between countries has all but disappeared.

The majority of nurses will readily state their belief that their faithfulness or first allegiance is to the patients/clients they serve. Blacks have been typically shown as slaves, nursemaids, and "nannies" who are ever-faithful to their charges. However, a minority group of nurses has dealt admirably with impediments from both society and nursing itself. They have worked constantly for the acceptance of Blacks in nursing, and for the promotion of equal opportunities for all minority persons. Numerous Black nurses have emerged as significant nursing leaders, made valuable contributions to nursing, and brought the concerns of Blacks to the attention of nurses and the general public.

The Managed Care Revolution

The movement toward managed care as a method to solve the issue of high health care costs began in the early 1990s, although it was pioneered in the mid-1930s. In this early stage of its development, emphasis was not on cost containment. Managed care was seen as a system of organizing care and providing comprehensive coverage, not just as a strategy for financial control. The potential cost-saving aspect of the plan would be the outcome or effect of an efficiently run system that incorporated a full range of services, continuity of care, emphasis on prevention, and early intervention. The original Kaiser shipbuilding company initiated managed care in response to employee health care concerns during World War II. Kaiser developed a health care plan for his employees that provided a comprehensive range of services from prevention to acute care. With this early approach, the Kaiser company ran its own hospitals and clinics and employed physicians, nurses, and other providers of care (Himali, 1995). This type of primary health care services was predicated on early, frequent entry into the system for treatment of small problems before they became large ones. Enrollees were enticed by low monthly premiums and convenient, accessible medical centers.

The early Kaiser prototype of managed care is no longer the only model; various forms have emerged that in many cases minimally resemble the original concept. Few are currently operating according to the original principles and strategies of managed care. The following are familiar types:

Home Is Where the Heart Is. (Copyright 1994 Andy Levin. All rights reserved.)

Maureen Raubert, a Mississippi nurse, drives about one hundred miles a day while visiting patients. She is one of nearly two hundred nurses who work for South Mississippi Home Health, a private agency credited with pioneering organized home health services in the late 1960s. As in prior decades, home visits by nurses can contribute to a reduction in health care costs.

- Health Maintenance Organization (HMO): Composed of hospitals and allied clinics; patients are enrolled as members for a fixed fee per year and receive all necessary health care services. Usually organized in a specific geographical area.

🖋 Preferred Provider Organization (PPO): Health care financing and delivery program comprising a group of providers such as hospitals and physicians under contract with a private indemnity insurance company for services on a fee-for-service basis. Customers use a select group of providers and pay less for services.

🖋 Independent Practice Association (IPA): Similar to an HMO in which physicians who are not salaried employees of the plan contract to provide services at a discounted fee. Physicians share risks and profits through an incentive system designed to achieve high standards of quality and remain within the budget.

🖋 Point of Service Systems: Similar to an HMO in which members are permitted to go outside the system to physicians not in the plan's network. Depending on the system, however, a patient using an outside provider may pay a percentage of the medical bill with a potentially high deductible.

— *Kalisch and Kalisch, 1995; Streef, 1994*

These models of managed care have had a profound, rapid influence on both the private insurance market and governmental insurance programs (Medicare and Medicaid) within the United States. In fact, many areas of the country are now dominated by managed care while other areas are attempting to follow suit. It will be interesting to observe the effect of managed care on other countries as they begin to incorporate some of the principles into their own health care systems in the face of a significant number of pressures. Failure to manage health care effectively may lead to further crises and collapse of systems. Organizational transformation appears to be the only solution and with it the challenge to nurses worldwide.

There is no doubt that the massive shift toward managed care has had a major impact on nursing. The nursing profession and the practice field are being bombarded on all sides by global, geopolitical, social, demographic, epidemiological, technological, political, and industrial forces. Cross-training of personnel, increased use of assistive personnel, and the emergence of new classes of workers are occurring at a rapid rate (Styles, 1993). Yet, most nurses would agree that managed care is good in principle and in practice if focused on quality and primary health care services. But as hospital restructuring and "downsizing" have escalated, managed care is being used as the rationale for the use of fewer nurses for patient care, layoffs, and job losses. Was it only a few years ago that hospitals were wooing nurses with cash and material bonuses? This has been a bitter pill for nurses to swallow who observe hospitals acquiring new equipment, continuing construction projects, and increasing salaries of chief executive officers and increasing numbers of administrators. Even more alarming is the lack of emphasis on high-quality patient care.

In response to this dramatic reversal more than twenty-five thousand registered nurses marched in protest in Washington, D.C., on March 31, 1995 (Himali, 1995b; McCrary, 1995). This was the first-ever national demonstration by nurses. It was the brainchild of Laura Gasparis Vonfrolio, owner and publisher of *Revolution: The Journal of Nurse Empowerment,* and was co-sponsored by the American Nurses' Association (ANA). As the nurses marched down Pennsylvania Avenue, members of Congress met in the U.S. Capitol with approximately two hundred of their nursing colleagues. Several state nurses' associations staged their own rallies in combination with the march on Washington. The purpose for the demonstration was not only to cite job cuts but also to protest the erosion of care in health care institutions. A strong message was given both to the public and to Congress about measures that have reduced the number of registered nurses caring for patients and creating, in many instances, an unsafe environment.

In the face of adversity, nurses acted in the role of advocates, even though some jeopardized their professional careers to attend. A number of hospitals had sent out memos prohibiting their nurses from taking the day of the rally

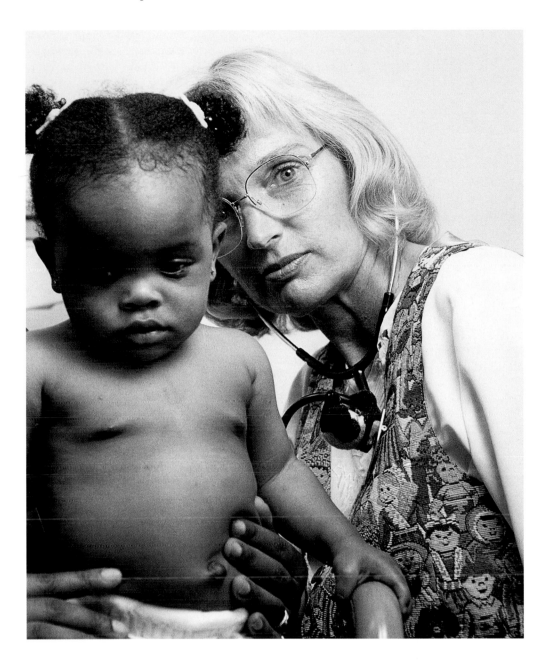

off. Using a variety of strategies, however, nurses have engaged and continue to engage in activities to demonstrate the critical link between nurses at the bedside and safe, high-quality care. State rallies and walks, press conferences, position statements, collective bargaining, and political involvement are all being used to strengthen nursing's position in health care delivery and take a proactive stand.

Case Management and Critical Paths

The term "managed care" in and of itself can at times be confusing. Managed care is frequently used to indicate health care plans in concert with facilities that are designed to contain the cost of services while upholding quality of care. Emphasis is on the achievement of specific patient outcomes within a fiscally responsible time frame. In other instances the phrase "managed care" is used to indicate a nursing model for patient care. In addition, managed care and case management are often used synonymously in the health care and nursing literature. Perhaps one of the more concise and comprehensible definitions of managed care is the following:

Managed care is unit-based care that is organized to achieve specific patient out-comes within fiscally responsible timeframes (length of stay) while utilizing

Cover photo, from *The Science of Caring,* Fall 1994. *(Courtesy of School of Nursing and Nursing Alumni Association, University of California San Francisco.)*

School of Nursing Professor Pat Jackson examines a patient at the Valencia Pediatric Practice in San Francisco's Mission District. This faculty-managed, bilingual, multicultural clinical practice provides primary care experience for advanced practice nursing students. The UCSF curriculum was restructured to focus on the role of the advanced practice nurse in anticipation of health care reform.

resources that are appropriate in amount and sequence to the specific case type and to the individual patient. Outcomes are the patient's discharge condition, stated in measurable terms, that result from the activities of nurses, physicians and other health care providers. The term 'unit' refers to the geographic area in which the patient receives care. The focus of managed care is on redesigning tools and systems, the outcomes and processes of care are identified on a daily basis; hourly in areas such as the Emergency Room or the Operating Room; by visit in ambulatory settings. This facilitates identifying those patients who are deviating from the expected early enough to take corrective action.

— *Bower, 1988, p. 1*

It is clear that a new language has been created that nurses, particularly those in advanced practice, will need to understand. But even more crucial is the question as to whether managed care has been a panacea to the ills of health care.

Managed care has provided an even greater impetus to the increased use of case management as a mechanism for the coordination and sequencing of care. Case management is not a new phenomenon but has emerged as a direct link to cost containment through the creation of an environment that attempts to control the quality and cost of patient care. Historically it has been used by a number of entities including social service agencies, insurance companies, rehabilitation centers, and public health nursing as a means of community service coordination. Although psychiatric–mental health nurses have used it for a number of years, only recently has it been evolving and begun to be incorporated into the practice of nurses in inpatient settings, including emergency care settings.

Confusion about case management may also occur because it is referred to by terms that are often used interchangeably: service management, care coordination, and care management. Some of the same arguments related to the use of patient versus client have surfaced here. To some, the label "case management" is not appropriate, since a patient is not a case, but a person or client who needs care. Case management may be described as a system, process, service, and a role, even as a technology. It may be defined in a variety of ways depending on the focus of the particular agency or institution. It is, however, broader in scope than primary nursing and can decrease fragmentation of care by crossing all departments.

Case management may involve many professional disciplines, including nursing, social work, mental health, and medicine. In fact, depending upon program policies and client needs, it is often preferable to have an interdisciplinary team participate in the planning and delivery of care. However, even if a team approach is used, one member of the team is usually designated as the case manager for a specific client. The manager then collaborates in the delivery of care with other professionals as well as family members, the client, and others providing services.

— *ANA, 1988*

Case management is built on the foundation of managed care. Theoretically any individual who possesses the appropriate knowledge and skills could be a case manager, since direct patient care might not be part of the role. It stands to reason, however, that physicians and nurses would be the most fitting managers because of their clinical expertise. Each organization, however, may put case management to use differently according to its environment. The nature of the population to be served seems currently to be the primary factor behind the designation of the case manager. Be that as it may, nurses are in a prime position to provide case management in collaboration with physicians. The nurse's self-satisfaction and sense of autonomy could only be enhanced through such an approach.

Tools considered to be essential for managed care and case management have also been evolving. Critical paths or their next generation, CareMaps (trademark and concept of The Center for Case Management, South Natick, Massachusetts), briefly and concisely map the sequence and timing of key tasks and technical aspects of the treatment plan and provide the framework for planning patient care. Originally developed at New England Medical Center in Boston, where the Nursing Case Management Model was pioneered in 1980, the critical paths specify daily events, tasks, and interventions that caregivers must provide (Zander, 1994). In other words, care is structured by critical pathways; care is achieved through collaboration of health care professionals. Processes and outcomes defined by expert physicians, nurses, and other interdisciplinary team members for the "usual" patient are generally reviewed by the patient and family members, thereby ensuring that all involved individuals are operating with the same time frame and process information. Variances can, of course, occur and mandate a review of the existing plan with the ultimate strategy for resolution of the problem.

There are numerous intricacies and ambiguities in managed care, case management, and the use of critical pathways. Whether managed care is here to stay remains to be seen, but emphasis on cost control and resource management will not disappear. Health care providers will continue to be asked to do more with less. In doing so, they will need to be more collaborative then ever and constantly remember that case management belongs to no one. This can be a disastrous time or a time of unique opportunity for nurses. As Ralph Waldo Emerson concluded, "This time, like all times, is a very good one, if we but know what to do with it."

Nursing Practice II student performing health assessment of a preschool child at the House of Peace Community Nursing Center in Milwaukee, 1991. *(Courtesy of The University of Wisconsin–Milwaukee, School of Nursing. Photograph, Alan Magayne-Roshak.)*

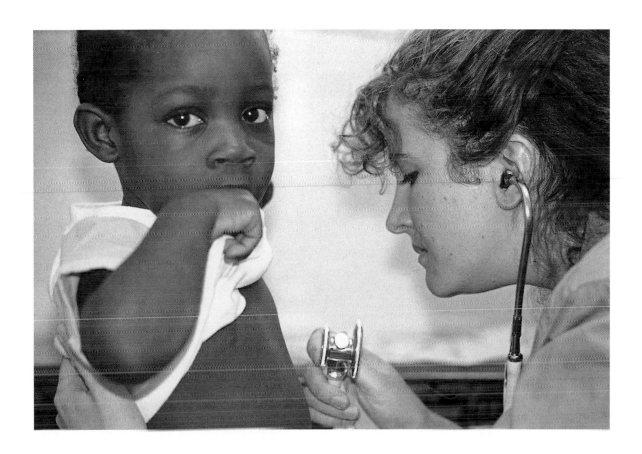

THE NURSING PERSPECTIVE: THE STATE OF THE ART

The last ten years in nursing have been intertwined with vast social problems, profound financial crises, and a health care arena in a state of turmoil. Essentially the issues of health care remain the same as when nursing was created and are related to accessibility, resources, division of labor, the caregiver pool, and reimbursement. Some of nursing's earlier issues have either improved or been resolved, or are no long problematic. The issue of entry-level education, for example, although not totally resolved, has improved along with greater numbers of nurses obtaining advanced degrees. Hospital diploma programs are continuing to close or become affiliated with colleges and universities. Educational programs across the world are being examined, and decisions are being made to move them into institutions of higher learning. Israel developed a twenty-five-year master plan to provide university education for nurses. A bachelor of arts (BA) degree program (post-basic) opened in 1968, a generic bachelor of science in nursing (BSN) program in 1975, and the master's degree program in 1982. Iceland is the only country that has mandated baccalaureate education as the basic form of nurse preparation. The issue is still, however, not without controversy and individuals who oppose educational change. A prime example occurred when Alice C. Ream (1982), a retired nurse, severely criticized the new generation of nurses who spend an "inadequate amount of time caring for patients." Nurse educators in particular were villains in her description of the situation:

> Nurse educators have a bug in their ears about being handmaidens to physicians. They are, for some unknown reason, ashamed of being nurses. Ashamed of

Student and client at the House of Peace Community Nursing Center in Milwaukee, 1992. *(Courtesy of The University of Wisconsin–Milwaukee, School of Nursing. Photograph, Alan Magayne-Roshak.)*

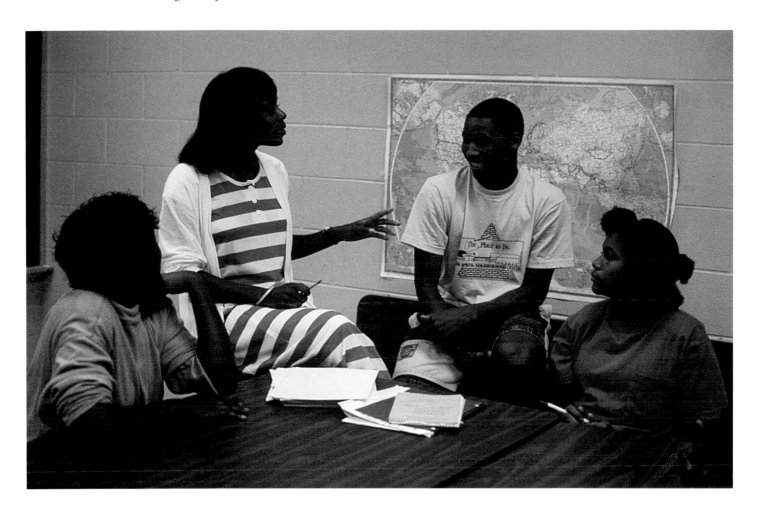

Teaching. Silver Spring Community Center. *(Courtesy of The University of Wisconsin–Milwaukee, School of Nursing.)*

bathing the sick? How else does one check for skin turgor, rashes and ulceration? Ashamed of handling excreta? How does one arrive at first hand knowledge of output or the possibility of intestinal bleeding? Not willing to carry a food tray? How does one assess the patient's appetite and potential need for supplemental nourishment? . . . So nurses end up as cocktail waitresses, clerks in stores or real-estate salesladies. That is called "burnout." Translated, it means that the nurse was not trained to cope, to organize or to perform and will, eventually, leave nursing for something she can handle. In the meantime, we face a stunning shortage of nurses. . . . When some of those nurses who can't measure up in a hospital reach burnout, they return to college, get another degree and become professors of nursing. One can only shudder at the thought of what their students will face one day (p. 17).

The primary difference in the nursing of today is its maturity that has evolved over the course of the twentieth century. Indeed, new concerns have arisen that may cause nurses to pause and deliberate, such as the increasing use of unlicensed assistive personnel, changed reimbursement systems, the presence of nursing information systems, and a return to alternative forms of health care and healing practices. What must constantly be remembered, however, is that change also brings opportunities.

To understand the nature of change is paramount to the progression and survival of nursing. Both external and internal forces are involved in the process of change and directly or indirectly affect the nursing discipline. External forces are generally believed to be the strongest, although internal forces may have a positive or negative effect. Bullough and Bullough (1994) have identified forces that are currently affecting the nursing profession and nursing roles:

External Forces

1. Development of science and technology has made a wider array of health care procedures possible.
2. The continued restriction by medicine of its numbers has resulted both in high incomes and the almost exclusive deployment of physicians into specialty roles (Office of Technology Assessment, 1986).
3. Changing demographic patterns created patterns of unmet needs, with an aging population, a decreasing birth rate, and increasing immigration of refugees and other Third World peoples.
4. Increased environmental hazards appeared and there was a growth in awareness of these problems.
5. A major pandemic of HIV/AIDS developed, along with epidemics of other sexually transmitted diseases.
6. The health care delivery system failed to keep pace with needs, although there is now some evidence that society may well be ready to deal with some of the inequities in the system.
7. Expanded nurse practice acts were enacted, providing at least limited increase in autonomy and responsibility for practice, although it is clear that further expansion of these acts would make better use of the talents of advanced practice nurses (Safriet, 1992).

Internal Forces

1. An increasing knowledge base and growing sophistication on the part of nurses.
2. A more functional and cost effective stratified system of nursing services, with educational systems that prepare a variety of nursing levels.
3. The development of a significant body of nursing research aimed at developing theory and improving nursing practice (pp. 3–4)

When nursing hesitates to fill the needs created by change, other individuals or groups move in. Numerous examples exist throughout history that attest to this phenomenon and are occurring once again. In the early 1970s, the American Medical Association (AMA) advocated that 100,000 nurses be upgraded to physician assistants. The ANA's rebuttal was that nurses were already assisting physicians and did not need to be upgraded to do so. The confrontation ended with the AMA creating the physician assistant (PA); the ANA created the nurse practitioner (NP). As recently as the late 1980s, an attempt was made by the AMA to introduce a new type of caregiver, the registered care technologist (RCT). This occurred at the peak of the nurse shortage in the United States and was proposed as a method to provide a new type of "bedside caregiver." According to some AMA members, the overemphasis on education by nurses had moved them away from the bedside. The AMA, without input from or discourse with organized nursing, approved plans for four pilot projects, with the first class to begin in July 1989. High school graduates would be trained to give patient care. They would take tests and be registered in their states. Basic RCTs would receive nine months of training; advanced RCTs would receive an additional nine months. The basic RCTs would learn some higher-level skills such as oral medication administration; the advanced RCTs would also be taught to care for cardiac monitors and ventilators and administer routine intravenous medication. Supervision of these activities was addressed, but the issue was not totally clarified.

This was one occasion that prompted unity in the nursing community. Professional nursing associations exerted enormous pressure in opposition to the proposal. They were joined by the American Osteopathic Association and the Florida Medical Association. Although one pilot project was initiated at a Kentucky nursing home, the enrolled RCTs evidently never finished the program.

Nursing and nurses must begin to direct educational, legislative, and organizational changes that will have an impact on the profession. Nurses must increasingly recognize their responsibility to be active, participating members in mandates for health care, initiating actions as problems emerge. The time to *react* to changes is long past; the time to be *proactive* has arrived.

The Practice Arena

Nursing changes and grows in response to perceived social need, parallels the development of the social welfare system, and reflects society's attitude toward sickness and health. Its history documents a detailed account of the growth of an occupation in its quest for professionalization, an intimate view of the work experiences of women in a culture traditionally dominated by men, and the impact of nursing on patient care in hospitals. "Perhaps the most important single element in reshaping the day-to-day texture of hospital life was the professionalization of nursing. In 1800, as today, nurses were the most important single factor determining ward and room environment. Nursing, like professional hospital administration changed modes of hospital financing, has played a key role in shaping the modern hospital" (Rosenberg, 1987, pp. 8–9). Historically, nurses have influenced patient care even in circumstances involving limited power, control, and resources.

During the past decade nursing practice has been characterized by rapidly increasing responsibility, accountability, autonomy, and authority in patient care. It is a decade of practice measurement and outcome research in health care. Potentially, further differentiation of roles will occur as relationships between nurses and physicians are transformed and new patterns of governance within the nursing hierarchy are established. Collaboration will be the byword as health professionals can no longer practice independently; boundaries are collapsing. The need for highly technically skilled nurses in hospitals will continue, but they will, in all probability, be accountable for their practice to a nurse with advanced preparation who will serve as the case manager for a group of patients. Departmental governance and the participation of nurse representatives in institutional, agency, and practice policies will continue and must escalate. But will nurses' redefined roles be formally recognized and adequately compensated? Will advanced practice nurses be permitted to function with the full spectrum of their abilities and capabilities?

The nurse practitioner movement has been one of the best illustrations of nursing's ingenuity in the face of societal upheaval and professional agitation. Created at a time of physician shortages in primary health care, it provided an opportunity for nurses to promote their professional agenda and embrace their service to society (Ford, 1992). One of the primary goals of the original pediatric nurse practitioner program in 1965 was to expand the nurse's scope of practice through an increased depth of knowledge; clinical judgment and management would be emphasized. It was, indeed, an avenue to advanced clinical expertise. The success of the practitioner movement has been demonstrated by the dramatic growth of practitioner specialties. In addition, rapidly increasing numbers of different types of practitioner programs are being initiated in nursing educational programs for a variety of reasons. Perhaps the most significant reason is the paradigm shift in health care.

Nurse specialists are here to stay. How they will fall out in terms of hierarchy remains to be seen. In the past, nurses in administrative positions ranked above those with specialized clinical expertise. Now clinical nursing expertise is usually equal to or ranked above administrative positions, and clinical nurse specialist positions may be equal to or above the traditional head nurse or supervisor positions. More and more attention is currently being given to defining and describing advanced practice nursing as dramatic increases are occurring in numbers of generalists, practitioners, and clinical specialists. Yet, there is still a difference of opinion regarding what Bullough (1992) refers to as two models for specialization. The first is the nursing model or clinical nurse specialist (CNS) with emphasis on advanced content from the behavioral sciences, education, and nursing. The focus of this model is the caring role of the nurse. The second model, the collaborative model, builds on acquired nursing skills with advanced knowledge of medicine and the behavioral and biological sciences. Nurse practitioners, nurse anesthetists, and nurse midwives are included in this model, which some nurses believed pushed nursing into a medical role. Styles (1992) has critically commented on spe-

Judy Waid, *Nursing: A Tradition of Caring,* 1994. *(Copyright Judy Waid and District Three, Ohio Nurses Association, Youngstown, Ohio.)*

This fifth edition medallion depicts a century of delivery of nursing care. Nurses' roles and images have changed to reflect the changing needs of society and culture. Nursing's philosophy of caring and advocacy has endured through time and will continue to light the way into the twenty-first century.

cialties, stating that ". . . it can be seen that (1) professional, practice, and market forces are accelerating the development of specialties in nursing; (2) this proliferation is not occurring in an orderly manner overall; and (3) there are no universally recognized specialties, no accepted standards, and no common principle or authority" (p. 33). Advanced practice nursing, for all practical purposes, has no common foundation: program admission criteria, educational preparation, credentialing standards, and regulatory mechanisms vary widely.

In the United States, nursing is the only profession that performs certification both internal and external to the professional association. The ANA and approximately twenty-five other groups act as certifying bodies. The American Nurses Credentialing Center (ANCC) was an internal unit of the ANA from 1982 until 1991, when it was established as a separately incorporated subsidiary of the ANA. Nurses in other countries are facing similar issues with regard to specialties and regulatory mechanisms. The development of specialties outside the United States, however, has for the most part been controlled by a centralized authority like a ministry of health or the professional association. In additional, several events have prompted a redefinition of nursing practice roles and functions: a twelve-member European Community was established that permits free movement of workers across national boundaries, international societies of nurse specialists are being developed, new groups of technicians are emerging, and nursing and postgraduate education is shifting into universities. In addition, the International Council of Nurses is addressing the definition, titling, and credentialing of specialists worldwide (Styles, 1992).

Nurses are making powerful contributions to health care with innovative community practices that promote health, accessibility, and lower costs and facilitate a high quality of care. Community nursing centers (CNCs) are key examples of these contributions to health care reform. The concept was conceived early in nursing's history with such nursing leaders as Lillian Wald at the Henry Street Settlement in New York and Mary Breckenridge at the Frontier Nursing Service in Kentucky. These two centers are classic examples of practice settings created and managed by nurses at the turn of the century. They established a precedent of direct access to professional nursing services by the consumer. The more recent CNC movement occurred in the middle to late 1970s in diverse geographical locations including Freeport, New York; Lehman College (Chicago); the University of Wisconsin–Milwaukee; Montana State University; and Arizona State University (Glass, 1989; Lundeen, 1994). As the number of CNCs steadily increased, two biennial conferences for nurse-managed centers were held in Milwaukee in 1982 and 1984. Since a variety of models of nursing centers were being developed, an effort was made to produce a consensus definition at the second conference. These centers covered a spectrum from individual nurse-established clinics and disease-specific clinics to academically based nursing centers. In 1986 an ANA task force reviewed and modified the definition that had been developed with the assistance of a Delphi survey at the 1984 conference, with the following result:

> Nursing centers—sometimes referred to as community nursing organizations, nurse-managed centers, nursing clinics, and community nursing centers—are organizations that give the client direct access to professional nursing services. Using nursing models of health, professional nurses in these centers diagnose and treat human responses to actual and potential health problems, and promote health and optimal functioning among target populations and communities. The services provided in these centers are holistic and client centered, and are reimbursable at a reasonable fee level. Accountability and responsibility for client care and professional practice remain with the professional nurse. Overall accountability and responsibility remain with the nurse executive.
>
> Nursing centers are not limited to any particular organizational configuration. Nursing centers may be freestanding businesses or may be affiliated with univer

Facing Page, P. Buckley Moss, *Miracle Workers,* 1990. Offset lithograph from watercolor, image size: 24.76 × 22.22 cm; paper size: 29.84 × 27.30 cm. *(The Moss Portfolio, Mathews, Virginia, copyright P. Buckley Moss.)*

Nurses, physicians, and others in health care are often regarded as "miracle workers," particularly when the outcomes of treatment and care result in prolongation of life and/or an improvement of health status.

Above, Photograph of a homeless man in Boston, pictured with Eunice MacAllister, BS, RN, as she dresses his leg in the Pine Street Inn Nurses' Clinic, Boston. *(Copyright 1995 Linda Haas. All rights reserved.)*

Right, Troy Spicer, RN, MS, CFNP, an AID Atlanta Nurse Practitioner, examines a patient at the Atlanta, Georgia clinic. *(By permission of AID Atlanta, Georgia. Photo by Susan Hixon.)*

Facing Page, The Sanctuary, 1993. *(Official U.S. Navy Photo by Don S. Montgomery, USN [Ret.])*

A port bow view of the former hospital ship *Sanctuary* moored at the Maryland Port Authority pier at Lambert Point. Life International, the non-profit organization that obtained the ship from the U.S. Navy in 1990 for fifteen dollars, has proposed a plan to use the ship as a shelter for homeless residents of Baltimore. The *Sanctuary* saw duty during the Vietnam war after joining the *Repose*.

its structure a number of programs have resulted, in keeping with its mission of advocacy, education, and service. AID Atlanta is run by a nurse and based on nursing theory. A nurse practitioner functions in the early intervention clinic, which provides care for patients who have the human immunodeficiency virus (HIV) but do not yet have AIDS. Issues of housing and other basic needs are addressed along with health care in this primary health care model. An interdisciplinary approach to case management provides for a continuum of care including hospital and community-based services. "This model seeks to fully integrate the nursing knowledge of the nurse practitioner into the overall case management model" (Sowell and Meadows, 1994).

It is apparent that the development of nursing centers puts nursing in a unique, important position to link hospital and community-based services. Nursing centers can also link nursing educators, schools of nursing, and nursing students with community practice settings where vital clinical experience and joint practice relationships can be achieved. Centers are consistent with the holistic care of patients, a philosophy long emphasized in nursing's history.

Standardized Language and Classification Systems

Now as never before has it become necessary for nurses to develop a standardized language of nursing. Concerns for the cost of health care and computerization will continue to force the nursing community to identify the structure and components of nursing practice. The clinical, theoretical, and research dimensions of nursing must be brought together in a unified whole with recognition of the influence of the political, economic, and ethical domains. It is believed that professional advancement of the discipline can be achieved only when a consistent language representing all settings and all levels can be used to communicate nursing activities. Nursing individuals, groups, and organizations have steadily moved toward that end with the development of classification systems that have been appearing in the nursing literature since the early 1970s.

Classification systems are often called taxonomies or taxonomic approaches. They are developed with particular goals or purposes in mind. The usefulness of classification systems cannot be denied: enhanced communication, generation of research hypotheses, projections of future trends, and other benefits can be realized. The classification system movement in nursing has led to the generation of various types. It would be well to remember, however, that nursing classification systems actually began in the late 1950s as patient classifications for nurse staffing.

The initial work toward the development of the Nursing Minimum Data Set (NMDS) began in the 1970s. Based on the concept of the Uniform Minimum Health Data Sets, the NMDS is an initial attempt to establish uniform standards for the collection of comparable, minimum, essential nursing data. According to Werley and others (1994), it is ". . . a standardized approach that facilitates the abstraction of essential, core minimum data to describe nursing practice. It is intended for use in any and all settings where nursing care is provided. The NMDS is unique in that it is the only data set whereby the practice of nursing can be described, resulting in a nursing database" (p. 113). Following the earlier work, the NMDS was developed in 1985 through the efforts of a national group of sixty-four experts. Three broad categories of elements were identified: nursing care (four elements), patient or client demographics (five elements), and service (seven elements). These sixteen elements include nursing diagnosis, intervention, outcome, and intensity of nursing care. As the title itself implies, the NMDS consists of a minimum set of items that have both uniform definitions and categories concerning nursing practice. Thus through the use of this system two primary aspects can potentially be achieved: the description of the essence of nursing and the development of a database.

Although individual nurses were involved in nursing diagnosis activities before the 1970s, the North American Nursing Diagnosis Association (NANDA) is considered the forerunner in this activity. Since 1973, members have diligently endeavored to develop nursing diagnoses and more recently a taxonomy for their classification. The NANDA Nursing Diagnosis Taxonomy has had great significance for both the discipline of nursing and the organization of its knowledge. This taxonomy is currently the best known and most widely used classification system in nursing. It is also, perhaps, one of the most controversial for a variety of reasons. Each NANDA-approved nursing diagnosis includes a definition of the diagnosis, defining characteristics, and related factors. Since the First National Conference on Classification of Nursing Diagnosis (October 1973) in St. Louis, a great number of nursing diagnoses have been approved for clinical testing. NANDA's Taxonomy I has been translated into the format used by the World Health Organization (WHO), the organization that revises and publishes the International Classification of Disease (ICD). This format provides for an organized international database for health care; the inclusion of nursing diagnoses assists the development of an international nursing database within the ICD framework (Warren, 1994). Ongoing work on the taxonomy involves the refinement and clinical testing of the existing nursing diagnoses, as well as the identification, development, and testing of new diagnoses. Movement toward a Taxonomy II is proceeding.

The Nursing Interventions Classification (NIC) was developed and is continuing at the University of Iowa College of Nursing by a large research team. The work of the team was begun in the late 1980s and has been facilitated by the help of nurse experts from many specialties. The primary usefulness of the classification of treatments that nurses perform is in the planning and documenting of nursing care, the communication of the nature of nursing, and the development of large databases for research related to the effectiveness of nursing care. In May 1992 the *Nursing Interventions Classification* was published with a standardized list of 336 direct-care nursing interventions. Each of these is elucidated by a definition, nurse activities necessary to carry out the intervention, and background readings. "NIC includes all direct care interventions that nurses do on behalf of patients, including both independent and collaborative interventions. The classification applies to nurses in all specialties and in all settings. While an individual nurse will have expertise in only a limited number of interventions, the entire classification is meant to capture the expertise of all nurses" (Bulechek and McCloskey, 1994, p. 133). The second edition of the book is in process and will contain 433 interventions. The book will include the revised NIC Taxonomy and a list of linkages with NANDA diagnoses.

The evaluation of health care effectiveness is one of the great challenges of the 1990s. Emphasis has thus been placed on the use of patient outcomes, which have been studied primarily in relation to specific diagnoses, whether medical or nursing, and specific interventions. The outcome models that have been generated, however, do not embrace the multivariate influences on patient outcomes. Going one step further, the models do not necessarily reflect nursing practice. The landmark research of Horn and Swain (1978) was a grand effort to organize nursing-sensitive patient outcomes. Their research was conducted to identify patient outcomes influenced by nursing care. Other research efforts have focused on the identification and categorization of those outcomes used to measure the effects of nursing care. Currently, a large research team at the University of Iowa College of Nursing is studying nursing-sensitive patient outcomes (Johnson and Maas, 1994). The overall purpose is to identify, label, define, and classify these outcomes and ultimately develop valid and reliable outcome measures. Although the project is painstaking and laborious, considerable work has been done.

North American Nursing Diagnosis Association Logo. (Courtesy of the North American Nursing Diagnosis Association (NANDA), Philadelphia, Pennsylvania.)

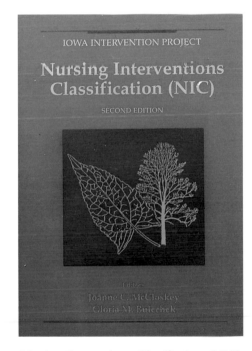

Nursing Interventions Classification (NIC), Second Edition, book cover, 1996. *(Courtesy of Mosby—Year Book, Inc.)*

Nursing Outcomes Classification Logo, 1995. (Courtesy of the Iowa Outcomes Project, Drs. Marian Johnson and Meridean Maas, Co-Principal Investigators. Photo: Steven Warner, The University of Iowa College of Nursing, Iowa City.)

The description of nursing practice remains at the forefront of nursing thought. A standardized language is believed to be the answer to facilitating that description and making it operational and measurable. The preceding examples of classification systems and, possibly, others that exist may provide the mechanism for achieving this goal as linkages between diagnoses, interventions, and outcomes are identified in the developmental processes. Perhaps most beneficial, standardized languages can be computerized. This is particularly significant since information system activities and the drive toward computer-based patient records are influencing, and will continue to influence, the day-to-day practice of nurses. The Institute of Medicine has set the year 2000 as the date for the actual achievement of a computer-based patient record and defined it in the following manner:

> . . . an electronic patient record that resides in a system specifically designed to support users through availability of complete and accurate data, practitioner reminders and alerts, clinical decision support systems, links to bodies of medical knowledge, and other aids. This definition encompasses a broader view of the patient record than is current today, moving from the notion of a location or device for keeping track of patient care events to a resource with much enhanced utility in patient care (including the ability to provide an accurate longitudinal account of care), in management of the health care system, and in extension of knowledge

> — *Dick and Stein, 1991*

Nurses must continue to focus their energy on developing a standardized language that will be comprehensive, yet flexible. Questions must still be addressed, however, such as whether nursing needs just one or more than one classification system.

Nursing Research

Research is not a new phenomenon in nursing. In its evolution, however, it has gone through numerous shifts and stages that have contributed to its overall development. At different periods in history the emphasis in nursing research was on the development of nursing education and administration, on the goals and the mission of nursing, and more recently on clinical practice. At different periods the idea of the replication of studies was viewed in a negative light. Current thought about replication is that it is needed, to build on the results of other studies and to confirm achieved results. Programs of research were either virtually unheard of or did not exist. Collaborative research with nursing colleagues or researchers from other disciplines was a rarity. Often the so-called research was not of a high caliber; nurse researchers were few or were not adequately prepared to conduct research. In retrospect, nursing has come a long way in its research endeavors. Nursing now has a sound research tradition; funding agencies give much more than lip service to nurse researchers, and federal funding has increased. Centers for nursing research have developed in various locations and the number of doctorally prepared nurses has significantly increased. Research is now accepted as legitimate in the eyes of the nursing community. But one thing remains clear: "There is no longer any question that the priorities and goals for nursing research must be based on predictions about future consumers of nursing services, evolving systems for health care delivery, and the context within which nurses practice" (Felton, 1989, p. 276).

A milestone was reached in the United States with the advent of the National Center for Nursing Research (NCNR) in 1986. The center became a reality through an intensive effort by nurses across the country and organized national, state, and specialty nursing associations. A congressional override of a presidential veto was necessary to enact legislation to establish the center at the National Institutes of Health (NIH) in Washington, D.C. The purpose of the center was threefold: to provide a focal point for promoting the growth and quality of research related to nursing and patient care, to provide leadership to expand the pool of experienced nurse researchers, and to promote closer interaction with other bases of health care research (NLN, 1985; *The American Nurse*, 1986). The center was elevated to the status of an institute in June 1993 by the National Institutes of Health Revitalization Act of 1993. The National Institute of Nursing Research (NINR) conducts and supports research and research training in universities and research centers across the country and at NIH. Its budget, however, has remained modest by NIH standards.

Nursing must not be satisfied with its accomplishments in research and its research efforts. Commentary can still be heard that there continues to be little evidence of the use of research in practice and little evidence of demand for research by practicing nurses. The acceptance and the valuing of nursing research cannot be mandated for the majority of nurses or the general public. It will be valued only when people see that it makes a difference. And what of the future for nursing research? Lindeman (1989) depicted the hypothetical challenges of nursing research for the late 1990s or early 2000s as reflected in the literature on the future:

1. Knowledge from health care research will double every two to three years. Researchers taking longer than two to three years to complete a study will produce knowledge that is obsolete.

2. Performance records on all health professionals will be maintained in a national data base. Those data will be used to determine research access to human subjects.

3. Telematics will link epidemiological and environmental data, enabling new understanding of the causes of illness, and reducing infectious disease by the very early detection of outbreaks.

4. Computer-applied quality assurance standards will determine who to treat with what means.

5. A small number of super-experts will update intelligent machines; other health professionals will use them.

6. People will become their own primary care practitioners and their own primary care system.

7. Automation and robotics will bring hospital staffing to less than two FTE per occupied bed.

8. Research is conducted through computer simulations and data banks controlled by the federal government.

9. Books, journals, and face to face conferences are obsolete; people network through computer systems or teleconferencing (p. 3).

Although this list was generated just six short years ago, a number of these hypothetical challenges have come to pass and the rest appear to be perfectly feasible and in the process of happening. Nursing research must not ever become an elitist endeavor. Researchers must not conduct research in isolation from practitioners but must continue to develop and increase partnerships in scholarly and scientific inquiry. It is the practitioners who are faced with the social realities involved in health care and must deal with them daily. Research, too, does not exist in a vacuum. Its focus must change as the economic, political, and ethical influences impinge on societal needs and the delivery of health care. Consequently the type of research that nurses must currently do more of is that concerned with primary health care issues and health care policy.

To be effective, research must be communicated, disseminated, tested, and adopted. Nurse researchers have a responsibility and an obligation to provide opportunities for practicing nurses to be involved in this process as participants in the discussion, testing, and use of research findings. A cautionary note: adoption of research findings can be time-consuming. A number of years ago Barnard (1982) commented that nursing is in the beginning phase of the dis-

"Nursing Approach" co-anchors on set. *Left,* Karlene Kerfoot, PhD, RN, CNAA, FAAN; *right,* Donna Hill Howes, MS, RN. *(Courtesy of Sigma Theta Tau International, Indianapolis, Indiana.)*

"Nursing Approach" was the first national television news series created for and about nurses. The show premiered on Sunday, January 3, 1993, on CNBC/ American Medical Television. It was produced by Sigma Theta Tau International and Samuel Merritt College's Studio Three Productions of San Francisco. The program co-anchors were Donna Hill Howes, executive vice-president of the Academy of Medical Film in San Francisco, and Karlene Kerfoot, executive vice-president, patient care, St. Luke's Episcopal Hospital, Houston, Texas. More than one hundred ten news stories were aired during the fourteen months the show was televised.

cipline of nursing. She said that we have a good beginning and that increasingly research is focusing on issues of practice. She continued:

> We must guard against impatience, expecting the answers from research to be instantly translated. History of other disciplines is instructive; it reveals the many years it takes for a science to build explanatory theories and have empirical evidence. Nurse researchers must continue with their creative work which deals with the most complex of all phenomena, the human being, and at the same time be encouraged to search for proof and the empirical evidence that will eventually lead to scientific bases for nursing practice (p. 11).

LEST WE FORGET: THINGS COULD BE WORSE!

Nursing has a long history of social activism. Its history is full of examples of nurses fighting against social injustices and fighting for positive social change. Many of these nurses are identified throughout this book, but their stories provide only a small sample of the many accomplishments that have been achieved, sometimes against overwhelming odds. The current events of the health care scene around the world can, indeed, leave us with a feeling of dread: so many changes, happening too fast, with chaos seemingly everywhere. Yet, nursing is always struggling with the challenges of change. Without question, nurses have become "tough" and in their toughness have continued a long legacy of humanitarian service. Yes, things could be better, but it is time that we herald nursing's glories.

The issue of the inaccurate image has long been among nursing's struggles. Few nurses would disagree that nursing is frequently misrepresented in the media, remembering Nurse Ratchet, Hot Lips Houlihan, nurses in soap operas, and one of the most recent television exposés, "The Nightingales." It is positive that nurses united in a common cause to eliminate some of these negative nurse stereotypes. "The Nightingales" was pulled from the air after protest from individual nurses and nursing organizations who believed that the negative portrayal of the nurses diminished public respect and discouraged talented people from seeking careers in nursing. Nurses and other "Women in White" were featured in the October 1983 issue of *Playboy* magazine. This display brought angry reactions from nurses in the form of letters to the editor. In addition, the nurses who were featured in the centerfold were criticized for betraying nursing and further contributing to the perpetuation of nurses as sex objects. Some people contend that nurses create their own images. In other words, information about nurses is acquired from their interactions with patients and visitors.

Various strategies can be used to inform the public of the "true" image of the nurse. This can be accomplished when nurses take the initiative in self-portrayal. Although many individual nurses and nursing organizations have been creative in attempts to educate the public about nursing, Sigma Theta Tau's *Nursing Approach* (1993) was unique. *Nursing Approach* was the first national television news series created for and about nurses. Co-produced by Sigma Theta Tau International and Samuel Merritt College's Studio Three Productions of San Francisco, the weekly half-hour show was billed as "the single most important national forum for nurses." It was televised on CNBC's American Medical Television. More than one hundred ten news stories were aired during the fourteen months the show was televised. Segments focused on the work of nurses and included updates on recent research findings. This was an exceptional example of nursing being proactive rather than reactive.

Although we cannot absolutely predict all the "tough" issues that nurses will face in the remaining years of this decade and into the next century, we can observe trends that will have a direct bearing on nursing and health care. Emphasis on cost containment will continue, and the allocation of scarce resources will prompt an even greater increase in ethical concerns. Managed care will continue to develop, along with shifting to outpatient services. Environmental concerns will escalate, along with consumer focus on personal physical and mental fitness. Consumers will be even more involved in decision making about their care and treatment and will strongly consider the use of alternative health care methods. Some hospitals are even now designing care units that combine traditional medicine with alternative techniques. The Planetree Model Hospital Unit at Beth Israel Medical Center in New York, established in 1992, is such a unit. On this unit, complementary modalities grounded in research and posing little risk to the patient are being used. Relationships between hospitals, health care providers, business, and industry will continue to be sought. In all this change, a vital place exists for nurses. Opportunities for nurses are limitless, if we but grasp them or create them. Nurses can be, are prepared to be, and should be, the front-runners in the primary health care movement.

Tim Porter-O'Grady, EdD, RN, CS, CNAA, FAAN. *(Courtesy of Sigma Theta Tau International, Indianapolis, Indiana. Wayne Scott Smith, Photographer.)*

Tim Porter-O'Grady donated his time for more than a year to consult on current events at the request of Sigma Theta Tau for news stories for "Nursing Approach." An eminent author and international health care consultant, he was a substitute news anchor and contributor of news interviews.

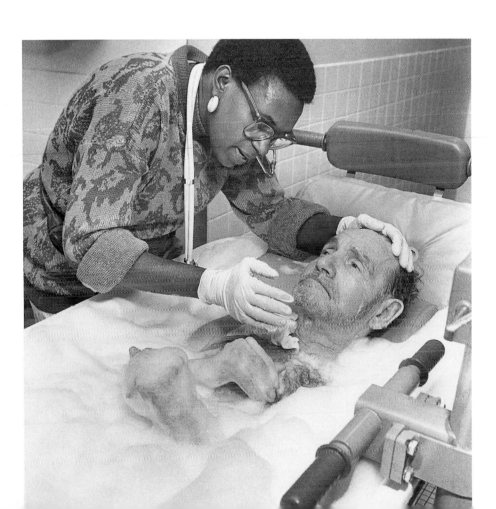

Massage of Hydrotherapy, 1994. (Courtesy of Beth Israel Medical Center, New York. Miller Photography, New Hyde Park, New York.)

At Beth Israel Medical Center, complementary modalities grounded in research and posing little, if any, risk to the patient are being used. Patients' responses to these modalities are being monitored through clinical data, patient verbal reports, and controlled studies. Here Elaine Davis, BSN, RN, comforts a hospice patient with a soothing tone of voice and the enveloping warmth and gentle massage of hydrotherapy.

471

Therapeutic Touch, 1994. (Courtesy of Beth Israel Medical Center, New York. Miller Photography, New Hyde Park, New York.)

The general public is seeking more humanistic health care that preserves human dignity, embraces caring and respect, and supports personal preferences related to health and recovery. The public is turning more and more to alternative medicine or holistic health care. At Beth Israel, the term *complementary modalities* is used to indicate that these non-mainstream approaches should be integrated into the traditional systems of care if appropriate. Here Aurora S. Ocampo, MA, RN, CS, clinical nurse specialist in surgery, performs therapeutic touch to create a balanced energy field and promote relaxation and healing.

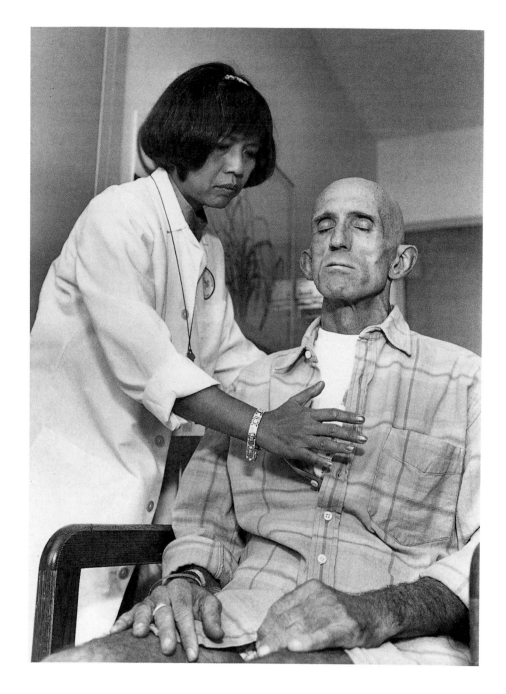

Planetree Model Hospital Unit, 1994. (Courtesy of Beth Israel Medical Center, New York. Miller Photography, New Hyde Park, New York.)

In September, 1992, the Samuels Planetree Unit was established at Beth Israel to provide a new model of inpatient care. The unit includes a redesign of the physical space to be more homelike, an emphasis on patient and family education, an approach to care that embraces the patient as its center, self-governance of staff, and the use of complementary modalities to support healing and recovery. It is a thirty-four–bed attending-oriented adult medical unit that includes a four-bed coronary care stepdown unit. A holistic, humanistic approach to patient care is stressed.

472

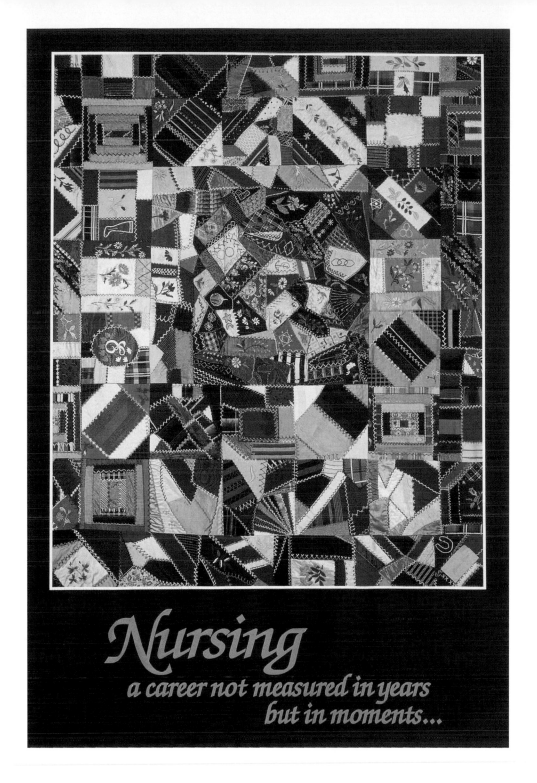

Melodie Chenevert, *Nursing: A Career Not Measured in Years But in Moments,* 1992. Poster, 60.96 × 91.44 cm. *(By permission of Pro-Nurse, Gaithersburg, Maryland.)*

"A Victorian crazy quilt. A nursing career. What do they have in common? Rich fabric. Fragmented. Held together by heart and hand. Elaborately embellished with unforgettable moments. Fine art. Painstakingly executed. A work in progress, often unfinished. Chaotic yet controlled. And synergy—the whole is greater than the sum of its parts. In the end we will not remember the years we spent in nursing. We will only remember the moments.

This was the third poster I created to commemorate nursing. For the first two, I had commissioned paintings to capture the theme. This one had me stumped. I couldn't visualize what I wanted put on canvas. I woke up in the middle of the night and knew exactly what to do. As a long-time quilt collector, I'm surprised it didn't occur to me sooner.

About the quilt: The only key to its origin is a yellowed scrap of paper basted in the lower right corner bearing the name, Myda Moar. Over 100 years old, mint condition, unfinished, found in Washington state. The quilt has been framed and now hangs in Sigma Theta Tau International Headquarters in Indianapolis."

—*Melodie Chenevert*

(Posters are available from Pro Nurse Headquarters.)

U N I T   11

Contact and Diversity

To accelerate the delivery of essential health services to the people of the world, particularly underserved populations, the transformation of the nursing profession is critical, and professional nurses must assume roles as leaders and active participants in change. 'Nurses must master the skills of visionary and strategic thinking to have an impact on institutional and political forces that control health development. The emergence of the phenomenon of transformation is providing a rare opportunity for nursing. Transformation provides a scenario for a new way of interacting, a new way of problem solving, and a means to developing a shared vision among health professionals in various settings.

– LILLIAN M SIMMS

Kitagawa Utamaro, *Mother and Child Before a Screen (Mother Playing With Her Child, and Nurse),* c. 1800, Polychrome woodblock print, 37.78 × 25.08 cm. *(The Metropolitan Museum of Art, Fletcher Fund, 1929. Copyright 1994 by The Metropolitan Museum of Art.)*

Utamaro frequently documents the day-to-day lives of women in a remarkably sensitive way. In this artwork, a willful little boy appears to be attempting to gain his mother's attention while at the same time scurrying away from his nurse. As the nurse tries to hold the child back with one hand, she covers her mouth with her kimono-sleeved hand, a sign of politeness when speaking. She may be giggling or scolding. Although the mother's back is to the observer, her reflection in the mirror depicts her impishly sticking her tongue out at the child.

ransformation is occurring everywhere—in organizations and corporations; in economic, political, social, educational, and religious institutions; in health care delivery systems. Transformation is occurring throughout the world. Each day the world becomes smaller and smaller. Individual countries can no longer remain isolated and concerned only with issues that arise within their own boundaries. International travel has become commonplace; this has facilitated a greater awareness of cultural similarities and differences, with the need for greater understanding and communication becoming apparent. Global interaction is progressing at a rapid pace that has been spurred by technological developments, particularly in the area of information systems. It will become even more important to understand and clarify language systems that are essentially developed not only to describe the world but also to define it. Languages represent a unique way of perceiving reality.

Helen Hardin, *Medicine Talk,* 1964. Casein, approximately 71.12 × 35.56 cm. *(Copyright Helen Hardin, 1964. Photo copyright Cradoc Bagshaw, 1995. All rights reserved. Helen Hardin Estate.)*

Medicine Talk was the painting in Hardin's first "formal" one-woman show at Enchanted Mesa in 1964 that proved to be significant to her career.

Introduction

The words currently being used to describe health care delivery systems are also being used to describe the world. Conflict, crisis, chaos, deterioration, and disintegration are part of the list that provides a picture of massive change and turmoil that is seemingly out of control and promoting human degradation. Societies are seeking new information, new knowledge, and new paradigms, new ways to help them understand and deal with the forces that are driving important decision making. Even more critical, societies are searching for ways to improve quality of life for present and future generations. Are societies also now in the process of *Creating a New Civilization* (1995) as suggested by the Tofflers? Although the United States is often the focus of much of their writings, their messages are applicable worldwide. The Tofflers have been writing about the future since 1970, when their first best seller, *Future Shock,* was published. This work discussed the impact of accelerated change that was overwhelming and disorienting people and their societies. *The Third Wave* (1980) was even more startling, since it contained a predictive framework. Here the information revolution was compared with the agricultural and industrial revolutions, two other great transformations in history. The Tofflers believe that the impact of this third historical wave of change is currently being felt and a new civilization is being created.

Worldwide, people are searching for new directions and alternatives to their current state of life, as numerous other titles of various types of literature attest. New paradigms are being created that seem to be leaning more toward a greater emphasis on human respect and human caring. Authors are proposing that an era of true spiritual awareness or a spiritual renaissance is occurring as people are attempting to find meaning in their lives. Redfield's *The Celestine Prophecy* (1993) provides one such view of the changing world. Its popularity is directly linked to predictions associated with relationships, international affairs, and insights that, if grasped, can provide a new image of human life and a vision for protecting and preserving the environment. All this current spiraling activity is also exhibited in a search for health-promotion therapies and a shift away from disease-oriented care. Health care reform is but one aspect of change; holistic and alternative approaches to care and cure are being investigated and accepted. In a number of instances people are returning to health care practices and systems that were used hundreds of thousands of years ago. An increasing emphasis on preventive medicine and health promotion is taking place.

Radioactive Mud Treatments. (Copyright Andy Levin. All rights reserved.)

Ukraine, Odessa. Treatments with radioactive mud from the Ukraine are thought to be beneficial in a variety of muscular and skeletal conditions. Patients are covered with mud or immersed in a bath like the one being drawn by the nurse in the photograph. Patients stay in the bath for up to one half hour, after which the mud is washed off in a shower.

Nursing is in a unique position to exercise courageous and visionary direction in creative health promotion practices and holistic care. Nursing is in a strategic position to help promote and facilitate this paradigm shift in health care. Nursing is in a key position to shape and provide primary health care. Nursing has been and still can be a strong social force and advocate for change. Thus it is essential that nursing create international links among nursing communities, since all nurses around the globe are facing common issues and experiencing increasing social pressures. The environments in which nurses work worldwide have drastically changed, presenting even greater challenges. Historically, nurses have risen to the task of overcoming barriers and meeting challenges. Their ultimate goal was concern and care for human beings, only some of whom were ill. For nurses to continue this humanitarian tradition will require a level of commitment and a degree of courage that will exceed previous circumstances. Nursing's vision for the future must embrace the building of a healthy international society in which adequate care is available to and provided for everyone. Nursing's choice for the twenty-first century remains clear: we can join in "health care for a few" or "health for all" (Maglacas, 1988; 1989). Nurses are strategically placed to support health care for all and to support one another in creating conditions for change.

Facing page, Mary Ericksen, *An Invitation to Dream,* 1993. Pastel, 26.67 × 41.91 cm. *(By permission of Mary Ericksen, Minnesota.)*

This beautiful painting graces the cover of the brochure announcing the eighteenth International Nursing Caring Conference in Rochester, Minnesota, in April 1996. International caring is portrayed through the spiraling figures united by human touch. Both the softness of the colors and the style of the art convey a sense of spirituality. One can imagine that the primary message is: "Let each of us reach out and care for one another as an international nursing community."

WORLD HEALTH ISSUES

At the thirtieth World Health Assembly in 1977, member states of the World Health Organization (WHO) established a broad common goal: "Health for All by the Year 2000." In Alma-Ata, Union of Soviet Socialist Republics, in 1978, primary health care was declared the mechanism for achieving this goal. A global strategy was formulated at the thirty-fourth World Health Assembly in 1981. Inherent in the strategy is the continuous, progressive improvement of the health status of populations through national health care systems that provide health promotion, disease prevention, and curative and rehabilitative services to all. The following were targeted:

1. All people in every country will have ready access at least to essential health care and first-level referral facilities.
2. All people will be actively involved in caring for themselves and their families as far as they can and in community action for health.
3. Communities throughout the world will share with Governments responsibility for the health care of their members.
4. All governments will assume overall responsibility for the health of their people.
5. Safe drinking water and sanitation will be available for all people.
6. All people will be adequately nourished.
7. All children will be immunized against the major infectious diseases of childhood.
8. Communicable diseases in the developing countries will be of no greater public health significance in the year 2000 than they were in developed countries in the year 1980.
9. All possible ways will be applied to prevent and control noncommunicable diseases and promote mental health through influencing lifestyles and controlling the physical and psychosocial environment.
10. Essential drugs will be available to all.

— UN Chronicle, *1992, p. 45*

Seventeen years have passed since the Alma-Ata Declaration on Primary Health Care. Although progress toward the goal has been made, barriers to its accomplishment still exist. Two reports regarding the implementation of the strategy were completed: the first was completed in 1984; the second covered 1985 through the middle of 1988. A substantial improvement was noted in the global health status, as demonstrated by decreasing infant mortality rates and increased life expectancy at birth. The WHO Expanded Programme on Immunization (EPI) has been successful in protecting the lives of children from vaccine-preventable deaths (poliomyelitis, measles, tuberculosis, diphtheria, whooping cough, and tetanus). Eighty percent of all infants worldwide have been vaccinated against the six diseases. Malaria remains one of the major and most serious of the world health problems; other tropical diseases (cholera, yellow fever, and dengue) continue to wreak havoc on human populations. Noncommunicable diseases such as cardiovascular disease, stroke, cancer, and chronic respiratory infection are decreasing in developed countries but increasing in developing countries. Since the common denominator of risk for these diseases is lifestyle, more healthful lifestyles continue to be promoted. Campaigns and programs for the provision of safe water and uncontaminated food continue, along with emphasis on better sanitation. Improvements have been made in these areas, particularly with safe water and rural water supply. Unfortunately achievements in access to health care are extremely uneven, and the health gap between the least developed countries and other developing countries is increasing. Downward economic trends have grossly affected the economic welfare and health status in the developing countries (Maglacas, 1989; *UN Chronicle,* 1992).

The world has, however, witnessed the eradication of a killer disease. Through the efforts of WHO, smallpox became the first disease ever eliminated by vaccination. The last case was diagnosed in the small coastal town of Merka in southern Somalia in 1977. Tuberculosis, however, is spiraling out of control. In the past ten years it has spread dramatically as a result of overcrowding and poverty, the spread of AIDS, and the resurgence of tuber-

P. Buckley Moss, *Heavenly Babe,* 1995. Offset lithograph from watercolor, image size: 21.11 × 18.25 cm; paper size: 31.27 × 28.41 cm. *(The Moss Portfolio, Mathews, Virginia, copyright P. Buckley Moss.)*

Heavenly Babe was printed in two editions of one thousand each and twenty-five artist's proofs. Of one edition of one thousand, seven hundred prints have been donated to the National SIDS (Sudden Infant Death Syndrome) Alliance and three hundred prints have been donated to the Iowa SIDS Alliance. The other edition was published for general distribution. This generous donation is not unusual for this artist, who has contributed greatly to fund raising for nursing organizations as well as for natural disaster relief as in the case of the Iowa floods in 1993.

Hans Baldung (called Grien), *The Witches' Sabbath*, 1510. Chiaroscuro woodcut, 37.78 × 26.03 cm. (block). *(Bequest of W.G. Russell Allen. Copyright 1995. Museum of Fine Arts, Boston. All rights reserved. Courtesy, Museum of Fine Arts, Boston.)*

During this period in history, prints and paintings of witches were popular. The great majority of witches were lay healers; the story of their persecution chronicles one of the initial struggles in the suppression of women as healers. Witch healers were frequently the only practitioners in communities in which poor and disease-ridden people had no doctors or hospitals.

culosis strains resistant to drugs. Tuberculosis and AIDS are currently deadly partners that are taking their toll globally. It is estimated that by the end of the 1990s, tuberculosis will speed the deaths of a third of AIDS sufferers; approximately fourteen percent of tuberculosis cases will be due to AIDS. The vast majority of the projected human immunodeficiency virus (HIV) infections and AIDS cases will be in developing countries by the year 2000. The world pandemic can be contained only through a strong commitment from all communities, national and international. Disease and ill health recognize no borders.

Advocacy Revisited

Societal trends, the complexities of life, technological innovations, and health care issues and dilemmas will force the need for advocates. It will be necessary for nurses to be staunch advocates for clients, families, and communities, as they were in the past. Early nurse leaders were patient advocates ". . . concerned about and committed to human rights, dignity, humanitarianism, and accountability" (Donahue, 1978, p. 146). Their definition of nursing included autonomy, advocacy, and independent practice that focused on the prevention of illness as well as the maintenance of health. Although the word *advocacy* might not have been used, nursing's history is rich with examples of the advocacy role.

> One need only to read about such individuals as Lavinia Dock and Lillian Wald to realize that nursing not only was concerned about patient advocacy but also practiced it. Delving even further into the roots of nursing, one cannot help but be impressed with the endeavors of Florence Nightingale, the founder of modern nursing. She was truly an independent practitioner who viewed herself as the patient's advocate. She thoroughly understood the importance of economics and the stratagems of power, and sought to establish a system whereby nurses themselves controlled nursing practice and nursing education. In her book, *Notes on Nursing: What It Is and What It Is Not* (1860), she set forth a clear concise charge to nurses for a broad definition of nursing; caring for and caring about, encompassing the care of the whole individual. It has taken the focus on consumer protection and human rights, however, for the emphasis on patient advocacy to resurface within nursing.
>
> — *Donahue, 1985, p. 341*

Nurse advocates also exist today and must exist, as society is faced with challenges and battles against enemies such as AIDS. Barbara Fassbinder, RN, was infected with HIV in 1986 while assisting with the treatment of a patient in the emergency room of Memorial Hospital in Prairie du Chien, Wisconsin. Her personal courage and her professional responsibility were the driving force behind her decision to make her story public. With the support of her family, she spent her remaining time as an outspoken advocate in the fights against AIDS. She traveled extensively, educating health care workers about HIV and its consequences for the U.S. health care system. In 1991 she spoke out against mandatory HIV testing of health care workers in her testimony before Congress. She received national recognition from the U.S. Surgeon General and the Department of Health and Human Services for her efforts in AIDS education in 1992. Her death in 1994 was a great loss to the nursing profession and to humankind.

The time is ripe for the nursing profession to once again make a difference in health care. In the face of dwindling and inadequate resources, however, different and more creative strategies must be developed to potentially achieve primary health care for all. New ideas, approaches, and knowledge in nursing must be shared with colleagues around the world; adaptations can be made for different health systems worldwide. Because of the humanistic approach and educational preparation of nurses in both areas of care and cure,

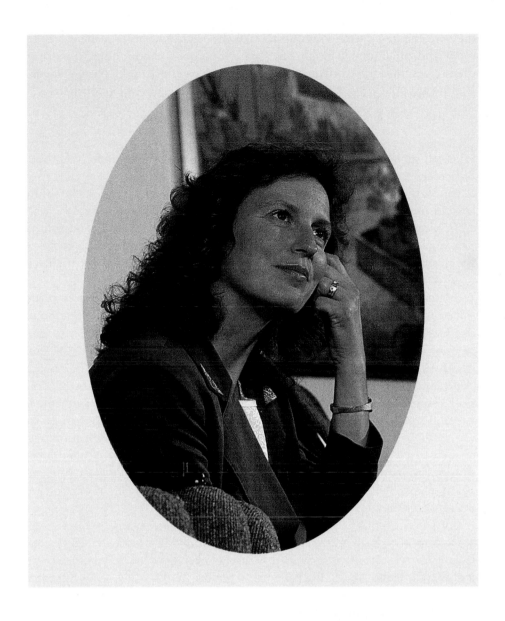

Barbara Fassbinder, November, 1990. *(Courtesy of The University of Iowa Hospitals and Clinics, Iowa City, Iowa/Warren Paris.)*

Barbara Fassbinder spoke out against mandatory HIV testing of health care workers in her testimony before Congress in September 1991. Fassbinder was infected with HIV in 1986 while assisting with the treatment of a patient in the emergency room of Memorial Hospital in Prairie du Chien, Wisconsin. She was recognized as the first health care professional to be infected with the AIDS virus while on the job. She died September 20, 1994. Fassbinder was an outspoken advocate of education, the use of universal precautions, and the need to protect the rights of health care workers. She traveled extensively to tell her story, which has had a lasting impact on health care, health care professionals, and the general public.

The Fassbinder Family, November, 1990. *(Courtesy of The University of Iowa Hospitals and Clinics, Iowa City, Iowa/Warren Paris.)*

Barbara Fassbinder is survived by her husband, David; two daughters, Eva and Emily; and a son, Joel. Throughout their devastating ordeal, the family demonstrated great courage and were extremely supportive of the important work of their wife and mother.

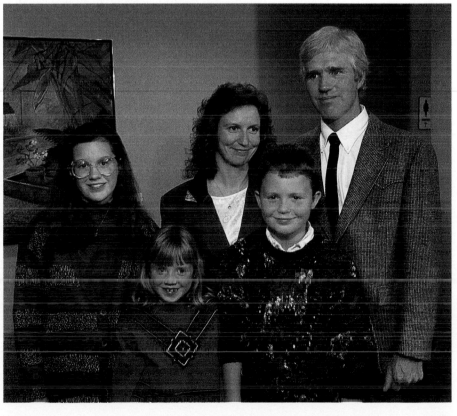

they might be asked to withhold their services; or in times of war, . . . or in caring for or refusing to care for people with certain diagnoses, such as AIDS" (p. 766). In addition to presenting a strong argument for all nurses to develop political savvy, Aroskar (1987) perhaps most effectively summarizes these points: "Dealing with ethical concerns in the world of nursing practice and service requires dealing with the political dimension as well. Ethics and politics interface and overlap. . . . Isn't ethics about right or good action and politics about power and manipulation?" (p. 268).

WORLDWIDE NURSING

Nursing was one of the first groups to understand the significance of primary health care and progress toward its implementation. This is true even though in some instances nurses were not enthusiastic about the movement. Yet, as gaps in primary health care have occurred, nurses have been willing and able to fill them and provide a highly cost-effective and high-quality service. The numbers of advanced practice nurses and their areas of clinical expertise have been steadily increasing since the 1960s. The number of "nursing specialty" areas is remarkable. Much to their credit, nurses have for some time emphasized preventive and primary health care rather than high-tech medical interventions. They have also been more prone to practice in disadvantaged areas with disadvantaged socioeconomic groups. Thus nursing is well positioned to lead the way toward the resolution of accessibility, quality of care, and cost issues in health care. The question is whether nurses are willing to intellectually view the future from a position of strength, for the time is ripe for creating a major impact on patient care. Are nurses willing to rise to the challenges of change and chaos and seize the opportunities available in

Mary Ellen Mark, *Mother Teresa Feeding Sick Man*, 1985. *(Mary Ellen Mark/Library.)*

This Calcutta photograph was originally reproduced in Mary Ellen Mark's book, *Photographs of Mother Teresa's Missions of Charity in Calcutta*. Mother Teresa Bojaxhiu was born in the Yugoslavian region of Skopje and joined the Sisters of Loreto order of the Roman Catholic church in 1928. After teaching in Calcutta for seventeen years, she left the Sisters and went to live and work among the poor in the slum district of Matizhi. There she founded The Missionaries of Charity organization; its first hospice opened in 1952.

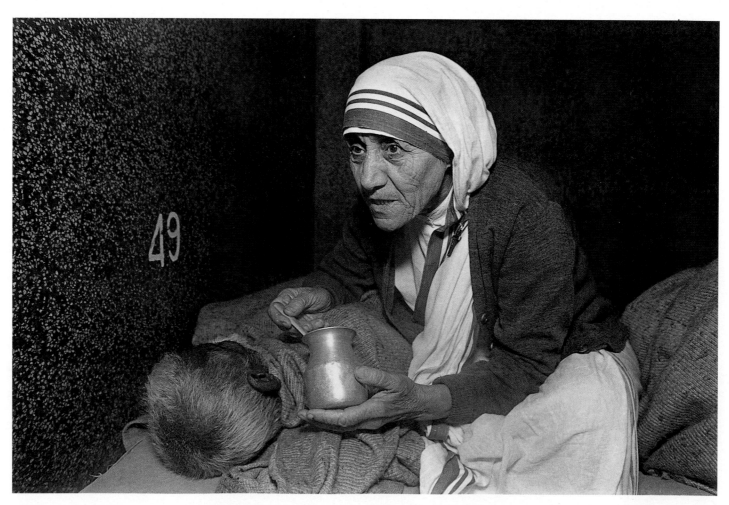

the current situation? Although things may currently appear bleak, Ferguson's words are significant:

> At first the idea of creating a new order by perturbation seems outrageous. . . . Yet our traditional wisdom contains parallel ideas. We know that stress often forces new solutions, that crisis often alerts us to opportunity; that the creative process requires chaos before form emerges; that individuals are often strengthened by suffering and conflict, and that societies need a healthy airing of dissent.
>
> — *Ferguson, 1980, p. 313.*

Health for All: Primary Health Care

A high priority was given to nursing in the early years of the WHO, which was established in 1948 as a specialized agency of the United Nations in Geneva, Switzerland. A nursing unit headed by a chief nursing officer was set up in 1949; nursing officer positions were later set up in six regional offices. Nurses from numerous specialty areas and countries provided the various services of consultation, conducted studies and research, and even engaged in nursing practice in several demonstration projects. But in 1972 both the nursing unit and chief nursing officer position were abolished. The nurses were transferred to functional units within the organization. For years thereafter the role of nursing was barely recognized. The re-emergence of the nursing influence was greatly assisted by Amelia Mangay Maglacas, a nurse from the Philippines, who held the position eventually designated as Chief Scientist for Nursing for fourteen years. Maglacas was experienced in the fields of teaching, administration, research, and international nursing. By the time of her retirement, nursing's status and influence within the organization had grown and flourished. By 1985, nursing's value to the Health for All objective and the strategy of primary health care to achieve it were recognized. According to Halfdan Mahler, then Director General:

> If the millions of nurses in a thousand different places articulate the same ideas and convictions about primary health care, and come together as one force, then they could act as a powerhouse for change. I believe that such a change is coming, and that nurses around the globe, whose work touches each of us intimately, will greatly help to bring it about. WHO will certainly support nurses in their efforts to become agents of change in the move towards Health for All. But if, the full potential of nursing contribution to primary health care is to be realized, it is paramount that governments accept and encourage the placement of nurse leaders where they can have a voice at the policy and decision-making levels.
>
> — *WHO, 1985*

International Nursing Educational Programs

The Health For All objective calls for an international view of nursing that has educational ramifications. A course or an elective on "international nursing" in curricula of programs of nursing education will no longer suffice. It will become necessary for an international dimension of health and nursing to be a vital component of all types of nursing education in all parts of the world. Much can be gained by understanding the merits of a variety of nursing education programs and of health care systems, including those that are nationalized of the Western European Welfare type and those in which privatization is operating. More countries are actually examining privatization as a possible way to provide greater efficiency and to provide services to immigrant workers from developing countries. The nursing literature more and more frequently reflects a growing commitment to such an endeavor. Models for identification of the conceptual components of both graduate and undergraduate international nursing programs and for the integration of international and transcultural content in nursing curricula are now available

(Andrews, 1988; Lindquist, 1990; May and Meleis, 1987; Salmon, Talashek, and Tichy, 1988). They can greatly facilitate the work of faculty who are involved in the revision or development of nursing curricula.

Equally important will be further development in the area of international exchange, which has occurred between schools of nursing for many years. Numerous models of international exchange in schools of nursing with wide structural variation currently exist. They range from formal to informal contacts; the sharing of courses, materials, and resources; and activities such as consultation and joint research and publication (Fenton, 1994; Lindquist, 1984, 1990). Student and faculty exchanges must be escalated, and additional avenues for funding international nursing activities investigated and obtained. International exchange will contribute to the development of nursing curricula and research consistent with contemporary societies and issues and will facilitate a collaborative effort to enhance worldwide health care.

Additional creative ventures involving the internationalization of nursing will continue and ultimately become standard components of educational programs. For example, Central Finland College of Health in Jyväskylä has become increasingly international. A joint International Nurse Program between the College and Lancashire College of Nursing and Health Studies in Preston, England, was designed with implementation beginning in August 1994. The four-year program conforms to the educational standards of both Finland and the United Kingdom; exchange visits are intended to occur in the fourth year. The Central Finland College of Health has international partners in Sweden, Norway, Denmark, Holland, Belgium, Great Britain, Estonia, and Hungary. It is currently seeking to establish contacts with health care educational institutions in the United States (Central Finland College of Health, 1994). This joint curriculum and collaborative effort may become the prototype for other explorations and developments in the field.

Organizational Efforts

Soon the International Council of Nurses (ICN) will be celebrating one hundred years of existence—its centennial. The organization is the international voice of nursing and stands strong beside other intergovernmental organizations like the WHO and the International Labour Organization (ILO). The ICN was organized in 1899 as an independent, nongovernmental federation of national nurses' associations. Emphasis was placed on education in the early years, as attempts were made to develop definitions of nursing and a "nurse." Although nursing education is still an important facet in the work of the ICN, other programs have contributed to its emergence as a primary societal force in many countries of the world. The ICN functions to promote the develop-

CONSEJO INTERNACIONAL DE ENFERMERAS

International Council of Nurses logo. (By permission of the International Council of Nurses, Geneva, Switzerland.)

EXECUTIVE DIRECTORS OF THE INTERNATIONAL COUNCIL OF NURSES

Name	Country	Year(s)
Lavinia L. Dock	United States	1900–1922
Christianne Reimann	Denmark	1922–1934
Anna Schwarzenberg	Austria	1934–1947
Daisy Bridges	United Kingdom	1948–1961
Helen Nussbaum	Switzerland	1961–1967
Sheila Quinn	United Kingdom	1967–1970
Adele Herwitz	United States	1970–1976
Barbara Fawkes	United Kingdom	1977–1978
Winnifred Logan	United Kingdom	1979–1981
Constance Holleran	United States	1981–

Source: Annual Reports, ICN

PRESIDENTS OF THE INTERNATIONAL COUNCIL OF NURSES

Name	Country	Years
Ethel Gordon Bedford Fenwick	United Kingdom	1900–1904
Susan McGahey	Australia	1904–1909
Agnes Karll	Germany	1909–1912
Annie Goodrich	United States	1912–1915
Henny Tscherning	Denmark	1915–1922
Sophie Mannerheim	Finland	1922–1925
Nina Gage	China	1925–1929
Leonie Chaptal	France	1929–1933
Alicia Lloyd Still	United Kingdom	1933–1937
Effie Taylor	United States	1937–1947
Gerda Hojer	Sweden	1947–1953
Marie Bihet	Belgium	1953–1957
Agnes Ohlson	United States	1957–1961
Alice Clamageran	France	1961–1965
Alice Girard	Canada	1965–1969
Margarethe Kruse	Denmark	1969–1973
Dorothy Cornelius	United States	1973–1977
Olive Anstey	Australia	1977–1981
E. Muringo Kiereini	Kenya	1981–1985
Nelly Garzon	Colombia	1985–1989
Mo-Im-Kim	Korea	1989–1993
Margretta Madsen Styles	United States	1993–1997

Source: Annual Reports, ICN

Chief among New Zealand's special-issue stamps were the annual Health stamps with premiums in aid of children's health camps and sanatoria. *(Stamp courtesy of Medical Economics Publishing, New Jersey.)*

The work of the Red Cross is depicted in this French stamp. The nurse holds a tray with needed supplies. Family members look on as the physician converses with the patient. *(Stamp courtesy of Medical Economics Publishing, New Jersey.)*

ment of nursing as a profession and to serve the health needs and promote the health status of humankind. International nursing leadership has been demonstrated throughout the years as the organization has had ten executive directors and twenty-two presidents.

The membership of ICN now comprises one hundred and eleven countries; it originated with three. Only one national nursing association per country can belong. The original purpose of the ICN remains the same: "to provide a medium through which the interests, needs, and concerns of member national nurses' associations can be addressed to the advantage of the public and nurses" (Ohlson and Styles, 1994, p. 408). It has the distinction of being the first international professional organization in the health care field. The ICN has served nursing well over the past century, particularly through its consultative status with the WHO. Close working relationships have also been developed with other United Nations agencies, other nongovernmental organizations, and international foundations.

The ICN quickly accepted nursing responsibility for primary health care in response to the Health For All global agenda. A number of activities were carried out to assist with nurse preparation and successful implementation. Between 1983 and 1985, seven regional workshops were organized to prepare nurse leadership. As another outcome of these workshops, a resource book for primary health care nursing was developed with guidelines for policy making, education, and practice. The response of the ICN to societal trends, health care crises, and varied challenges has been phenomenal. Its strength and timing have proven to be particularly significant to the progression of nursing's role in health care.

The ICN is also currently involved in a far-reaching project, the International Classification for Nursing Practice (ICNP). In a 1989 Council of National Representatives meeting in Seoul, Korea, the American Nurses Association and the Canadian Nurses Association proposed the resolution to the ICN that led to the project's development. Essentially, the resolution

This Romanian stamp is indicative of nursing's assistance during times of war, a scene that is frequently illustrated on postage stamps. The nurse cradles the soldier in her arms and renders physical and emotional support. *(Stamp courtesy of Medical Economics Publishing, New Jersey.)*

This 1954 stamp issued by Turkey demonstrates the close bond between nurses and children. The facial expression of the beautiful child seems to indicate contentment and trust. The nurse's smile is one of joy and happiness as she holds the child close. *(Stamp courtesy of Medical Economics Publishing, New Jersey.)*

expressed "nurses' concerns about the effects of nursing's inability to define the problems to which it addressed its activities and the distinctive contribution it makes to solving them. The resolution asked that ICN encourage member nurses' associations (NNAs) to become involved in developing classification systems for nursing care, nursing information management systems, and nursing data sets to provide tools that nurses in all countries could use to describe nursing and its contributions to health" (Clark, 1994, p. 146). Thus considerable activity has been taking place to develop a common language that can be used across borders to describe and organize nursing data. Such a tool will greatly enhance the work of nursing in all endeavors: teaching, research, practice, organization and management, and policy development (Fitzpatrick and Zanotti, 1995). Major contributors to the work of the ICNP are the North American Nursing Diagnosis Association (NANDA); Nursing Interventions Classification (NIC); Saba's (1992) Home Health Classification; and The Omaha System (Martin and Scheet, 1992). In addition, major collaborative work within the European Nursing Diagnosis Group is ongoing.

Other types of professional nursing groups and organizations have also been extensively involved in numerous enterprises that include international conferences, participation in the development of public policy, development of strategies to improve nursing's image, and the protection of the economic and general welfare of nurses. National nursing organizations are collaborating and coordinating efforts to ensure the future of the nursing profession and continually emphasizing quality and cost-efficient care. The American Nurses' Association established an International Nursing Center in 1991 in its Washington, D.C., office. Two significant developments led to its institution: "—increasing trends throughout the world toward regionalism and globalism in political, economic, and labor sectors, and—a realization among ANA leadership of ANA's need to respond to these trends with renewed focus on its international activities" (*The American Nurse,* 1991). Sigma Theta Tau International Honor Society of Nursing became an international organization in 1988.

The Global Scene

Nursing and nurses around the world are the same yet different. Nursing personnel in most countries represent a potentially powerful force capable of initiating changes in health care delivery and arousing public opinion. Most importantly, they are in constant contact with the people they care for in every type of environment imaginable. Nurses in different countries are not alone in facing challenges that have occurred as a result of organizational changes and economic constraints. The majority of local, regional, or national issues are also global issues. It may well be that the emphasis on primary health care will be the motivating force that will unify nurses nationally and internationally.

The nursing profession will continue to be bombarded by giant forces of a political, sociological, technological, epidemiological, and ethical nature. Some of these forces will even escalate, but others will change direction. Nurses must be flexible; they must be prepared to change course as the situation warrants. Nurses must be visionary and anticipate the waves of the future. Styles (1993) projects the following macrotrends—a combination of forecasts from professional futurists and personal observation—to occur: health care reform; motivation of the workforce; gender issues; quality care and the empowerment of the consumer; and organizational transformation. These are consistent with other projections that appear in the literature. They are also compatible with the major implications for nurses as a result of health care reform identified by Buchan (1993): ". . . employment opportunities will grow more slowly; shift of care from acute sector to outpatient and commu-

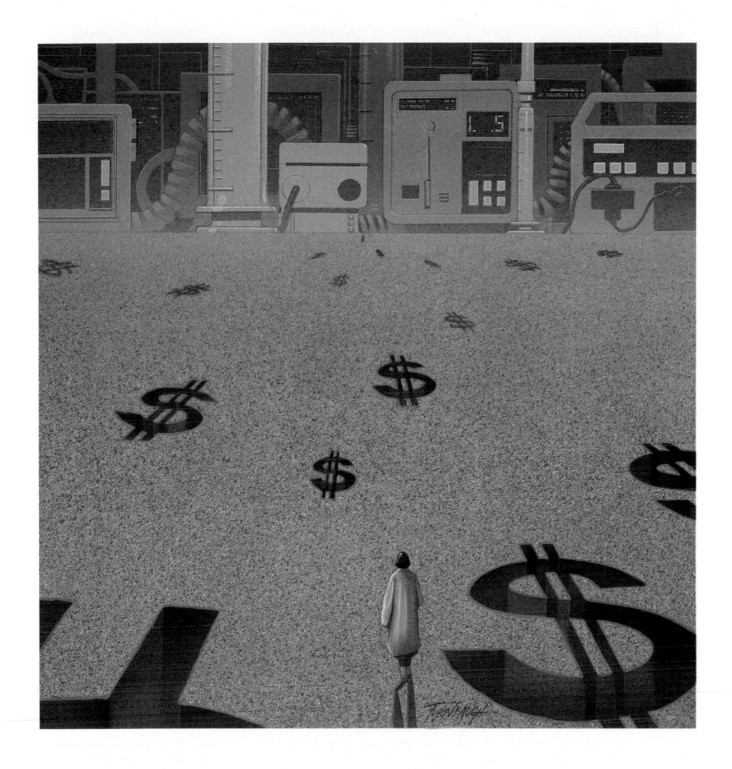

nity care; more appropriate use of nursing staff; greater potential for autonomous health practice; and increasing emphasis on management skills" (p. 21). Although speaking of Canadian and United Kingdom nurses, the implications are applicable to nurses everywhere and are discussed frequently. Other trends are taking their toll on the nursing workforce—the increasing use of unlicensed assistive personnel, the cross-training of personnel, and the regulation and licensure of new types of technical workers. The rationale for these trends may not be universal, nonetheless, they have ramifications for nursing. In addition, as the macrotrends, major implications, and workplace trends are examined, it becomes apparent that nurses worldwide share common concerns about their workplaces and practices.

Paul D. Turnbaugh, *Material Management: Nurses' Involvement*, 1990. (*By permission of Paul D. Turnbaugh, West Dundee, Illinois.*)

Paul D. Turnbaugh, *Modular Nursing: Partners in Professional Practice,* 1990. *(By permission of Paul D. Turnbaugh, West Dundee, Illinois.)*

Modular nursing is an approach in which patients are generally grouped geographically. The module consists of a small group of patients that varies in size, patient acuity, and nursing skill levels. Assigned staff share responsibility for the total care of all patients in the module. The use of this system has been shown to provide improved quality of care and greater nursing satisfaction, to promote professional practice, to support the nursing process and continuity of care, and to grant flexibility to adapt to daily changes in the patients' need for nursing intensity.

Because of continually changing statistics, it is often difficult to adequately, accurately ascertain at any given moment the global picture of nursing. What follows is a **brief overview** of the nursing workplace according to specific regions (International Labour Office, 1994; International Nursing Foundation of Japan, 1977; Ketter, 1994; Maglacas, 1989; Rosenthal and Frenkel, 1992).

Region of Africa.   Nursing shortages are being experienced in many of the African nations consistent with the overall picture of limited numbers of all types of health workers. An average estimate of nursing numbers is 2.5 per 10,000 population. Most are employed in urban areas, since environmental, educational, and family and working conditions in rural areas are less than desirable. The majority of nurses are women, although nursing used to be a predominantly male profession. Salaries are extremely low.

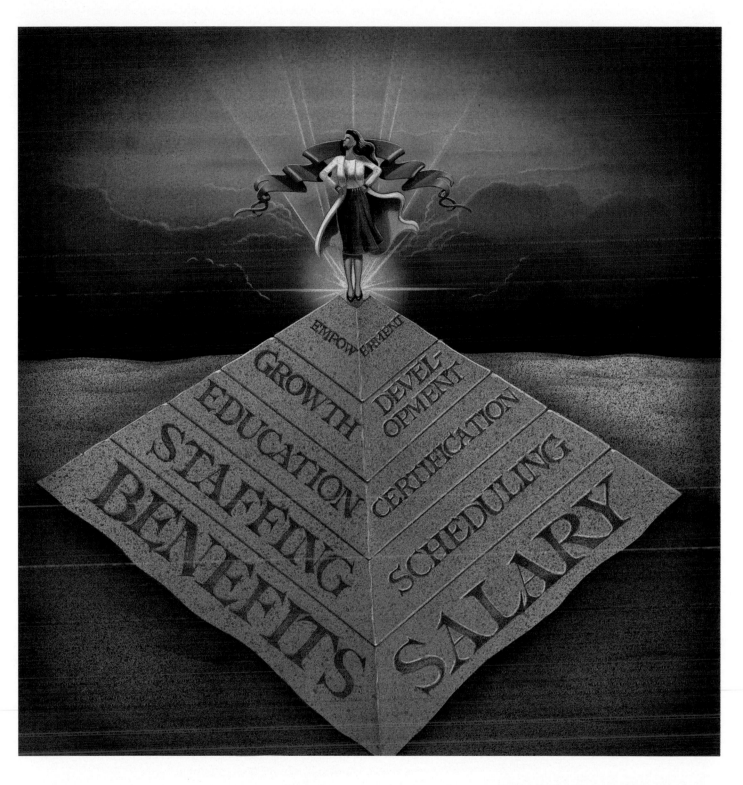

Paul D. Turnbaugh, *Staffing and Scheduling: Empowering Nurses*, 1993. *(By permission of Paul D. Turnbaugh, West Dundee, Illinois.)*

Nurse managers are faced with collecting information, measuring unit activity, and justifying appropriate budgets and controlling costs.

Facing page, Siobhan Manger talks with ninety-four-year-old Neta Shortall at St. Vincent's in Dublin, Ireland. Manger, one of three hundred nurses in training at St. Vincent's, became a practicing nurse in May of 1991. *(Photo by Nick Kelsh.)*

Region of the Americas. The supply of nurses varies considerably within the Americas. Countries in North America are well supplied with nurses, whereas Latin American countries are not, although the situation varies among these countries. The Caribbean countries have a higher proportion of nurses, except Haiti, where there are 1.9 per 10,000 population. A number of areas have resorted to the use of unlicensed assistive personnel to perform nursing tasks.

Region of Eastern Mediterranean. A gross imbalance of nurses exists between oil-producing countries and the rest in the Eastern Mediterranean region. Oil-producing countries often have 20 to 30 per 10,000 population; other countries have less than 5, and in others there are less than 2 per 10,000 population. For example, Afghanistan has 1 per 10,000 population and Pakistan, 1.8 per 10,000 population. The immigration of nurses from India, Egypt, and the Far East account for the highest density of nurses in the oil-producing countries. The heavy migration of nurses out of Egypt is due to low financial and moral rewards and poor working conditions.

Region of Europe. The European region has the highest density of nurses. The highest ratios occur in the Nordic countries with 85 to 87 per 10,000 population. Lower ratios are present in the southern countries such as Greece with 37 and Spain with 20 per 10,000 population. Differences in health care coverage are the least noticeable in this region. For example, working conditions have been favorable in Denmark, where most nurses who want to work, do so, and enjoy comfortable benefit packages. The majority of nurses in Denmark work under a collective bargaining agreement.

Region of Southeast Asia. Human resources in Southeast Asia are generally poor. There is an extremely low ratio of nurses: 1 to 5 per 10,000 population. In some countries the number of nurses per 10,000 population is much less: Bangladesh, 0.5; Bhutan, 0.4; and Nepal, 0.3. Thailand, the exception, has 10 per 10,000 population. There are well-developed nursing programs in Thailand, and nurses are leaders in primary health care.

Region of Western Pacific. A number of countries in the Western Pacific enjoy a high nurse-to-population ratio as compared with other regions of the world. The highest ratios occur in Australia, Japan, and New Zealand, with 54 to 124 per 10,000 population. Australian nurses have improved their conditions through the united voices of strong nursing unions that have made them effective in lobbying. Nurses' wages are low in Japan, where they work long hours, but efforts are being made to improve their economic and general welfare. The nursing ratio in the Philippines is 3.7 per 10,000 population; in the Republic of Korea, 16.9 per 10,000 population. The Philippines continue to lose nurses to countries that are willing to pay higher salaries. Filipino nurses receive no health benefits, have no job security, and work under extremely stressful conditions. China has 7 nurses/midwives per 10,000 population. Since the 1980s Chinese nurses have been rebounding from the effects of communism, which cut off their contact with the West. Nurses are currently controlled by the medical profession.

Vung Dao Clinic. (Copyright Andy Levin. All rights reserved.)

Photograph taken at the Vung Dao Clinic in Vung Dao, Vietnam, about fifty miles from Ho Chi Minh City, or Saigon. Due to the high cost of plastic gloves, the gloves are washed and reused. These gloves are drying in the corridor of the maternity ward as a Vietnamese nurse tries one on for fit.

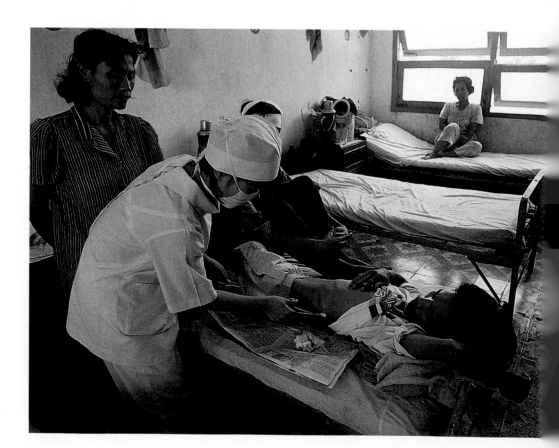

Vung Dao Clinic. (Copyright Andy Levin. All rights reserved.)

Photograph taken at the Vung Dao Clinic in Vung Dao, Vietnam. Here a nurse dresses the wound of a patient in one of the wards.

THE INFORMATION REVOLUTION

It is almost an impossible task to determine the total impact of information technology on society, let alone on health care and nursing. At first, many people did not know what to make of the "new technology." Some were confused; others realized that it would help people communicate in ways they never dreamed possible. Currently, not a day goes by without some type of publication appearing about the wonders of the new information age and the development of new hardware and software. It is even difficult to keep up with the evolution of terminology that is coming forth so rapidly. For example, the term *cyberspace* has now caught on to describe not a science-fiction fantasy but today's increasingly interconnected computer systems, particularly those plugged into the Internet. *Cyberspace* has come to be synonymous with other terms—such as the *Net,* the *Web,* the *Cloud,* the *Matrix,* the *Electronic Frontier,* and the *information superhighway*—bestowed on that nebulous space where all computer data reside. Some individuals go so far as to embrace cyberspace as the land of knowledge.

Cyberspace encompasses millions of personal computers connected by modems to local area networks, e-mail systems, commercial online services, and the Internet. Contrary to what some think, cyberspace is not the wires and the cables. It is about people using the new technology to communicate with one another. So advanced is the transformation that several of the most recent innovations are already being taken for granted. The prominent Internet exemplifies the paradigm shift into this information society, a world owing to electronics. Physical presence is no longer necessary for communication. Internet began more than twenty years ago in the United States as a Department of Defense experiment. On its release in 1984 it spread rapidly, nearly doubling every year. Approximately thirty to forty million people in more than one hundred and sixty countries have, as a minimum, e-mail access to the Internet. The last three years have witnessed more than a thousand-percent increase in users in New Zealand, Japan, and parts of Europe. Part of the success of the Internet is that it is open, or nonproprietary. It is owned by no one, and no single organization controls it. It crosses national and international boundaries.

Information technology has, in a sense, also revolutionized health care delivery. It comprises hardware and software that is used to manage and process information. Information systems in the field of health care are labeled to specify the discipline or purpose(s) they serve. Hospital information systems thus support hospital functions. Information is managed for financial or other operational aims of the institution. Nursing and medical information systems manage information that is necessary for clinical practice. Data are stored that are relevant and necessary in bolstering practice and decision making. Computerized information systems are increasingly replacing the patient's paper chart and various other types of paper and telephone communication such as requisitions and memos. Computerization has entered health care and will continue to survive. In addition to hospitals, insurance companies, payors, regulators, and health care personnel have seen benefits resulting from computerized medical and patient information data. Correspondingly, the specialized field of nursing informatics has become a reality with the development of courses and entire programs of study in nursing education. Nursing informatics combines computer science, information science, and nursing science to support the practice of nursing and the delivery of nursing care.

With the use of advanced computer technology a significant contribution to nursing was made through the joint effort of Sigma Theta Tau Interna-

Paul D. Turnbaugh, *Automating the Patient Chart*, 1990. *(By permission of Paul D. Turnbaugh, West Dundee, Illinois.)*

Computer technology and information systems have greatly influenced nursing practice. Nurses now must learn techniques to help them use computers effectively and understand their relationship to practice and research.

tional and the Online Computer Library Center (OCLC) Electronic Journals Online Service with the publication in 1994 of *The Online Journal of Knowledge Synthesis for Nursing.* This is the first peer-reviewed electronic journal to be published in the field of nursing; it is the second in the health care field. The journal, which transmits via computer linkages, provides critical reviews of research literature that are pertinent to clinical practice problems. It is of primary consideration that knowledge is disseminated more rapidly and knowledge is continuously available. The potential for additional innovations in nursing exists and is limitless. Conferences, "list-serves," bulletin boards, and courses for credit have already found their way into the information revolution of nursing.

Consumers of health care have also entered the age of information. Individuals and families are turning to computers for advice on everyday illnesses. The practice of thumbing through clumsy, heavy reference books is becoming obsolete. With computer technology the search for medical, health, and fitness information is not only possible but rapid, and the information is generally more extensive and easier to read. The question being raised, however, pertains to the reliability of the programs, which should be regarded as another form of educational tool. Titles of a few of the programs include *Mayo Clinic Family Health Book, The Doctor's Book of Home Remedies, Health Desk, Medical HouseCall,* and *The Family Doctor.* The difficulty with the increase in this type of program lies in the fact that laypeople are providing some of this information. Their advice may or may not contain a cautionary statement that directs users to consult their physicians for more information and to not substitute software information for professional treatment.

The use of computer technology is, indeed, reordering the health care system as envisioned by Lesse (1981) in *The Future of the Health Sciences.* His discussion envisioned a system in which consumers will monitor their own care, that technology will be the primary care modality, and that vast storage banks of scientific data will be available to ensure that each person's health will become a certainty. The impact of such a system on health care professionals would be profound. Intense competition for employment would potentially occur as the number of people needed to provide care would greatly decrease, and only the most competent would be retained and advanced. There have already been significant effects on nursing, since computer-assisted nursing practice has mandated changes in knowledge acquisition. Nurses now need additional knowledge in mathematics and statistics and in the biophysical and behavioral sciences. In addition, they will need to learn techniques in order to use computers effectively and understand their relationship to practice and research.

Major problems exist with the use of computer information systems of any type: confidentiality, security, and liability. Currently these are particularly sensitive issues in health care, since the identification and resolution of ethical issues and the legislation of laws related to the use of such information are still in their infancy. As time passes, the criticism that this technology is potentially dangerous because of the loss of the human element may also be laid to rest in one way or another. Nurses will need to be constantly vigilant for possible misuse or misinterpretation of information that is retained in various types of databases. In addition, they will need to help ensure that technology does not become an end in itself that results in the dehumanization of patients in the health care system.

The inevitability of remarkable change in health care systems will continue to confront the nursing profession worldwide. This is a reality that must be understood by nurses, along with an awareness that through contact with one another, through unity, and through diversity, they can be advocates and a primary force for changes that are consistent with nursing's traditional values and will lead to health care for all.

Judith R. Graves, Nursing Informatics Director of the Virginia Henderson International Nursing Library at Sigma Theta Tau International. *(Courtesy of Sigma Theta Tau International, Indianapolis, Indiana.)*

. . . IN CONCLUSION

Early and contemporary leaders in nursing have consistently referred to nursing as an art as well as a science. Art in this context, however, is more than a static, linear concept. It involves a type of perception that is active, dynamic, and developing. An emotional quality guides the transformation of the material in art, but the role of intelligence or thinking is stressed. Thus art is a form of qualitative inquiry that draws its substance from the aesthetic insight. Isabel M. Stewart frequently wrote about nursing as an art. She stressed that the nurse as a "true artist" was essential to the progression of nursing into something other than a highly skilled trade. Stewart realized that numerous individuals thought of art and technique as a single entity, but she emphasized that a piece of work could be technically perfect, yet fall short of being a work of art. Technique, soul, mind, and imagination were all essential in the formation of a true artist.

> The real essence of nursing, as of any fine art, lies not in the mechanical details of execution, nor yet in the dexterity of the performer, but in the creative imagination, the sensitive spirit, and the intelligent understanding lying back of these techniques and skills. Without these, nursing may become a highly skilled trade, but it cannot be a profession or a fine art. All the rituals and ceremonials which our modern worship of efficiency may devise, and all our elaborate scientific equipment will not save us if the intellectual and spiritual elements in our art are subordinated to the mechanical, and if the means come to be regarded as more important than ends.
>
> — *Stewart, 1929, p. 1*

The heritage of nursing is a rich one. Its history is a record of pioneering that reflects new advancements with each generation. Although the entire story of the development of nursing has not been told in these pages, it is hoped that the reader will be able to envision the beauty and essence of its art as captured by some of the greatest masters in the world. This wide range of artwork adds significantly to an understanding of nursing itself because the history of nursing portrayed through art demonstrates the most valuable aspect of nursing: care and caring. Caring is an essential component of nursing—caring for, caring with, and caring about. The pages of this book, through discussion and artwork, reflect the history of that caring as it has varied according to societal events and needs throughout the ages. No one, however, through pen or canvas, will ever be able to entirely capture the true art and the caring spirit of nursing. Both defy expression.

*Nursing is an art; and if it is to be made an art,
it requires as exclusive a devotion, as hard a preparation,
as any painter's or sculptor's work;
for what is the having to do with dead canvas or cold
marble, compared with having to do with the living
body—the temple of God's spirit?
It is one of the Finest Arts;
I had almost said, the finest of the Fine Arts.*

—FLORENCE NIGHTINGALE

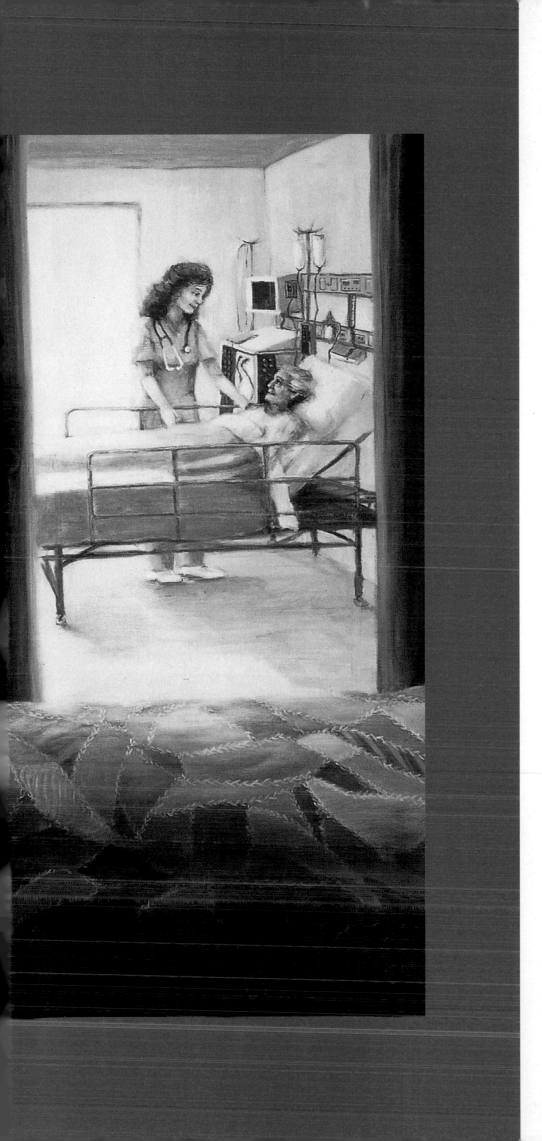

Winona Chenevert, *Nursing: Yesterday, Today, Forever*, 1989. Oil on canvas, 91.44 × 121.92 cm. *(By permission of Pro-Nurse, Gaithersburg, Maryland.)*

In the foreground a turn-of-the-century nurse tends a patient at home in a quilt-covered bed. Light spills across the foot of the bed from the doorway where today's nurse tends a patient in the hospital. Beyond is another doorway opening to an intense light—the promise of an even brighter future for nursing. The original painting hangs in Pro-Nurse headquarters in Gaithersburg, Maryland, from which posters are available.

List of Plates

UNIT 11

References

UNIT 1

Alexander W: *The history of women from earliest antiquity to the present time,* London, 1782, C Dilly.

Berdoe E: *The origin and growth of the healing art,* London, 1893, Swan, Sonnenschein & Co.

Catlin G: *North American Indians,* vol 1, Edinburgh, 1926, John Grant.

Davison WC: Nursing as the foundation of medicine, *North Carolina Medical Journal* p. 141, April 1943.

Dock LL, Stewart IM: *A short history of nursing,* ed 2, New York, 1925, GP Putnam's Sons.

Dolan JA, Fitzpatrick ML, and Hermann EK: *Nursing in society: A historical perspective,* ed 15, Philadelphia, 1983, WB Saunders Co.

Jamieson EM, Sewall MF: *Trends in nursing history,* Philadelphia, 1950, WB Saunders Co.

Mason OT: *Woman's share in primitive culture,* New York, 1894, D Appleton & Co.

Nutting MA, Dock LL: *A history of nursing,* vol 1, New York, 1937, GP Putnam's Sons.

Robinson V: *White caps: The story of nursing,* Philadelphia, 1946, JB Lippincott Co.

Shryock RH: *The history of nursing: An interpretation of the social and medical factors involved,* Philadelphia, 1959, WB Saunders Co.

Stewart IM: How can we help to improve our teaching in nursing schools? *Canadian Nurse* 22:1593, 1918.

Stewart IM: Popular fallacies about nursing education, *The Modern Hospital* 18:1, November 1921

Stewart IM, Austin AL: *A history of nursing,* ed 5, New York, 1962, GP Putnam's Sons.

Jones WHS: *Malaria and Greek history,* Manchester, 1909, Manchester University Press.

Kaviratna AC, trans: *Charaka-Samhita,* Calcutta, n.d.

Lewis F: Quantum mechanics of politics and life, *Des Moines Sunday Register* p. 1C, November 13, 1983.

Lyons AS: Ancient China. In Lyons AS, Petrucelli RJ: *Medicine: An illustrated history,* New York, 1978, Harry N Abrams, Inc.

Lyons AS: Ancient Hebrew medicine. In Lyons AS, Petrucelli RJ: *Medicine: An illustrated history,* New York, 1978, Harry N Abrams, Inc.

Lyons AS: Hippocrates. In Lyons AS, Petrucelli RJ: *Medicine: An illustrated history,* New York, 1978, Harry N Abrams, Inc.

Lyons AS: Medicine in Roman times. In Lyons AS, Petrucelli RJ: *Medicine: An illustrated history,* New York, 1978, Harry N Abrams, Inc.

Nutting MA, Dock LL: *A history of nursing,* vol 1, New York, 1937, GP Putnam's Sons.

Reinach S: *Orpheus: A history of religions,* New York, 1930, Liveright, Inc.

Rosen G: *A history of public health,* New York, 1958, MD Publications, Inc.

Sellew G, Nuesse CJ: *A history of nursing,* St Louis, 1946, The CV Mosby Co.

Seymer LR: *A general history of nursing,* London, 1932, Faber & Faber Ltd.

Shryock RH: *The history of nursing: An interpretation of the social and medical factors involved,* Philadelphia, 1959, WB Saunders Co.

Stewart IM, Austin AL: *A history of nursing,* ed 5, New York, 1962, GP Putnam's Sons.

Taylor HO: *Greek biology and medicine,* Boston, 1922, Marshall Jones Co.

UNIT 2

Berdoe E: *The origin and growth of the healing art,* London, 1893, Swan, Sonnenschein & Co.

Bhishagratna KKL, trans: *The Sushruta Samhita,* Calcutta, 1907, JN Bose.

Castiglioni A: *A history of medicine,* ed 2, trans. EB Krumbhaar, New York, 1947, Alfred A Knopf.

Dolan JA, Fitzpatrick ML, and Hermann EK: *Nursing in society: A historical perspective,* ed 15, Philadelphia, 1983, WB Saunders Co.

Edwards AB: *Pharaohs, fellahs, and explorers,* New York, 1892, Harper & Brothers.

Frank CM, Sr: *The historical development of nursing,* Philadelphia, 1953, WB Saunders Co.

Goodnow M: *Nursing history,* Philadelphia, 1942, WB Saunders Co.

Hermann P: *Conquest by man,* New York, 1954, Harper & Brothers.

Jamieson EM, Sewall MF: *Trends in nursing history,* Philadelphia, 1950, WB Saunders Co.

UNIT 3

Christy TE: Historical perspectives on accountability. In Williamson JA (Ed): *Current perspectives in nursing education,* St Louis, 1976, The CV Mosby Co.

Dock LL, Stewart IM: *A short history of nursing,* ed 2, New York, 1925, GP Putnam's Sons.

Dolan JA, Fitzpatrick ML, and Hermann EK: *Nursing in society: A historical perspective,* ed 15, Philadelphia, 1983, WB Saunders Co.

Frank Sister CM: *The historical development of nursing,* Philadelphia, 1953, WB Saunders Co.

Garrison FH: *An introduction to the history of medicine,* Philadelphia, 1913, WB Saunders Co.

Goodnow M: *Nursing history,* Philadelphia, 1942, WB Saunders Co.

Haeser H: *Geschichte Christlicher Krankenpflege und Pflegerschaften,* Berlin, 1857, Anmerkungen.

Jamieson EM, Sewall MF: *Trends in nursing history*, Philadelphia, 1950, WB Saunders Co.

Kingsley C: *Hypatia*, New York, n.d., Lovell, Coryell & Co.

Lord J: *Beacon lights of history*, vol 5, Great women, New York, 1885, Fords, Howard, & Hulbert.

Lyons AS: Medicine under Islam (Arabic medicine). In Lyons AS, Petrucelli RJ: *Medicine: An illustrated history*, New York, 1978, Harry N Abrams, Inc.

Nutting MA, Dock LL: *A history of nursing*, vol 1, New York, 1937, GP Putnam's Sons.

Petrucelli RJ: The dark ages. In Lyons AS, Petrucelli RJ: *Medicine: An illustrated history*, New York, 1978, Harry N Abrams, Inc.

Putnam EJ: *The lady*, New York, 1921, GP Putnam's Sons.

Robinson V: *White caps: The story of nursing*, Philadelphia, 1946, JB Lippincott Co.

Saint Jerome: Letters. In *Nicene and post-Nicene fathers of the Christian church*, vol 6, New York, 1893, The Christian Literature Co.

Sellew G, Nuesse CJ: *A history of nursing*, St Louis, 1946, The CV Mosby Co.

Seymer LR: *A general history of nursing*, London, 1932, Faber & Faber Ltd.

Shryock RH: *The history of nursing: An interpretation of the social and medical factors involved*, Philadelphia, 1959, WB Saunders Co.

Stewart IM: *The education of nurses*, New York, 1943, The Macmillan Co.

Stewart IM, Austin AL: *A history of nursing*, ed 5, New York, 1962, GP Putnam's Sons.

Tuker MAR, Malleson H: *Handbook to Christian and ecclesiastical Rome*, New York, 1900, Macmillan & Co.

Walsh JJ: *The history of nursing*, New York, 1929, PJ Kenedy & Sons.

UNIT 4

Austin AL: *History of nursing source book*, New York, 1957, GP Putnam's Sons.

Butler A: *The lives of the saints*, 12 vols, ed. and rev. by H Thurston and D Attwater, London, 1934, Burns, Oates & Wasbourne, Ltd.

Chesterton GK: *St. Francis of Assisi*, New York, 1924, George H Doran Co.

Eckenstein L: *Women under monasticism*, Cambridge, 1896, Cambridge University Press.

Frank Sister CM: *The historical development of nursing*, Philadelphia, 1953, WB Saunders Co.

Fuller J: *The days of St. Anthony's fire*, New York, 1968, Macmillan Publishing Co., Inc.

Garrison FH: *An introduction to the history of medicine*, Philadelphia, 1913, WB Saunders Co.

Griffin GJ, Griffin HJ: *History and trends of professional nursing*, St Louis, 1973, The CV Mosby Co.

Haggard HW: *Devils, drugs, and doctors*, New York, 1929, Harper & Brothers.

Jamieson EM, Sewall MF: *Trends in nursing history*, Philadelphia, 1950, WB Saunders Co.

Lamb H: *The crusades: Iron men and saints*, New York, 1930, Doubleday, Doran & Co.

Nutting MA, Dock LL: *A history of nursing*, vol 1, New York, 1937, GP Putnam's Sons.

Robinson V: *White caps: The story of nursing*, Philadelphia, 1946, JB Lippincott Co.

Sellew G, Nuesse CJ: *A history of nursing*, St Louis, 1946, The CV Mosby Co.

Seymer LR: *A general history of nursing*, London, 1932, Faber & Faber Ltd.

Shryock RH: *The history of nursing: An interpretation of the social and medical factors involved*, Philadelphia, 1959, WB Saunders Co.

Zinsser H: *Rats, lice and history*, New York, 1934, Blue Ribbon Books, Inc.

UNIT 5

Cohen IB: Florence Nightingale, *Scientific American* 250:128, March 1984.

Cook, Sir Edward: *The life of Florence Nightingale*, vols 1 and 2, London, 1914, The Macmillan Co.

Devane RS: *The failure of individualism*, Dublin, 1948, Browne & Nolan, Ltd.

Dickens C: *Martin Chuzzlewit*, New York, 1910, The Macmillan Co.

Dolan JA, Fitzpatrick ML, and Hermann EK: *Nursing in society: A historical perspective*, ed 15, Philadelphia, 1983, WB Saunders Co.

Evans AD, Howard LGR: *The romance of the British voluntary hospital movement*, 1930.

Frank Sister CM: *The historical development of nursing*, Philadelphia, 1953, WB Saunders Co.

Goldsmith M: *Florence Nightingale: The woman and the legend*, London, 1937, Hodder & Stoughton.

Haggard HW: *Mystery, magic and medicine*, New York, 1933, Doubleday, Doran & Co., Inc.

Howard J: *An account of the principal lazarettos in Europe*, London, 1791, Johnson, Dilly & Cadel.

Hunt L: *Essays—The monthly nurse*, London, 1889, Fredericke Warne & Co.

Jamieson EM, Sewall MF: *Trends in nursing history*, Philadelphia, 1950, WB Saunders Co.

Nightingale F: *Notes on nursing*, New York, 1860, D Appleton & Co.

Nutting MA, Dock LL: *A history of nursing*, vol 1, New York, 1937, GP Putnam's Sons.

On the genius and character of Hogarth, In *The Works of Charles Lamb*, vol 1, 1818.

Petrucelli RJ: Art and science. In Lyons AS, Petrucelli RJ: *Medicine: An illustrated history*, New York, 1978, Harry N Abrams, Inc.

Robinson V: *White caps: The story of nursing*, Philadelphia, 1946, JB Lippincott Co.

Sellew G, Nuesse CJ: *A history of nursing*, St Louis, 1946, The CV Mosby Co.

Seymer LR: *A general history of nursing*, London, 1932, Faber & Faber Ltd.

Shryock RH: *The history of nursing: An interpretation of the social and medical factors involved*, Philadelphia, 1959, WB Saunders Co.

Smith FB: *Florence Nightingale: Reputation and power*, London, 1982, Croom Helm.

Stewart IM: Florence Nightingale—educator, *Teachers College Record* 41:208, December 1939.

Strachey GL: Florence Nightingale. In *Eminent victorians*, London, 1918, GP Putnam's Sons.

Whitney J: *Elizabeth Fry*, Boston, 1936, Brown & Co.

Woodham-Smith C: *Florence Nightingale*, New York, 1951, McGraw-Hill Book Co.

UNIT 6

Andrews CM: *The fathers of New England*, vol 6, The chronicles of America, New Haven, Conn, 1918, Yale University Press.

Ashley J: *Hospitals, paternalism, and the role of the nurse*, New York, 1976, Teachers College Press.

Austin AL: *History of nursing source book*, New York, 1957, GP Putnam's Sons.

Baker NB: *Cyclone in calico: The story of Mary Ann Bickerdyke*, Boston, 1952, Little, Brown & Co.

Boardman MT: *Under the Red Cross flag at home and abroad*, Philadelphia, 1915, JB Lippincott Co.

Bradford S: *Harriet Tubman: The Moses of her people*, New York, 1961, Corinth Books.

Bush LP: Reminiscences of the Philadelphia Hospital and remarks on oldtime doctors and medicine, *Philadelphia General Hospitals Reports* 1:68, January 1890.

Carlisle R: *An account of Bellevue Hospital,* New York, 1893, Society of Alumni of Bellevue Hospital.

Cheney ED (Ed): *Louisa May Alcott: Her life, letters, and journals,* Boston, 1889, Little, Brown & Co.

Davis MB: *The woman who battled for the boys in blue—Mother Bickerdyke,* San Francisco, 1886, Pacific Press Publishing House.

Dock LL: History of the reform in nursing in Bellevue Hospital, *American Journal of Nursing* 2:90, 1901.

Donahue MP: Isabel Maitland Stewart's philosophy of education, doctoral dissertation, Iowa City, 1981, The University of Iowa.

Frank Sister CM: *The historical development of nursing,* Philadelphia, 1953, WB Saunders Co.

Gibbon JM, Mathewson MS: *Three centuries of Canadian nursing,* Toronto, 1947, The Macmillan Co. of Canada Ltd.

Goodnow M: *Nursing history,* Philadelphia, 1942, WB Saunders Co.

Grippando GM: *Nursing perspectives and issues,* Albany, 1983, Delmar Publishers, Inc.

Hahn RE: A history of nursing scrapbook, *American Journal of Nursing* 27:279, 1927.

Hale S: Lady nurses, *Godey's Lady's Book and Magazine* 82:188, 1871.

Henrietta, Sister: A famous New Orleans hospital, *American Journal of Nursing* 39:249, March 1939.

Hine DC: *Black women in white,* Bloomington, 1989, Indiana University Press.

Jamieson EM, Sewall ME: *Trends in nursing history,* Philadelphia, 1950, WB Saunders Co.

Kane JN: *Famous first facts,* New York, 1934, The HW Wilson Co.

Kenton E (Ed): *The Jesuit relations and allied documents (1610-1791),* New York, 1925, A & C Boni.

Lyons AS: The nineteenth century (The beginnings of modern medicine). In Lyons AS, Petrucelli RJ: *Medicine: An illustrated history,* New York, 1978, Harry N Abrams, Inc.

Miller HS: *The history of Chi Eta Phi Sorority, Inc., 1932-1967,* Washington, DC, 1968, Negro Life and History, Inc.

Munson HW: Linda Richards, *American Journal of Nursing* 48:552, 1948.

Nightingale F: Nurses, training of. In Richard Quain (Ed): *A dictionary of medicine,* New York, 1883, Appleton and Co.

Nutting MA, Dock LL: *A history of nursing,* vol 2, New York, 1907, GP Putnam's Sons.

Pilcher JE: The Red Cross, *Military Surgery* 20:230, April 1907.

Preston A: *Nursing the sick and the training of nurses,* Philadelphia, 1863, King & Baird.

Proceedings of the American Medical Association, New Orleans, May 1869. Reprinted in *Medical News* 20:339, 351, 1869.

Robinson V: *White caps: The story of nursing,* Philadelphia, 1946, JB Lippincott Co.

Roddis LH: The U.S. Hospital Ship *Red Rover* (1862-1865), *Military Surgeon* 77:92, August 1935.

Selections from Leaves of Grass by Walt Whitman, New York, 1961, Menel Books (Crown Publishers, Inc.).

Shryock RH: *The history of nursing: An interpretation of the social and medical factors involved,* Philadelphia, 1959, WB Saunders Co.

Sigerist HE: *American medicine,* New York, 1934, WW Norton & Co., Inc.

Stewart IM: The hospital economics course from the students' standpoint, Paper presented before the Maryland Nurses' Association, 1909.

Stimson JC: Earliest known connection of nurses with Army hospitals in the United States, *American Journal of Nursing* 25:18, 1925.

Walsh JJ: *The history of nursing,* New York, 1929, JP Kenedy & Sons.

Woolsey JS: *Hospital days,* New York, 1868, Van Nostrand.

UNIT 7

American Medical Association, House of Delegates: Proceedings of the eighty-first annual session of the House of Delegates, June 1930, pp 35-41, Chicago, The Association.

American Nurses Association: Proceedings of convention, 1950, The Association.

American Nurses Association: *The A.N.A. and you,* New York, 1941, The Association.

Ashley J: Nursing and early feminism, *American Journal of Nursing* 75:1465, September 1975.

Association of Collegiate Schools of Nursing: Proceedings of the tenth annual meeting, 1943, The Association.

Brown EL: *Nursing for the future,* New York, 1948, Russell Sage Foundation.

Burgess MA: Nurses, patients, and pocketbooks, Proceedings of the thirty-fourth annual convention of the National League of Nursing Education, June 1928, 34:237.

Christy TE: *Cornerstone for nursing education,* New York, 1969a, Teachers College Press.

Christy TE: Portrait of a leader: M. Adelaide Nutting, *Nursing Outlook* 17:20, January 1969b.

Christy TE: Portrait of a leader: Isabel Maitland Stewart, *Nursing Outlook* 17:44, October 1969c.

Christy TE: The fateful decade, 1890-1900, *American Journal of Nursing* 75:1163, July 1975.

Committee for the Study of Nursing Education: *Nursing and nursing education in the United States,* New York, 1923, The Committee.

Committee on the Grading of Nursing Schools: *Nurses, patients, and pocketbooks,* New York, 1928, The Committee.

Dock LL: Secretary's report of the meeting of the International Council of nurses, Buffalo, New York, *American Journal of Nursing,* 2:51, December 1901.

Dock L, Stewart IM: *A short history of nursing,* ed 4, New York, 1938, GP Putnam's Sons.

Dolan JA, Fitzpatrick ML, and Hermann EK. *Nursing in society: A historical perspective,* ed 15, Philadelphia, 1983, WB Saunders Co.

Fitzpatrick ML: *Prologue to professionalism,* Bowie, Md, 1983, Robert J Brady Co.

Gibbon JM, Mathewson MS: *Three centuries of Canadian nursing,* Toronto, 1947, The Macmillan Co. of Canada Ltd.

Hine DC: *Black women in white,* Bloomington, 1989, Indiana University Press.

Kansas State Nurses' Association: *Lamps on the prairie: A history of nursing in Kansas,* Kansas, 1942, Emporia Gazette Press.

Moilett W: On the necessity of legal registration for nurses, *Nursing Record,* June 28, 1888.

Nutting MA: *American Journal of Nursing* 5:654, 1905.

Nutting MA: Greetings. In Souvenir programme of the annual convention of the New York State Nurses' Association, the New York State League for Nursing, the New York Organization for Public Health Nursing, Albany, October 27-29, 1925.

Nutting MA: *A sound economic basis for schools of nursing,* New York, 1926, GP Putnam's Sons.

Nutting MA, Dock LL: *A history of nursing,* vol 3, New York, 1912, GP Putnam's Sons.

Rathbone W: *History and progress of district nursing,* New York, 1890, The Macmillan Co.

Roberts MM: *American nursing: History and interpretation,* New York, 1954, The Macmillan Co.

Roberts MM: Lavinia Lloyd Dock—Nurse, feminist, internationalist, *American Journal of Nursing* 56:176, February 1976.

Robinson V: *White caps: The story of nursing,* Philadelphia, 1946, JB Lippincott Co.

Seymer LR: *A general history of nursing,* London, 1932, Faber & Faber Ltd.

Stewart IM: Popular fallacies about nursing education, *The Modern Hospital* 18:1, November 1921.

Stewart IM: *The education of nurses,* New York, 1943, The Macmillan Co.

Stewart IM: *Reminiscences of Isabel M. Stewart,* New York, 1961, Oral History Research Office, Columbia University.

Stewart IM, Austin AL: *A history of nursing,* ed 5, New York, 1962, GP Putnam's Sons.

The State Board Test Pool Examination, *American Journal of Nursing* 52:613, May 1952.

Wald LD: *The house on Henry Street,* New York, 1915, Henry Holt & Co.

Woolf SJ: Miss Wald at 70 sees her dreams realized, *New York Time Magazine,* March 7, 1937.

UNIT 8

Aynes EA: *From Nightingale to eagle,* Englewood Cliffs, NJ, 1973, Prentice-Hall, Inc.

Beeber LS: To be one of the boys: Aftershocks of the World War I nursing experience, *Advances in Nursing Science* 12:39, 1990.

Bureau of Medicine and Surgery: Navy Nurse Corps observes forty-fifth anniversary (release), *Military Surgeon* 113:45, July 1953.

Chow RK and others: Historical perspectives of the U.S. Air Force, Army, Navy, Public Health Service, and Veterans Administration Nursing Services, *Military Medicine* 143:457, July 1978.

Christy TE: Portrait of a leader: Annie Warburton Goodrich, *Nursing Outlook* 18:46, 1970.

David P: *Triumph in the desert,* New York, 1991, Random House.

Dreves KD: Nurses in American history: Vassar Training Camp for nurses, *American Journal of Nursing* 75:2000, November 1975.

Fischer J: *Images of war,* Boston, 1990, Boston Publishing Company.

Flikke JO: *Nurses in action: The story of the Army Nurse Corps,* Philadelphia, 1943, JB Lippincott Co.

Freedman D, Rhoads J (Eds): Nursing in Vietnam: The forgotten veterans, Austin, 1987, *Texas Monthly.*

Goodrich AW: The school of nursing and the future, Proceedings of the thirty-eighth annual convention of the National League of Nursing Education, New York, 1932, National Headquarters.

Goostray S: Isabel Maitland Stewart, *American Journal of Nursing* 54:302, March 1954.

Hardaway RM: *Care of the wounded in Vietnam,* 1988, Manhattan, Kansas, Sunflower University Press.

Headline News: Military nurses rally for Operation Desert Shield, *American Journal of Nursing* 90:7, October 1990.

Holm JM, Wells SP: Air Force women in the Vietnam War, in *Celebration of Patriotism and Courage: Dedication of the Vietnam Women's Memorial,* November 10-12, 1993, Vietnam Women's Memorial Project.

Joint Committee on Nursing in National Security: Mobilization of nurses for national security, *American Journal of Nursing* 51:78, February 1951.

Judson H: *Edith Cavell,* New York, 1941, The Macmillan Co.

Kalisch PA, Kalisch BJ: *The advance of American nursing,* Boston, 1978, Little, Brown & Co.

Kalisch PA, Kalisch BJ: *Changing of the image of the nurse,* Menlo Park, Calif, 1987, Addison-Wesley Publishing Company.

Lippard LR: *A different war,* Seattle, 1990, Wahtcom Museum of History and Art and Real Comet Press.

Lippmann W: American women and our wounded men, *Washington Post,* December 19, 1944. Reprinted in *The Congressional Record* as an extension of the remarks of Hon. Edith Nourse Roberts, December 19, 1944.

Norman EM: *Women at war: The story of fifty military nurses who served in Vietnam,* Philadelphia, 1990, University of Pennsylvania Press.

The nurses have not lagged behind, editorial, *The Saturday Evening Post,* April 28, 1945.

Nurses monument unveiled in Arlington, *American Journal of Nursing* 39:90, 1993.

Proceedings of the eighteenth annual convention of the American Society of Superintendents of Training Schools for Nursing, New York, 1912, The Society.

Roberts MM: *American nursing: History and interpretation,* New York, 1954, The Macmillan Co.

Robinson V: *White caps: The story of nursing,* Philadelphia, 1946, JB Lippincott Co.

Shields EA (Ed): *Highlights in the history of the Army Nurse Corps,* Washington, DC, 1981, U.S. Army Center of Military History.

Smith MM: Message from Sharon—A reading, *The Connection* 8:3, June 1984.

Song of the Army Nurse Corps. Music by Lou Singer. Words by Hy Zaret. Copyright 1944 by MCA Music, a division of MCA Inc., 445 Park Avenue, New York, New York 10022.

Spelts D: Nurses who served—And who did not return, *American Journal of Nursing* 86:1037, 1986.

Taft WH: A distinct call to women, *Ladies Home Journal* 34:5, September 1917.

Vreeland EM: Fifty years of nursing in the federal government nursing services, *American Journal of Nursing* 50:626, October 1950.

With the Army Nurse Corps in Korea, *American Journal of Nursing* 51:387, June 1951.

U.S. Council of National Defense: First annual report of the Council of National Defense, fiscal year 1917, Washington, DC, 1917, U.S. Government Printing Office.

Vietnam Veterans' Association: Women vets profiled in new VA study, *Veteran,* October 1984.

Walsh J, Aulich J (Eds): *Vietnam images: War and representation,* New York, 1989, St. Martin's Press.

UNIT 9

American Nurses Association: First position paper on education for nurses, *American Journal of Nursing* 65:106, 1965.

American Nurses Association: *Nursing: A social policy statement,* Kansas City, Mo, 1980, The Association.

Dennison C: Nursing service in the emergency room, *American Journal of Nursing* 42:777, July 1942.

Dock LL: Editorial, *American Journal of Nursing,* vol 2, December 1901.

Fitzpatrick ML: *Prologue to professionalism,* Bowie, Md, 1983, Robert J Brady Co.

Grace HK: The development of doctoral education in nursing: A historical perspective. In Chaska NL (Ed): *The nursing professional—Views through the mist,* New York, 1978, McGraw-Hill Book Co.

Grippando GM: *Nursing perspectives and issues,* Albany, NY, 1977, Delmar Publishers, Inc.

Haldeman JC, Abdellah FG: Concepts of progressive patient care, *Hospitals* 33:38, 1959.

Hall L: A center for nursing, *Nursing Outlook* 11:805, 1963.

Henderson V: *The nature of nursing,* New York, 1966, Macmillan Publishing Co., Inc.

Kalisch PA, Kalisch BJ: *The advance of American nursing,* Boston, 1978, Little, Brown & Co.

King IM: *Toward a theory of nursing,* New York, 1971, John Wiley & Sons, Inc.

Krampitz SD: Clinical specialization: Historical antecedents of today's issues. In McCloskey JC, Grace HK: *Current issues in nursing,* Boston, 1981, Blackwell Scientific Publications, Inc.

Lambertson EC: *Nursing team organization and functioning,* New York, 1953, Teachers College, Columbia University.

Marram G, Barrett M, and Bevis E: *Primary nursing: A model for individualized care,* ed 2, St Louis, 1979, The CV Mosby Co.

McManus RL: Isabel M. Stewart—Foremost researcher, *Nursing Research* 2:6, Winter 1962.

Metarazzo JD, Abdellah FH: Doctoral education for nurses in the United States, *Nursing Research* 20:404, 1971.

National Federation for Specialty Nursing Organizations Public Relations Committee: *NFSNO: The first ten years,* Washington, DC, 1984, The Federation.

Newton ME: Florence Nightingale's philosophy of life and education, unpublished dissertation, 1949, Leland Stanford Junior University.

Nightingale F: *Notes on nursing,* New York, 1860, D Appleton & Co.

Reeder SJ: The social context of nursing. In Chaska NL (Ed): *The nursing profession: Views through the mist,* New York, 1978, McGraw-Hill Book Co.

Rogers ME: *An introduction to the theoretical basis of nursing,* Philadelphia, 1970, FA Davis Co.

Shaw E: The black nurse—Then, now and ? Paper presented for continuing education, Nashville, Tenn, 1973, Meharry Medical College.

Smith GR: From invisibility to Blackness: The story of the National Black Nurses' Association, *Nursing Outlook* 23:225, April 1975.

Styles MM: Doctoral education in nursing: The current situation in historical perspective. In National Conference on Doctoral Education in Nursing, Philadelphia, 1977, University of Pennsylvania.

Styles MM: *On nursing: Toward a new endowment,* St Louis, 1982, The CV Mosby Co.

Whitehead AN: *The aims of education and other essays,* New York, 1929, The Macmillan Co.

UNIT 10

American Nurses Association: *The nursing center: Concept and design,* Kansas City, Mo, 1986, The Association.

American Nurses Association: *Nursing case management,* 1988, Kansas City, Mo, 1988, The Association.

Bower K: Managed care: Controlling costs, guaranteeing outcomes, *Definition* 3:1, 1988.

Buchan J: The same but different, *Nursing Standard* 7:21, 1993.

Bulechek GM, McCloskey J: Nursing interventions classification (NIC). Defining nursing care. In J McCloskey, HK Grace (Eds): *Current issues in nursing,* ed 4, pp. 129-135, St Louis, 1994, Mosby.

Bulger RJ: *Technology, bureaucracy, and healing in America: A Postmodern paradigm,* Iowa City, 1988, University of Iowa Press.

Bullough B: Alternative for specialty nursing practice, *Nursing and Health Care* 13:254, 1992.

Bullough VL, Bullough B: *History, trends, and politics of nursing,* Norwalk, Connecticut, 1984, Appleton-Century-Crofts.

Bullough B, Bullough VL: *Nursing issues for the nineties and beyond,* New York, 1994, Springer Publishing Company.

Dick RS, Stein EB (Eds): *The computer-based patient record: An essential technology for health care,* Washington, DC, 1991, National Academy Press.

Duffield C: Nursing in the 1980s and 1990s—A challenge for managers, *International Journal of Nursing Studies* 25:125, 1988.

Felton G: Nursing: A profession to celebrate, *Journal of Professional Nursing* 5:273, 1989.

Ford LC: Advanced nursing practice: Future of the nurse practitioner. In L Aiken, C Fagin: *Charting Nursing's Future Agenda for the 1990s,* pp. 287-297, Philadelphia, 1992, JB Lippincott Company.

Glass LK: The historic origins of nursing centers. In A Arvonio (Ed): *Nursing Centers: Meeting the demand for quality health care* (NLN Pub No. 21-2311), New York, 1989, National League for Nursing.

Himali U: Managed care: Does the promise meet the potential? *The American Nurse* 27:1, 1995a.

Himali U: More than 25,000 RNs march on Washington, issuing a wake-up call to consumers and lawmakers, *The American Nurse* 27:1, 1995b.

Horn BJ, Swain MA: *Criterion measures of nursing care* (DHEW Pub. No. HS78-3187) Hyattsville, Md, 1978, National Center for Health Services Research.

Johnson M, Maas M: Nursing-focused patient outcomes. Challenge for the nineties. In J McCloskey, HK Grace (Eds.): *Current issues in nursing,* ed 4, pp. 136-142, St Louis, 1994, Mosby.

Kalisch PA, Kalisch BJ: *The advance of American nursing,* ed 3, Philadelphia, 1995, JB Lippincott Company.

Lindeman CA: Choices within challenges, *Communicating Nursing Research* 22:1, 1989.

Lundeen SP: Comprehensive, collaborative, coordinated, community-based care: A community nursing center model, *Family and Community Health* 16:57, 1993.

Lundeen SP: Community nursing centers. Implications for health care reform. In J McCloskey and H Grace (Eds.) *Current Issues in Nursing,* ed 4, pp. 382-387, St Louis, 1994, Mosby.

McCrary L: Nurses to protest in DC, saying job cuts erode care, *The Philadelphia Inquirer,* pp. A1, A20, March 31, 1995.

Moloney TW, Rogers DE: Medical technology—A different view of the contentious argument over costs, *New England Journal of Medicine* 305:1413, 1979.

National League for Nursing: Legislative update, p. 1, December 5, 1985.

Ream AC: Our undertrained nurses, *Newsweek* p.17, October 25, 1982.

Rosenberg CE: *The care of strangers,* New York, 1987, Basic Books, Inc.

Sowell RL, Meadows TM: An integrated case management model: Developing standards, evaluation, and outcome criteria, *Nursing Administration Quarterly* 18:53, 1994.

Streef MB: Third-party reimbursement issues for advanced practice nurses in the '90s. In J McCloskey, HK Grace (Eds.): *Current issues in nursing,* ed 4, pp. 437-449, St Louis, 1994, Mosby.

Styles MM: Macrotrends in nursing practice: What's in the pipeline, *Journal of Continuing Education in Nursing* 24:7, 1993.

Styles MM: Specialization and credentialing. In L Aiken, C Fagin: *Charting Nursing's Future Agenda for the 1990s,* pp. 29-39, Philadelphia, 1992, JB Lippincott Company.

The American Nurse: Congress overrides veto, nursing gets center for research, pp. 1, 24, January, 1986.

van Maanen HMT: Nursing in transition: An analysis of the state of the art in relation to the conditions of practice and society's expectations, *Journal of Advanced Nursing* 15:914, 1990.

Warren JJ: Nursing diagnosis taxonomy development. Overview and issues. In J McCloskey, HK Grace (Eds.): *Current issues in nursing,* ed 4, pp. 122-128, St Louis, 1994, Mosby.

Werley H, Ryan P, Zorn CR, and Devine EC: Why the nursing minimum data set (NMDS)? In J McCloskey, HK Grace (Eds.): *Current issues in nursing,* ed 4, pp. 113-122, St Louis, 1994, Mosby.

Zander K: Nurses and case management. To control or to collaborate? In J McCloskey, HK Grace (Eds.): *Current issues in nursing,* ed 4, pp. 254-260, St Louis, 1994, Mosby.

UNIT 11

ANA starts center for international nursing, *The American Nurse* 23:5, April 1991.

Andrews MM: Education preparation for international nursing, *Journal of Professional Nursing* 4:430, 1988.

Aroskar MA: The interface of ethics and politics in nursing, *Nursing Outlook* 5:268, 1987.

Buchan J: The same but different, *Nursing Standard* 7:21, 1993.

Central Finland College of Health and Lancashire College of Nursing and Health Studies: Preliminary plan for joint curriculum year 1994, Author.

Clark J: The international classification of nursing. In J McCloskey and HK Grace (Eds): *Current issues in nursing,* ed 4, pp. 143-147, St Louis, 1994, Mosby.

Donahue MP: The nurse: A patient advocate? *Nursing Forum* 17:143, 1978.

Donahue MP: Advocacy. In GM Bulechek, JC McCloskey (Eds.): *Nursing Interventions. Treatments for Nursing Diagnoses,* pp. 338-351, Philadelphia, 1985, WB Saunders Company.

Fenton MV: Development of models of international exchange to upgrade nursing education. In J McCloskey, HK Grace (Eds.): *Current issues in nursing,* ed 4, pp. 202-206, St Louis, 1994, Mosby.

Ferguson M: *The Aquarian conspiracy,* Los Angeles and New York, 1980, TP Tarcher, Inc. and St. Martin's Press.

Fitzpatrick JJ, Zanotte R: Where are we now? Nursing diagnosis internationally, *Nursing Diagnosis* 6:42, 1995.

Health for all by the year 2000, *UN Chronicle* 29:44, September 1992.

International Labour Office: The remuneration of nursing personnel: An international perspective, Geneva, 1994, Author.

Ketter J: Nurses worldwide speak the same language, *The American Nurse* 26:8, 1994.

Lesse S: *The future of the health sciences,* New York, 1981, Irvington.

Lindquist GJ: A cross-cultural experience: Comparative study in nursing and health care, *Journal of Nursing Education* 23:212, 1984.

Lindquist GJ: Integration of international and transcultural content in nursing curricula: A process for change, *Journal of Professional Nursing 6:272, 1990.*

Maglacas AM: Health for all: Nursing's role, *Nursing Outlook* 36:66, 1988.

Maglacas AM: Close encounters in international nursing: Impact on health policy and research, *Journal of Professional Nursing* 5:304, 1989.

Martin KS, Scheet NJ: The Omaha System: Applications for community health nursing, Philadelphia, 1992, WB Saunders.

May KA, Meleis AI: International nursing: Guidelines for core content, *Nurse Educator* 12:36, 1987.

Ohlson VM, Styles MM: International nursing. The role of the International Council of Nurses and the World Health Organization. In J McCloskey and HK Grace (Eds.): *Current issues in nursing,* ed 4, pp. 407-415, St Louis, 1994, Mosby.

Redfield J: *The celestine prophecy,* New York, 1993, Warner Books.

Rosenthal MM, Frenkel M: *Health care systems and their patients. An international perspective,* Boulder, San Francisco, Oxford, 1992, Westview Press.

Saba V: The classification of home health care nursing: Diagnoses and interventions, *Caring Magazine* 3:50, 1992.

Salmon M, Talashek M, Tichy A: Health for all: A transnational model for nursing, *International Nursing Review* 35:107, 1988.

Simms LM: The professional practice of nursing administration, *Journal of Nursing Administration* 21:37, 1991.

Stewart IM: The science and art of nursing, editorial, *Nursing Education Bulletin* 2:1, 1929.

Styles MM: Macrotrends in nursing practice: What's in the pipeline, *The Journal of Continuing Education in Nursing* 24:7, 1993.

The International Nursing Foundation of Japan: *Nursing in the world. The needs of individual countries, and their programmes,* Japan, 1977, Author.

Toffler A, Toffler H: *Creating a new civilization. Politics of the third wave,* Atlanta, 1995, Turner Publishing, Inc.

Toffler A, Toffler H: *Future shock,* New York, 1970, Random House.

Toffler A, Toffler H: *The third wave,* New York, 1980, Morrow.

World Health Organization: *Nurses lead the way,* Geneva, June 1985, Author.

Selected Bibliography

Abdellah FG, Levine E: *Better patient care through nursing research,* New York, 1979, Macmillan Publishing Co., Inc.

Abdellah FG and others: *Patient centered approaches to nursing,* New York, 1960, Macmillan Publishing Co., Inc.

Adams F: *The genuine words of Hippocrates,* Baltimore, 1939, Williams & Wilkins Co.

Addams J: *Forty years at Hull House,* New York, 1935, The Macmillan Co.

Aiken LH, Fagin CM: *Charting nursing's future. Agenda for the 1990s,* Philadelphia, 1992, JB Lippincott Company.

Albert J: Air evacuation from Korea—a typical flight, *Military Surgeon* 112:256, 1953.

Alcott LM: *Hospital sketches,* Boston, 1885, Roberts Brothers.

Alcott LM: *Hospital sketches, camp and fireside stories,* Boston, 1963, James Redpath.

Alexander W: *The history of women from earliest antiquity to the present time,* London, 1782, C Dilly.

Alger RA: *The Spanish-American War,* New York, 1901, Harper & Brothers.

Allen TB, Berry FC, and Polmar N: *CNN. War in the Gulf.* Atlanta, 1991, Turner Publishing, Inc.

American Foundation for Mental Hygiene: *The mental hygiene movement: Origin, objects and work of the National Committee and of the American Foundation for Mental Hygiene,* New York, 1938, The Foundation.

American Journal of Nursing: *The story of the journal,* New York, 1950, The Journal.

American Journal of Nursing: Headline news. Military nurses rally for Operation Desert Shield, *American Journal of Nursing* 22:7, October, 1990.

ANA starts center for international nursing, *The American Nurse* 23:5, April 1991.

American Nurses Association: *The A N.A. and you,* New York, 1941, The Association.

American Nurses Association: Proceedings of convention, 1950, The Association.

American Nurses Association: First position paper on education for nurses, *American Journal of Nursing* 65:106, 1965.

American Nurses Association: *Nursing: A social policy statement,* Kansas City, Mo, 1980, The Association.

American Nurses Association: *The nursing center: Concept and design,* Kansas City, Mo, 1986, The Association.

American Nurses Association: *Nursing case management,* Kansas City, Mo, 1988, The Association.

Andrews CM: *The fathers of New England,* vol 6, The chronicles of America, New Haven, Conn, Yale University Press.

Andrews MM: Education preparation for international nursing, *Journal of Professional Nursing* 4:430, 1988.

Armstrong G: *The summer of pestilence: A history of yellow fever,* Philadelphia, 1856, JB Lippincott & Co.

Aroskar MA: The interface of ethics and politics in nursing, *Nursing Outlook* 5:268, 1987.

Ashley J: Nursing and early feminism, *American Journal of Nursing* 75:1465, September 1975.

Ashley J: *Hospitals, paternalism, and the role of the nurse,* New York, 1976, Teachers College Press.

Association of Collegiate Schools of Nursing: Proceedings of the tenth annual meeting, 1943, The Association.

Auel JM: *The clan of the cave bear,* New York, 1980, Bantam Books, Inc.

Austin AL: *History of nursing source book,* New York, 1957, GP Putnam's Sons.

Austin AL: *The Woolsey sisters of New York: 1860-1900,* Philadelphia, 1971, American Philosophical Society.

Aynes EA: *From Nightingale to eagle,* Englewood Cliffs, NJ, 1973, Prentice-Hall, Inc.

Bache D: The place of the female nurse in the Army, *Journal of the Military Service Institution* 25:307, 1899.

Bacon F: Founding of the Connecticut training school for nurses, *Trained Nurse* 15:187, 1895.

Baker NB: *Cyclone in calico: The story of Mary Ann Bickerdyke,* Boston, 1952, Little, Brown & Co.

Baker R: *The first woman doctor: The story of Elizabeth Blackwell, M.D.,* New York, 1944, Julian Messner.

Baker R: *America's first trained nurse, Linda Richards,* New York, 1959, Julian Messner.

Barrus C: *Nursing the insane,* New York, 1908, The Macmillan Co.

Barton G: *Angels of the battlefield: A history of the labors of the Catholic sisterhoods in the late Civil War,* Philadelphia, 1897, Catholic Publishing Co.

Barton WE: *Life of Clara Barton,* Boston, 1922, Houghton-Mifflin Co.

Beckett B: *The illustrated history of the Vietnam War,* Poole, Dorset, 1985, Blandford Press.

Bedford WKR, Holbeche R: *The order of the Hospital of St. John of Jerusalem,* London, 1902, FF Robinson & Co.

Beeber LS: To be one of the boys: Aftershocks of the World War I nursing exprience, *Advances in Nursing Science* 12:39, 1990.

Berdoe E: *The origin and growth of the healing art,* London, 1893, Swan, Sonnenschein & Co.

Bessey M: *Magic and the supernatural,* London, 1966, Spring Books.

Bhishagratna KKL, trans: *The sushruta samhita,* Calcutta, 1907, JN Bose.

Billings JS, Hurd HM (Eds): *Hospitals, dispensaries, and nursing, International Congress of Charities, Correction and Philanthropy,* sec 3, Baltimore, 1894, Johns Hopkins Press.

Blackwell E: *Pioneer work in opening the medical profession to women: Autobiographical sketches,* New York, 1895, Longmans, Green & Co.

Blair AH: *At war in the gulf,* College Station, Texas, 1992, Texas A&M University Press.

Boardman MT: *Under the Red Cross flag at home and abroad,* Philadelphia, 1915, JB Lippincott Co.

Bonds R (Ed): *The Vietnam War: The illustrated history of the conflict in Southeast Asia,* New York, 1979, Crown Publishers, Inc.

Bower K: Managed care: Controlling costs, guaranteeing outcomes, *Definition* 3:1, 1988.

Boyd LC: *State registration for nurses,* ed 2, Philadelphia, 1915, WB Saunders Co.

Bradford S: *Harriet Tubman: The Moses of her people,* New York, 1961, Corinth Books.

Brainard AM: *The evolution of public health nursing,* Philadelphia, 1922, WB Saunders Co.

Breasted JH: *The conquest of civilization,* New York, 1938, Harper & Brothers.

Breay M, Fenwick EG: *The history of the International Council of Nurses, 1899-1925,* Geneva, 1931, The International Council of Nurses.

Breckinridge M: *Wide neighborhoods,* New York, 1952, Harper & Brothers.

Bridges DC: *A history of the International Council of Nurses,* 1899-1964, Philadelphia, 1967, JB Lippincott Co.

Bridgman M: *Collegiate education for nursing,* New York, 1953, Russell Sage Foundation.

Brown AF: *Research in nursing,* Philadelphia, 1958, WB Saunders Co.

Brown EL: *Nursing as a profession,* New York, 1936, Russell Sage Foundation.

Brown EL: *Nursing for the future,* New York, 1948, Russell Sage Foundation.

Brown EL: *Nursing reconsidered: A study of change.* I. The professional role in institutional nursing, Philadelphia, 1970, JB Lippincott Co.

Brown EL: *Nursing reconsidered: A study of change.* II. The professional role in community nursing, Philadelphia, 1971, JB Lippincott Co.

Buchan J: The same but different, *Nursing Standard* 7:21, 1993.

Bulechek GM, McCloskey J: Nursing interventions classification (NIC). Defining nursing care. In J McCloskey, HK Grace (Eds): *Current issues in nursing,* ed 4, pp. 129-135, St Louis, 1994, Mosby.

Bulger RJ: *Technology, bureaucracy, and healing in America: A postmodern paradigm,* Iowa City, 1988, The University of Iowa Press.

Bullough B: Alternative for specialty nursing practice, *Nursing and Health Care* 13:254, 1992.

Bullough VL, Bullough B: *History, trends, and politics of nursing,* Norwalk, Conn, 1984, Appleton-Century-Crofts.

Bullough VL, Bullough B, and Stanton, MP (Eds): *Florence Nightingale and her era: A collection of new scholarship,* New York, 1990, Garland.

Bullough B, Bullough VL (Eds): *Nursing issues for the nineties and beyond,* New York, 1994, Springer Publishing Company.

Bulwer-Lytton E: *The last days of Pompeii,* New York, 1834, Dodd, Mead, & Co.

Bureau of Medicine and Surgery: Navy Nurse Corps observes forty-fifth anniversary (release), *Military Surgeon* 113:45, July 1953.

Burgess MA: *Nurses, patients and pocketbooks,* New York, 1928, National League of Nursing Education.

Burgess MA: *Nursing schools today and tomorrow,* New York, 1934, National League of Nursing Education.

Butler A: *The lives of the saints,* 12 vols, ed. and rev. by H Thurston and A Attwater, London, 1934, Burns, Oates & Wasbourne, Ltd.

Caldwell T: *Dear and glorious physician,* New York, 1959, Doubleday & Co.

Carlisle R: *An account of Bellevue Hospital,* New York, 1893, Society of Alumni of Bellevue Hospital.

Carnegie ME: *Historical perspectives of nursing research,* Boston, 1976, Nursing Archive of Boston University.

Carnegie ME: *The path we tread: Blacks in nursing, 1854-1984,* Philadelphia, 1986, JB Lippincott.

Carnegie ME: *The path we tread: Blacks in nursing, 1854-1990,* ed 2, New York, 1991, National League for Nursing.

Carnegie ME: *The path we tread: Blacks in nursing worldwide, 1854-1994,* ed 3, New York, 1995, National League for Nursing Press.

Castiglioni A: *A history of medicine,* ed 2, trans. EB Krumbhaar, 1947, New York, Alfred A. Knopf.

Catlin G: *North American Indians,* vol 1, Edinburgh, 1926, John Grant.

Caulfield E: *The infant welfare movement in the eighteenth century,* New York, 1931, Paul B Hoeber.

Central Finland College of Health and Lancashire College of Nursing and Health Studies: Preliminary plan for joint curriculum year 1994, Author.

Cheney ED (Ed): *Louisa May Alcott: Her life, letters, and journals,* Boston, 1889, Little, Brown & Co.

Chesterton GK: *St. Francis of Assisi,* New York, 1924, George H Doran Co.

Chow RK and others: Historical perspectives of the U.S. Air Force, Army, Navy, Public Health Service, and Veterans Administration Nursing Services, *Military Medicine* 143:457, July 1978.

Christy TE: *Cornerstone for nursing education: A history of division of nursing education of Teachers College, Columbia University, 1899-1947,* New York, 1969, Teachers College Press.

Christy TE: Portrait of a leader: Isabel Hampton Robb, *Nursing Outlook* 17:26, 1969.

Christy TE: Portrait of a leader: Isabel Maitland Stewart, *Nursing Outlook* 17:44, 1969.

Christy TE: Portrait of a leader: Lavinia Lloyd Dock, *Nursing Outlook* 17:72, 1969.

Christy TE: Portrait of a leader: M. Adelaide Nutting, *Nursing Outlook* 17:20, 1969.

Christy TE: Portrait of a leader: Annie Warburton Goodrich, *Nursing Outlook* 18:46, 1970.

Christy TE: Portrait of a leader: Lillian D. Wald, *Nursing Outlook* 18:50, 1970.

Christy TE: Equal rights for women: Voices from the past, *American Journal of Nursing* 71:288, 1971.

Christy TE: The fateful decade, 1890-1900, *American Journal of Nursing* 75:1163, July 1975.

Christy TE: Historical perspectives on accountability. In JA Williamson (Ed): *Current perspectives in nursing education,* St Louis, 1976, The CV Mosby Co.

Christy TE: Clinical practice as a function of nursing education: A historical analysis, *Nursing Outlook* 28:493, 1980.

Churchill F: *On the theory and practice of midwifery,* Philadelphia, 1851, Blanchard & Lea.

Clark J: The international classification of nursing. In J McCloskey, HK Grace (Eds): *Current issues in nursing,* ed 4, pp. 143-147, St Louis, 1994, Mosby.

Clay RM: *Medieval hospitals of England,* London, 1909, Methuen & Co.

Cohen IB: Florence Nightingale, *Scientific American* 250:128, March 1984.

Commission on Nursing Research, American Nurses Association: *Priorities for research in nursing,* Kansas City, Mo, 1976, The Association.

Committee on Nursing and Nursing Education in the United States: *Nursing and nursing education in the United States,* New York, 1923, The Macmillan Co.

Committee on the Structure of National Nursing Organizations: *New horizons in nursing,* New York, 1950, The Macmillan Co.

Congress overrides veto, nursing gets center for research, *The American Nurse,* pp. 1, 24, January 1986.

Cook, Sir Edward: *The life of Florence Nightingale,* vols 1 and 2, London, 1914, The Macmillan Co.

Cooper P: *Navy nurse,* New York, 1946, McGraw-Hill Book Co.

Cope Z: *Florence Nightingale and the doctors,* Philadelphia, 1958, JB Lippincott Co.

Crawford R: *The plague and pestilence in literature and art,* New York, 1914, Oxford University Press.

Croutier AL: *Taking the waters. Spirit, art, sensuality,* New York, 1992, Abbeville Press.

Cunningham JT: *Clara Maass—a nurse—a hospital—a spirit*, New Jersey, 1976, Rae Publishing Co.

Curtayne A: *St. Catherine of Siena*, New York, 1935, Sheed & Ward.

Curtis, Denny: Early history of the Boston Training School, *American Journal of Nursing* 2:331, 1902.

Damel-Rops H: *Monsieur Vincent*, New York, 1961, Hawthorn Books.

David P: *Triumph in the desert: The challenge, the fight, the legacy*, New York, 1991, Random House.

Davison WC: Nursing as the foundation of medicine, *North Carolina Medical Journal*, April 1943.

Defoe D: *A journal of the plague year (1721)*, New York, 1966, Penguin Books.

Delano JA: Nursing as it relates to the war, *American Journal of Nursing* 18:1064, 1918.

Delano JA: How American nurses helped win the war, *Modern Hospital* 12:7, 1919.

Dennison C: Nursing service in the emergency room, *American Journal of Nursing* 42:777, July 1942.

Deutsch A: *Mentally ill in America: A history of their care and treatment from colonial times*, New York, 1937, Doubleday.

Deutsch A: *The mentally ill in America*, ed 2, New York, 1946, Columbia University Press.

Devane RS: *The failure of individualism*, Dublin, 1948, Browne & Nolan, Ltd.

Dewar M and the Press Association: *The Gulf War: A photographic history*, London, 1992, Robert Hale.

Dick RS, Stein EB (Eds): *The computer-based patient record: An essential technology for health care*, Washington, DC, 1991, National Academy Press.

Dickens C: *A tale of two cities*, New York, 1859, EP Dutton & Co.

Dickens C: *Martin Chuzzlewit*, New York, 1910, The Macmillan Co.

Dock LL: *Textbook of materia medica for nurses*, New York, 1890, GP Putnam's Sons.

Dock LL: Editorial, *American Journal of Nursing*, vol 2, December 1901.

Dock LL: History of the reform in nursing in Bellevue Hospital, *American Journal of Nursing* 2:90, 1901.

Dock LL: *Hygiene and morality*, New York, 1912, GP Putnam's Sons.

Dock LL and others: *History of American Red Cross nursing*, New York, 1922, The Macmillan Co.

Dock LL, Stewart IM: *A short history of nursing*, ed 2, New York, 1925, GP Putnam's Sons.

Dock LL, Stewart IM: *A short history of nursing*, ed 4, New York, 1938, GP Putnam's Sons.

Dolan JA, Fitzpatrick ML, and Hermann EK: *Nursing in society: A historical perspective*, ed 15, Philadelphia, 1983, WB Saunders Co.

Donahue MP: Advocacy. In GM Bulechek, JC McCloskey (Eds): *Nursing interventions: Treatments for nursing diagnoses*, pp. 338-351, Philadelphia, 1985, WB Saunders Company.

Donahue MP: Isabel Maitland Stewart's philosophy of education, doctoral dissertation, 1981, The University of Iowa.

Donahue MP: The nurse: A patient advocate? *Nursing Forum* 17:143, 1978.

Douglas M (Ed): *Witchcraft: Confessions and accusations*, London, 1970, Tavistock Publications.

Dreves KD: Nurses in American history: Vassar Training Camp for nurses, *American Journal of Nursing* 75:2000, November 1975.

Duffield C: Nursing in the 1980s and 1990s: A challenge for managers, *International Journal of Nursing Studies* 25:125, 1988.

Duffus RL: *Lillian Wald, neighbor and crusader*, New York, 1938, The Macmillan Co.

Eckenstein L: *Women under monasticism*, Cambridge, 1896, Cambridge University Press.

Edwards AB: *Pharaohs, fellahs, and explorers*, New York, 1892, Harper & Brothers.

Ehrenreich B, English D: *Witches, midwives, and nurses: A history of women healers*, New York, 1973, The Feminist Press.

Ehrhart WD (Ed): *Carrying the darkness: The poetry of the Vietnam War*, Lubbock, Texas, 1989, Texas Tech University Press.

Elgood C: *A medical history of Persia*, London, 1951, Cambridge University Press.

Elmore JA: Black nurses: Their service and their struggle, *American Journal of Nursing* 76:435, 1976.

Evans AD, Howard LGR: *The romance of the British voluntary hospital movement*, 1930.

Faddis MO: *A school of nursing comes of age*, Cleveland, 1973, The Alumni Association of The Frances Payne Bolton School of Nursing.

Faulkner HV: *The quest for social justice, 1899-1914*, New York, 1931, The Macmillan Co.

Faxon NW: *The hospital in contemporary life*, Cambridge, 1949, Harvard University Press.

Felton G: Nursing: A profession to celebrate, *Journal of Professional Nursing* 5:273, 1989.

Fenton MV: Development of models of international exchange to upgrade nursing education. In J McCloskey, HK Grace (Eds): *Current issues in nursing*, ed 4, pp. 202-206, St Louis, 1994, Mosby.

Ferguson M: *The Aquarian conspiracy*, Los Angeles and New York, 1980, TP Tarcher, Inc. and St. Martin's Press.

Fischer J, Stone R: *Images of war*, Boston, 1986, Boston Publishing Company.

Fiske A: *Structure and functions of the body: A handbook of anatomy and physiology for nurses and others desiring a practical knowledge of the subject*, Philadelphia, 1911, WB Saunders Co.

Fitzpatrick ML: *The National Organization for Public Health Nursing, 1912-1952: Development of a practice field*, New York, 1975, National League for Nursing.

Fitzpatrick ML: *Prologue to professionalism*, Bowie, Md, 1983, Robert J Brady Co.

Fitzpatrick JJ, Zanotte R: Where are we now? Nursing diagnosis internationally, *Nursing Diagnosis* 6:42, 1995.

Flanagan LC: *One strong voice: The story of the American Nurses Association*, Kansas City, Mo, 1976, The Association.

Flikke JO: *Nurses in action: The story of the Army Nurse Corps*, Philadelphia, 1943, JB Lippincott Co.

Foran JK, Morrissey SH: *Jeanne Mance; or, the angel of the colony*, Montreal, 1931, Sisters of the Hôtel Dieu.

Ford LC: Advanced nursing practice: Future of the nurse practitioner. In L Aiken, C Fagin (Eds): *Charting Nursing's Future Agenda for the 1990s*, pp. 287-297, Philadelphia, 1992, JB Lippincott Company.

Frank, Sister CM: *The historical development of nursing*, Philadelphia, 1953, WB Saunders Co.

Freedman D, Rhoads J (Eds): *Nurses in Vietnam: The forgotten veterans*, Austin, Texas, 1987, Texas Monthly Press.

Friedrich O: *Desert storm: The war in the Persian Gulf*, Boston, 1991, Little, Brown and Company.

Fuller J: *The days of St. Anthony's fire*, New York, 1968, Macmillan Publishing Co., Inc.

Gadon EW: *The once and future goddess*, San Francisco, 1989, Harper.

Garrison FH: *An introduction to the history of medicine*, Philadelphia, 1913, WB Saunders Co.

Gelinas A: *Nursing and nursing education*, New York, 1946, The Commonwealth Fund.

Gibbon E: *The decline and fall of the Roman Empire*, New York, 1900, Viking Press.

Gibbon JM, Mathewson MS: *Three centuries of Canadian nursing*, Toronto, 1947, The Macmillan Co. of Canada Ltd.

Ginzberg E: *A pattern of hospital care*, New York, 1949, Columbia University Press.

Giordani I: *Catherine of Siena*, Milwaukee, 1959, Bruce Publishing Co.

Glass LK: The historic origins of nursing centers. In A Arvonio (Ed): *Nursing Centers: Meeting the demand for quality health care* (NLN Pub. No. 21-2311), 1989, New York, National League for Nursing.

Goldsmith M: *Florence Nightingale: The woman and the legend*, London, 1937, Hodder & Stoughton.

Goodnow M: *Nursing history*, Philadelphia, 1942, WB Saunders Co.

Goodrich AW: The school of nursing and the future, Prodeedings of the thirty-eighth annual convention of the National League of Nursing Education, New York, 1932, National Headquarters.

Goodrich AW: *The social and ethical significance of nursing*, New York, 1932, The Macmilliam Co.

Goodstray S: Isabel Maitland Stewart, *American Journal of Nursing* 54:302, March 1954.

Grace HK: The development of doctoral education in nursing: A historical perspective. In NL Chaska (Ed): *The nursing profession: Views through the mist*, New York, 1978, McGraw-Hill Book Co.

Grattan JHG, Singer C: *Anglo-Saxon magic and medicine*, New York, 1952, Oxford University Press.

Griffin GJ, Griffin HJ: *History and trends of professional nursing*, St Louis, 1973, The CV Mosby Co.

Grippando GM: *Nursing perspectives and issues*, Albany, 1977, Delmar Publishers, Inc.

Grosvenor G and others: *Everyday life in ancient times*, Washington, DC, National Geographic Society.

Haeser H: *Geschichte Christlicher Krankenpflege und Pflegerschaften*, Berlin, 1857, Anmerkungen.

Haggard HW: *Devils, drugs, and doctors*, New York, 1929, Harper & Brothers.

Haggard HW: *Mystery, magic and medicine*, New York, 1933, Doubleday, Doran & Co., Inc.

Hahn RE: A history of nursing scrapbook, *American Journal of Nursing* 27:279, 1927.

Haldeman JC, Abdellah FG: Concepts of progressive patient care, *Hospitals* 33:38, 1959.

Hale S: Lady nurses, *Godey's Lady's Book and Magazine* 82:188, 1871.

Hall L: A center for nursing, *Nursing Outlook* 11:805, 1963.

Hampton IA: *Nursing: Its principles and practice for hospital and private use*, Philadelphia, 1893, WB Saunders Co.

Hampton IA and others: *Nursing of the sick: 1893*, New York, 1949, McGraw-Hill Book Co.

Hanaford P: *Daughters of America, or women of the century*, Augusta, Me, 1882, True & Co.

Hardaway RM: *Care of the Wounded in Vietnam*, Manhattan, Kansas, 1988, Sunflower University Press.

Harnack A: *Luke, the physician*, New York, 1909, GP Putnam's Sons.

Headline News: Military nurses rally for Operation Desert Shield, *American Journal of Nursing* 90:7, October 1990.

Health for all by the year 2000, *UN Chronicle* 29:44, September 1992.

Henderson V: *The nature of nursing*, New York, 1966, Macmillan Publishing Co., Inc.

Henrietta, Sister: A famous New Orleans hospital, *American Journal of Nursing* 39:249, March 1939.

Hermann P: *Conquest by man*, New York, 1954, Harper & Brothers.

Hill D: *Magic and superstition*, London, 1968, Hamlyn Publishing Group.

Himali U: *Managed care: Does the promise meet the potential? The American Nurse* 27:1, 1995a.

Himali U: More than 25,000 RNs march on Washington, issuing a wake-up call to consumers and lawmakers, *The American Nurse* 27:1, 1995b.

Hine DC: *Black women in the nursing profession: A documentary history*, New York, 1985, Garland.

Hine DC: *Black women in white: Racial conflict and cooperation in the nursing profession, 1890-1950*, Bloomington, 1989, Indiana University Press.

Hiro D: *Desert shield to desert storm*, New York, 1992, Routledge.

Hobson W: *World health and history*, Bristol, 1963, John Wright & Sons.

Holland MA: *Our Army nurses*, Boston, 1895, B Wilkins & Co.

Holloran CA: What are the ethical issues from a worldwide viewpoint? In J McCloskey, HK Grace (Eds): *Current issues in nursing*, ed 4, pp. 763-770, St Louis, 1994, Mosby.

Holm JM, Wells SP: Air Force women in the Vietnam War. In *Celebration of Patriotism and Courage: Dedication of the Vietnam Women's Memorial*, November 10-12, 1993.

Horn BJ, Swain MA: *Criterion measures of nursing care* (DHEW Pub. No. HS78-3187), Hyattsville, Md, 1978, National Center for Health Services Research.

Hovis B: *Station hospital Saigon, A navy nurse in Vietnam, 1963-1964*, Annapolis, Md, 1991, Naval Institute Press.

Howard J: *An account of the principal lazarettos in Europe*, London, 1791, Johnson, Dilly & Cadel.

Hughes EC, Hughes HM, and Deutscher I: *Twenty thousand nurses tell their story*, Philadelphia, 1958, JB Lippincott Co.

Hunt L: *Essays—the monthly nurse*, London, 1889, Frederick Warne & Co.

International Labour Office: *The remuneration of nursing personnel. An international perspective*, Geneva, 1994, Author.

International Nursing Foundation of Japan: *Nursing in the world. The needs of individual countries, and their programmes*, Japan, 1977, The Foundation.

Jacobs JB: Elizabeth Fry, Pastor Fliedner and Florence Nightingale, *Annals of Medical History* 3:17, 1921.

Jamieson EM, Sewall MF: *Trends in nursing history*, Philadelphia, 1950, WB Saunders Co.

Johns E, Pfefferkorn B: *An activity analysis of nursing*, New York, 1934, New York Committee on the Grading of Nursing Schools.

Johns E, Pfefferkorn B: *The Johns Hopkins Hospital School of Nursing, 1889-1949*, Baltimore, 1954, Johns Hopkins University Press.

Johnson M, Maas M: Nursing-focused patient outcomes. Challenge for the nineties. In J McCloskey, HK Grace (Eds): *Current issues in nursing*, ed 4, pp. 136-142, St Louis, 1994, Mosby.

Joint Committee on Nursing in National Security: Mobilization of nurses for national security, *American Journal of Nursing* 51:78, February 1951.

Jolly ER: *Nuns of the battlefield*, Providence, RI, 1927, Providence Visitor Press.

Jones WHS: *Malaria and Greek history*, Manchester, 1909, Manchester University Press.

Judson H: *Edith Cavell*, New York, 1941, The Macmillan Co.

Kalisch PA, Kalisch BJ: *The advance of American nursing*, Boston, 1978, Little, Brown & Co.

Kalisch PA, Kalisch BJ: *The politics of nursing*, Philadelphia, 1982, Lippincott.

Kalisch PA, Kalisch BJ: *The changing image of the nurse*, Menlo Park, Calif, 1987, Addison-Wesley Publishing Company.

Kalisch PA, Kalisch BJ: *The advance of American nursing*, ed 3, Philadelphia, 1995, JB Lippincott Company.

Kane JN: *Famous first facts*, New York, 1934, The HW Wilson Co.

Kansas State Nurses' Association: *Lamps on the prairie: A history of nursing in Kansas*, Kansas, 1942, Emporia Gazette Press.

Kavanagh J: *Women of Christianity*, New York, 1852, D Appleton Co.

Kaviratna AC, trans: *Charaka-Samhita*, Calcutta, n.d.

Kellogg FS: *Mother Bickerdyke as I knew her*, Chicago, 1907, Unity Publishing.

Kelly HA: *Walter Reed and yellow fever*, New York, 1923, GP Putnam's Sons.

Kenton E, (Ed): *The Jesuit relations and allied documents (1610-1791)*, New York, 1925, A & C Boni.

Kernodle PB: *Red Cross nurse in action: 1882-1948*, New York, 1949, Harper & Brothers.

Ketter J: Nurses worldwide speak the same language, *The American Nurse* 26:8, 1994.

Kimber DC, Gray CE: *Anatomy and physiology for nurses*, New York, 1893, The Macmillan Co.

King IM: *Toward a theory of nursing*, New York, 1971, John Wiley & Sons, Inc.

King LS: *The medical world of the eighteenth century*, Chicago, 1958, University of Chicago Press.

Kingsley C: *Hypatia*, New York, n.d., Lovell, Coryell & Co.

Kramer M: *Reality shock: Why nurses leave nursing*, St Louis, 1974, The CV Mosby Co.

Krampitz SD: Clinical specialization: Historical antecedents of today's issues. In JC McCloskey, HK Grace: *Current issues in nursing,* Boston, 1981, Blackwell Scientific Publications, Inc.

Lamb H: *The crusades: Iron men and saints,* New York, 1930, Doubleday, Doran & Co.

Lambertsen EC: *Nursing team organization and functioning,* New York, 1953, Teachers College, Columbia University.

Lambertsen EC: *Education for nursing leadership,* Philadelphia, 1958, JB Lippincott Co.

Lazaro AR: The role of the flight nurse in air evacuation, *Military Surgeon* 105:60, 1949.

Leake CD: *The old Egyptian medical papyri,* Lawrence, 1952, University of Kansas Press.

Lear LE: Coping of nurses who served in the Vietnam conflict, thesis, Iowa City, 1989, The University of Iowa.

Lee E: *History of the School of Nursing of the Presbyterian Hospital, 1892-1942,* New York, 1942, GP Putnam's Sons.

Lesnik MJ, Anderson BL: *Legal aspects of nursing,* Philadelphia, 1947, JB Lippincott Co.

Lesse S: *The future of the health sciences,* New York, 1981, Irvington.

Lewis EP: A collection of editorials from Nursing Outlook *1971-1980,* 1980, American Journal of Nursing Company.

Lewis F: Quantum mechanics of politics—and life, *Des Moines Sunday Register,* p. 1C, November 13, 1983.

Lin Y: *The wisdom of China and India,* New York, 1942, Random House.

Lindeman CA: Choices within challenges, *Communicating Nursing Research* 22:1, 1989.

Lindquist GJ: A cross-cultural experience: Comparative study in nursing and health care, *Journal of Nursing Education* 23:212, 1984.

Lindquist GJ: Integration of international and transcultural content in nursing curricula: A process for change, *Journal of Professional Nursing* 6:272, 1990.

Link EP: Elizabeth Blackwell, citizen and humanitarian, *Woman Physician* 26:451, 1971.

Lippard LR: *A different war,* Co-publication of the Whatcom Museum of History and Art, Bellingham, Washington, and Seattle, 1990, The Real Comet Press.

Lippmann W: American women and our wounded men, *Washington Post,* December 19, 1944. Reprinted in the *Congressional Record* as an extension of the remarks of Hon. Edith Nourse Rogers, December 19, 1944.

Longmore T: *The sanitary contrasts of the British and French armies during the Crimean War,* London, 1883, C Griffin & Co.

Lord J: *Beacon lights of history,* vol 5, Great women, New York, 1885, Fords, Howard, & Hulbert.

Loshak D: *Munch,* New York, 1994, Smithmark Publishers, Inc.

Lowenfels W: *Walt Whitman's Civil War,* New York, 1961, Alfred A Knopf, Inc.

Lundeen SP: Comprehensive, collaborative, coordinated, community-based care: A community nursing center model, *Family and Community Health* 16:57, 1993.

Lundeen SP: Community nursing centers. Implications for health care reform. In J McCloskey, HK Grace (Eds.): *Current issues in nursing,* ed 4, pp. 382-387, St Louis, 1994, Mosby.

Lyons AS: Ancient China. In AS Lyons, RJ Petrucelli: *Medicine: An illustrated history,* New York, 1978, Harry N Abrams, Inc.

Lyons AS: Ancient Hebrew medicine. In AS Lyons, RJ Petrucelli: *Medicine: An illustrated history,* New York, 1978, Harry N Abrams, Inc.

Lyons AS: Hippocrates. In AS Lyons, RJ Petrucelli: *Medicine: An illustrated history,* New York, 1978, Harry N Abrams, Inc.

Lyons AS: Medicine in Roman times. In AS Lyons, RJ Petrucelli: *Medicine: An illustrated history,* New York, 1978, Harry N Abrams, Inc.

Lyons AS: Medicine under Islam (Arabic medicine). In AS Lyons, RJ Petrucelli: *Medicine: An illustrated history,* New York, 1978, Harry N Abrams, Inc.

Lyons AS: The nineteenth century (The beginnings of modern medicine). In AS Lyons, RJ Petrucelli: *Medicine: An illustrated history,* New York, 1978, Harry N Abrams, Inc.

Lyons AS, Petrucelli RJ: *Medicine: An illustrated history,* New York, 1978, Harry N Abrams, Inc.

Maglacas AM: Health for all: Nursing's role, *Nursing Outlook* 36:66, 1988.

Maglacas AM: Close encounters in international nursing: Impact on health policy and research, *Journal of Professional Nursing* 5:304, 1989.

Mannino AJ: Men in nursing, *American Journal of Nursing* 51:198, 1951.

Marram G, Barrett M, and Bevis E: *Primary nursing: A model for individualized care,* ed 2, St Louis, 1979, The CV Mosby Co.

Marshall HE: *Dorothea Dix, forgotten Samaritan,* Chapel Hill, 1937, University of North Carolina Press.

Marshall HE: *Mary Adelaide Nutting,* Baltimore, 1972, Johns Hopkins University Press.

Marshall K: *In the combat zone, an oral history of American women in Vietnam, 1966-1975,* Boston, 1987, Little, Brown and Company.

Martin KS, Scheet NJ: *The Omaha System: Applications for community health nursing,* Philadelphia, 1992, WB Saunders.

Mason OT: *Woman's share in primitive culture,* New York, 1894, D Appleton & Co.

May KA, Meleis AI: International nursing: Guidelines for core content, *Nurse Educator* 12:36, 1987.

Maynard T: *Apostle of charity: The life of St. Vincent de Paul,* New York, 1939, Dial Press.

Maynard T: *St. Benedict and his monks,* London, 1956, Staples Press.

McCrary L: Nurses to protest in D.C., saying job cuts erode care, *The Philadelphia Inquirer,* pp. A1, A20, March 31, 1995.

McIsaac I: *Bacteriology for nurses,* New York, 1909, The Macmillan Co.

McJunkin JN, Crace MD: *Visions of Vietnam,* Novato, Calif, 1983, Presidio Press.

McKenzie JL, Chrisman NL: Healing herbs, gods and magic, *Nursing Outlook* 25:326-329, 1977.

McMahon N: *The story of the Hospitallers of St. John of God,* Westminster, Md, 1959, Newman Press.

McManus RL: Isabel M. Stewart—Foremost researcher, *Nursing Research* 2:6, Winter 1962.

Mead KC: *History of women in medicine,* New York, 1938, Haddam Press.

Merejkowski D: *The romance of Leonardo da Vinci,* New York, 1902, Random House.

Merton RK: *Issues on the growth of a profession,* New York, 1958, American Nurses Association.

Metarazzo JD, Abdellah FG: Doctoral education for nurses in the United States, *Nursing Research* 20:404, 1971.

Middleton J (Ed): *Magic, witchcraft and curing,* New York, 1967, The Natural History Press.

Miller HS: *The history of Chi Eta Phi Sorority, Inc., 1932-1967,* Washington, DC, 1968, Negro Life and History, Inc.

Millett AR (Ed): *A short history of the Vietnam War,* Bloomington & London, 1978, Indiana University Press.

Mollett W: On the necessity of legal registration for nurses, London, *Nursing Record* June 28, 1888.

Moloney TW, Rogers DE: Medical technology—a different view of the contentious argument over costs, *New England Journal of Medicine* 305:1413, 1979.

Montag ML: *The education of nursing technicians,* New York, 1951, GP Putnam's Sons.

Montag ML: *Community college education for nursing: An experiment in technical education for nursing,* New York, 1959, McGraw-Hill Book Co.

Morison SE: *The Oxford history of the American people,* New York, 1965, Oxford University Press.

Morison SE, Commager HS: *The growth of the American republic,* vols 1 and 2, New York, 1942, Oxford University Press.

Morten H: *Nurse's dictionary of medical terms and nursing treatment,* Philadelphia, 1894, WB Saunders Co.

Styles MM: Specialization and credentialing. In L Aiken, C Fagin: *Charting nursing's future agenda for the 1990s,* pp. 29–39, Philadelphia, 1992, JB Lippincott Company.

Taft WH: A distinct call to women, *Ladies Home Journal* 34:5, September 1917.

Talley C: *Ethics: A textbook for nurses,* New York, 1925, GP Putnam's Sons.

Taylor EJ: The school of nursing at the Yale University, *American Journal of Nursing* 25:9, 1925.

Taylor HO: *Greek biology and medicine,* Boston, 1922, Marshall Jones Co.

Thatcher VS: *History of anesthesia with emphasis on the nurse specialist,* Philadelphia, 1953, JB Lippincott Co.

Thibodeau JA: *Nursing models: Analysis and evaluation,* Belmont, Calif, 1983, Wadsworth Health Sciences.

Thompson J: *The ANA in Washington,* Kansas City, Mo, 1972, American Nurses Association.

Thompson M: *The cry and the covenant,* New York, 1954, Doubleday & Co.

Thoms AB: *Pathfinders: A history of the progress of colored graduate nurses,* New York, 1929, Kay Printing House.

Thoms AB, Bullock CE: Developing of facilities for colored nurse education, *Trained Nurse and Hospital Review* 80:722, 1928.

Thorwald J: *Science and secrets of early medicine,* New York, 1963, Harcourt, Brace, & World, Inc.

Tiffany F: *Life of Dorothea Lynde Dix,* Boston, 1937, Houghton.

Tinkham C, Voorhees E: *Community health nursing—evolution and process,* New York, 1972, Appleton-Century-Crofts.

Toffler A, Toffler H: *Creating a new civilization. Politics of the third wave,* Atlanta, 1995, Turner Publishing, Inc.

Toffler A, Toffler H: *Future shock,* New York, 1970, Random House.

Toffler A, Toffler H: *The third wave,* New York, 1980, Morrow.

Tuker MA., Malleson H: *Handbook to Christian and ecclesiastical Rome,* New York, 1900, The Macmillan Co.

Tuttle GT: The male nurse, *American Journal of Insanity* 63:192, 1906.

Uhlhorn G: *Christian charity in the ancient church,* New York, 1883, Charles Scribner.

U.S. Council of National Defense: First annual report of the Council of National Defense, fiscal year 1917, Washington, DC, 1917, U.S. Government Printing Office.

Vallery-Radot D: *Life of Pasteur,* Garden City, NY, 1923, Doubleday.

Van Doren M: *Walt Whitman,* New York, 1945, Viking Press.

Van Loon HW: *RVR: The life and times of Rembrandt,* New York, 1931, Liveright Publishing Co.

van Maanen HMT: Nursing in transition: An analysis of the state of the art in relation to the conditions of practice and society's expectation, *Journal of Advanced Nursing* 15:914, 1990.

Vietman Veterans' Association: Women vets profiled in new VA study, *Veteran,* p. 5, October 1984.

Vreeland EM: Fifty years of nursing in the federal government nursing services, *American Journal of Nursing* 50:626, October 1950.

Wakeford C: *The wounded soldiers' friends: The story of Florence Nightingale, Clara Barton, and others,* London, 1917, Headley-Brothers.

Wald LD: *The house on Henry Street,* New York, 1915, Henry Holt & Co.

Wald L: *Windows on Henry Street,* Boston, 1934, Little, Brown & Co.

Walsh J, Aulich J (Eds): *Vietnam images: War and representation,* Houndmills, Basingstoke, Hampshire, England, 1989, Macmillam Press Ltd.

Walsh JJ: *The history of nursing,* New York, 1929, PJ Kenedy & Sons.

Waltari M: *The Egyptian,* New York, 1949, GP Putnam's Sons.

Warren JJ: Nursing diagnosis taxonomy development. Overview and issues. In J McCloskey, HK Grace (Eds): *Current issues in nursing,* ed 4, pp. 122–128, St Louis, 1994, Mosby.

Waters Y: *Visiting nursing in the United States,* New York, 1909, Charities Publication Committee.

Weeks-Shaw CS: *A textbook of nursing for the use of training schools, families, and private students,* New York, 1885, Appleton.

Weinreb N: *The Babylonians,* New York, 1953, Doubleday & Co.

Wells C: *Bones, bodies, and disease,* New York, 1964, Frederick A Praeger.

Werley H, Ryan P, Zorn CR, and Devine EC: Why the nursing minimum data set (NMDS)? In J McCloskey, HK Grace (Eds), *Current issues in nursing,* ed 4, pp. 113–122, St Louis, 1994, Mosby.

West M, Hawkins C: *Nursing schools at the mid-century,* New York, 1950, National Committee for the Improvement of Nursing Services.

Wheeler H: *Deaconesses, ancient and modern,* New York, 1889, Hunt & Eaton.

Whitehead AN: *The aims of education and other essays,* New York, 1929, The Macmillan Co.

Whitman W: *The works of Walt Whitman,* New York, 1968, Funk & Wagnall's, Inc.

Whitman W: *The wound-dresser, a series of letters written from the hospitals in Washington during the war of the rebellion,* Boston, 1898, Small, Maynard.

Whitney J: *Elizabeth Fry,* Boston, 1936, Brown & Co.

Wilson F: *Crusader in crinoline: The life of Harriet Beecher Stowe,* Philadelphia, 1941, JB Lippincott Co.

With the Army Nurse Corps in Korea, *American Journal of Nursing* 51:387, June 1951.

Woelful N: *Molders of the American mind,* New York, 1933, Columbia University Press.

Wong KC, Wu Lieu-Teh: *History of Chinese medicine,* Shanghai, 1936, National Quarantine Service.

Woodham-Smith C: *Florence Nightingale,* New York, 1951, McGraw-Hill Book Co.

Woody T: *A history of women's education in the United States,* 2 vols, New York, 1929, The Science Press.

Woolf SJ: Miss Wald at 70 sees her dreams realized, *New York Times Magazine,* March 7, 1937.

Woolley L: *History unearthed,* London, 1963, Ernest Benn Ltd.

Woolsey JS: *Hospital days,* New York, 1868, Van Nostrand.

World Health Organization: *Nurses lead the way,* Geneva, June 1985, WHO.

Wylie WG: *Hospitals: Their history, organization and construction,* New York, 1877, Appleton.

Zander K: Nurses and case management. To control or to collaborate? In J McCloskey, HK Grace (Eds): *Current issues in nursing,* ed 4, pp. 254–260, St Louis, 1994, Mosby.

Zielger P: *The black death,* New York, 1969, John Day Co.

Zimmermann A: ANA: Its record on social issues, *American Journal of Nursing* 76:588, 1976.

Zinsser H: *Rats, lice and history,* New York, 1934, Blue Ribbon Books, Inc.

Index

Health for All objective of, 479
World War I, 354–369
   Army School of Nursing and, 360–361
   nursing at front, 361–369
   Vassar Training Camp and, 358
World War II, 369–380
   Nurse Draft Bill and, 378–380
   nursing at front, 373–378
   nursing organizations and, 328–329
   United States Cadet Nurse Corps in, 370–373
Worldwide nursing, 486–496
Wounded Cavalier (Burton), 149
Wylie, Gill, 275

X

Xenodocheion, 93
Xenodochium
   Greek, 54
   Hebrew, 45

Y

Yajur-Veda, 46
Yale University, 237, 277, 361
Yellow Emporer, 50
Yellow fever, 283
Yin and yang, 50

Young Men's Christian Association, 298
Young Woman and Winged Child (Rodin), 438
Young Women's Christian Association, 298
Your Red Cross Needs You (Flagg), 380

Z

Zakrzewska, Marie, 269–270
Zaret, Hy, 377
Zoroastrianism, 34
Zurbarán, Francisco de, *St. Jerome With Saint Paula and Saint Eustochium,* 88